HUMAN SEXUALITY
& the Holy Spirit

SPIRIT-EMPOWERED
PERSPECTIVES

Explore These Other Empowered21 Titles

Global Renewal Christianity: Spirit-Empowered Movements Past, Present, and Future. Vinson Synan, Amos Yong, general editors.
  Volume 1: Asia and Oceania.
    ISBN: 978-1-62998-688-3
  Volume 2: Latin America, with Miguel Álvarez, editor.
    ISBN: 978-1-62998-767-5
  Volume 3: Africa, with J. Kwabena Asamoah-Gyadu, editor.
    ISBN: 978-1-62998-768-2
  Volume 4: Europe and North America.
    ISBN: 978-1-62998-943-3

The Truth about Grace: Spirit-Empowered Perspectives. Vinson Synan, editor. ISBN: 978-1-62999-504-5

HUMAN SEXUALITY
& the Holy Spirit

SPIRIT-EMPOWERED
PERSPECTIVES

Edited by
Wonsuk Ma *and* **Kathaleen Reid-Martinez**
Annamarie Hamilton, *Associate Editor*

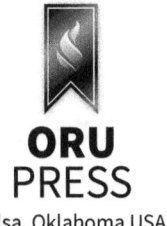

ORU
PRESS
Tulsa, Oklahoma USA

Copyright © 2019 Oral Roberts University

Published by ORU Press
7777 S. Lewis Ave., Tulsa, OK 74171 USA

ORU.edu/ORUPress

ORU Press is the book-and-journal-publishing division of Oral Roberts University.

All rights reserved. No part of this publication may be reproduced, stored in a retrieval system, or transmitted in any form or by any means without the prior permission of the publisher. Brief quotation in book reviews and in scholarly publications is excepted.

Published in the United States of America with permission from Empowered 21, Tulsa, Oklahoma

Empowered21 aims to help shape the future of the global Spirit-empowered movement throughout the world by focusing on crucial issues facing the movement and connecting generations for intergenerational blessing and impartation. Its vision is that every person on Earth would have an authentic encounter with Jesus Christ through the power and presence of the Holy Spirit by Pentecost 2033. Get more information about Jerusalem 2020 at www.empowered21.com. Empowered21 is a Kingdom initiative served by Oral Roberts University, www.oru.edu.

Cover design by Jiwon Kim
Composed at Pressbooks.com using the Clarke design by Angela Sample
Design & Production Editor: Mark E. Roberts

ISBN: 978-1-950971-00-8 (softcover)
ISBN: 978-1-950971-01-5 (ebook)

Printed in the United States of America
C05/20

Contents

Part I. Laying a Foundation

	Introduction *Wonsuk Ma and Kathaleen Reid-Martinez*	3
1.	God's Original Design for Human Sexuality and Spirit-Empowered Leaders in the Old Testament *Lian Mung*	9
2.	A Historical and Hermeneutical Approach to the Vice-Lists: A Pauline Perspective Concerning Homosexuality and the Holy Spirit *Mark Hall*	25
3.	Leaving the Past Behind: A Historical Survey of the Church's Response to Homosexuality *Clayton Coombs*	37
4.	Querying Queer Theory: Gender Expression and Transgender Identity in Manifold Perspective *Michael McClymond*	53

Part II. Learning from Real Life

5.	Sexuality, Gender, and Marriage: Pentecostal Theology of Sexuality and Empowering the Girl-Child in India *Brainerd Prince and Atula Walling*	101
6.	Girls' Education and Sexuality in Burkina Faso: The Contribution from Pentecostal Churches and NGOs *Philippe Ouedraogo*	115
7.	Sexual Exploitation of Children in the Philippines and the Role of Pentecostal Churches *Lulu Suico and Joseph Suico*	129

8.	Resilience and Spirit-Empowered Communities: Stories of Overseas Filipino Women Workers in Pentecostal-Charismatic Churches	153
	Doreen Alcoran-Benavidez and Edwardneil Benavidez	
9.	African Sexuality in the Context of HIV/AIDS	165
	Joshua Banda	
10.	Good News from Africa: Is a Person's Sexual Behavior Influenced by Their Attitude and Behavior towards God? A Voice of Evidence	181
	Joshua Banda	
11.	A Transformational Work of the Holy Spirit For Freedom from Gender Inequality In Nepal	199
	Bal Krishna Sharma and Karuna Sharma	
12.	Holy Sex: A Sermon	215
	William Wilson	
13.	Marriage, Human Sexuality, and the Body	223
	Timothy Tennent	
14.	A Case Study from Malaysia: Struggling Pastor Who Pastors Strugglers	239
	Teresa Chai and Tryphena Law	
15.	Spirit Baptism as a Framework for Ministry to the Struggling	251
	Megan Grondin	
16.	Women at Yoido Full Gospel Church: Pentecostalism in a Confucian Context	267
	Julie Ma	
17.	Postscript: A Reflection	285
	Annamarie Hamilton	
	Notes	299
	Contributors	349
	Select Bibliography	353
	Scripture Index	359

I

Laying a Foundation

Introduction

Wonsuk Ma and Kathaleen Reid-Martinez

Introduction

Empowered21 is a global network of Spirit-empowered churches and ministries. Since its inception in 2010, the Scholars' Consultation has been a prominent standing program of the network. As a pilot project, in 2012, a dozen global Pentecostal scholars were brought to Oxford to share regional theological landscapes. Under the leadership of Harold Hunter, its studies have subsequently been published.[1] When the inaugural congress was explored and finally held in 2015 in Jerusalem, under the co-chairship of Drs. Vinson Synan and Kathaleen Reid-Martinez, scores of Spirit-empowered scholars gathered from around the world. The enthusiasm and inspiration of this first meeting eventually gave birth to the five-volume series of Global Renewal Movement.[2]

Since then, the annual consultation has been held in conjunction with a regional congress which also hosts the global council meeting. A theological and ministerial issue pertinent to the global Spirit-empowered movement is identified by the Global Council. The consultation is to explore the underlying theological assumptions, the contemporary expressions, and the response of Spirit-empowered communities to the theme. The first of such, under the continuing leadership of Drs. Synan and Reid-Martinez, was hosted in London (2016) to deal with the issue of hyper-grace. This international gathering later resulted in the publication of *The Truth about Grace*.[3]

2017 Theme

The Global Council deliberated that the 2017 Scholars' Consultation would deal with the issue of human sexuality which churches in various social settings were facing, e.g., theological and pastoral challenges of homosexuality. The Consultation team decided to compose a theme description to elaborate on the theme and to provide useful guidance to the presenters. To broaden the scope of service, the Theme Description took two directions. Firstly, it expanded the theme to human sexuality, thus, the theme was modified to "The Gift of Human Sexuality and the Holy Spirit."

Secondly, as seen in the revised theme, the studies were to begin with the giftedness of sexuality, which was then corrupted by the sin. The corrupted state is countered by the restorative work of the Holy Spirit, illustrated by the ministry of contemporary Spirit-empowered communities. The full text of the Theme Description is found below:

> Chosen through carefully surveying world leaders of the Spirit-Empowered Movement (hereafter "SEM"), this theme invites scholars in this movement (and others wishing to help) to help SEM members minister the gospel in the Spirit's power more effectively with regard to issues arising from our creation as male and female beings. The following description of the theme aims to inform E21 leaders of how the Forum intends to approach the topic and to suggest to scholars how broadly the Forum views the theme so they may offer scholarship that aligns with it.
>
> E21 leaders and ministers in the SEM ask for help in meeting pressing challenges; the Scholars' Forum will help by focusing reverent and rigorous scholarship first on biblical and theological foundations that support examining today's specific challenges. The result all Forum participants seek is a deeper understanding of such issues in order to promote effective Spirit-empowered ministry.

Foundations

Our male-female differentiation is a gift among the many gifts of Creation. Genesis teaches that God created humanity uniquely, among all beings, in the divine image (1.26–27). This divine image is borne by "man" as "male and female," with no hint of one sex's imaging the divine more fully than—or apart from—the other. This teaching and the Genesis description of divine reasoning in creating man as male and female (with other biblical witnesses) invite scholarly probing to grasp God's intention not only for the existence of humanity (in contrast with other ancient accounts) but also and especially for the gifts of sexual differentiation, of sexual acts and marriage, and of family. After Creation, the Bible records the Fall, which is the Christian premise for all that is wrong in Creation, including human suffering and especially, for this Forum, the many harms the gift of sexuality has suffered: the Creation ideal persists in our yearnings, but the Fall pervades human living, with sin marring all divine gifts, and especially so the unique gift of sexuality. The present evil age bears down even upon believers, who are living the new life of the Spirit that is reordered by Redemption, yet continuing to contend with the brokenness of this fallen world. The Bible, with the Holy Spirit within believers agreeing, looks forward to the Consummation of Redemption, begun by the Second Coming of Jesus Christ. To what extent does the partial presence of this Age to Come—for which the Holy Spirit is a down payment for believers (2 Cor 1.22; Eph 1.14)—impinge on our differentiation as male and female, on sexual acts and marriage, and on gender roles that cohere with the orders of the original Creation and of the New Creation in which believers already participate?

Just these brief statements and questions pertaining to the foundations of this topic invite scholarly investigation that can promote effective ministry. Such studies cross and draw from multiple disciplines: Bible, theology, and history (also Christian worldview); anthropology; psychology and sociology; philosophy; gender and marriage-and-family studies; and more. A major aim of such foundational studies is to synthesize for the topic specially revealed truths (Scripture interpreted within the church relying on the Holy Spirit) with truths discovered by human means and revised by new evidence. Such studies may, in this Forum, propose answers to foundational questions, such as these:

- What is the human person, male and female?
- What are God's explicit and implicit purposes for the gift of humanity as male and female, for sexual acts, for marriage, for family?
- To what extent do these purposes define gender roles, especially for believers?
- How do sin and the Fall affect all these, especially in communities and in the ways religion and culture shape communities?
- In what ways are believers and communities redeemed now from the effects of sin and the Fall on these realities?
- What practices of gospel ministry in the power of the Holy Spirit lead to the greatest deliverance and healing for those suffering violations of this gracious gift (both perpetrators and victims)?

Challenges, Gospel Responses, and Opportunities

From Foundations, the Forum focuses on specific challenges to Christian teaching about human sexuality and to ministry to those suffering from sexual malpractice and its effects in the forms known today. A general pattern for topics in this part of the Forum begins with understanding the challenge; then identifying a wholistic gospel response that includes but, as is pertinent, goes beyond proclaiming the gospel in the power of the Holy Spirit to grappling with the networks of issues that accompany an effective ministry of healing from sexual abuse and brokenness; studies may also sketch the opportunity for such healing ministry that exists regionally or globally.

The topics will likely include these and others, as scholars are invited and confirm their contributions to the Forum:

- Issues defining "sex" and "gender," especially in the West, including understanding and responding to gender studies and gender theory
- Is marriage and family a vocation? How church teaching can help believers understand and practice godly sexuality

- Assessing gender roles and redressing gender inequalities
- Prophetic and pastoral approaches toward persons struggling with same-sex attractions
- The church combating gender-related crimes, such as human trafficking
- Case studies of Spirit-empowered ministries responding effectively to various harms resulting from cultural and religious forces.

Singapore Consultation

The formation of the presenter group for the Singapore consultation was the first involvement of the two organizers, Wonsuk Ma and Mark Roberts, under the co-chairs Drs. Synan and Reid-Martinez. Under the warm support and able leadership of Drs. William M. Wilson and George Wood, the co-chairs of the Global Council, and the late Rev. Ossie Mills, Executive Director of Empowered21, the organizers drafted the Theme Description and began to assemble the Consultation participants The team also decided to take advantage of the region where the Consultation was to take place. This decision was motivated by two reasons. Firstly, the team wished to encourage the regional scholar-practitioners to showcase their experiences and reflections to the world. To bring the field experiences and their theological reflections in each study, all the presentations from Asia were done by wife-husband, friend-friend, or daughter-father teams. Ma's extensive previous teaching work in the Philippines and Great Britain proved to be useful. The active role that women play has been the hallmark of Pentecostal mission, and the very high number of women participation is the reflection of this value. Secondly, the team designed the Consultation in order for the Consultation participants to learn more about and engage with the local environment of the Spirit-empowered theological institutions and churches. Throughout the Consultation, local leaders of theological education and ministries were invited in the sessions and meal fellowships. After one-and-half-day sessions, the participants were hosted by two Singaporean theological institutions of the Spirit-empowered movement: ACTS College and TCA Asia.

The Global Council of the Empowered21 was extremely supportive of the Consultation. The Cochairs of the Council joined selected presentation and fellowship sessions. Several members of the Global Council also visited the proceedings to render their support. At the end of the Consultation, the organizers were invited to bring a report to the entire Global Council, which illustrated the weight that the Council had for the Consultation. Providing too-good-to-be-true accommodation in Singapore, the frontline fieldworkers among the poor and marginalized were rarely treated with such niceties.

From the Papers to a Book

The process of transforming the conference papers into a book has required a new editorial team. Ms. Annamarie Hamilton joined the editorial team as Associate Editor. She signed up for a one-student directed course custom-made for this editorial process. As a student of the Counseling Program of Oral Roberts University, she proved to be deeply interested in the subject matter.

As the editorial team was preparing the process, the goal of the book was also clarified. First, the book is to explore theoretical reflection on human sexuality: biblical, historical, and contemporary philosophical discussions. This group of studies is intended to prepare the readers to approach various issues of human sexuality with an informed mind. Second, the book is to illustrate the real-life experiences to learn the devastating impact that sins have had on the gift of human sexuality. Cultures, religions, or social systems represent the fallenness of the gift. Placing the challenge securely grounded in the given context, the case studies also accentuate the work of the Holy Spirit in restoring the giftedness of human sexuality through the agency of Spirit-empowered communities. The Spirit-filled friends brought their unique experiences and valuable insights to the table. Five studies from Asia formed the core of the contextual studies, joined by three from Africa, two from North America, and one from Europe. This section is presented by the age-bracket of the subjects. Thus, three studies on children first appear, followed by the studies exploring the issue among youths and young adults in various social settings. The last three studies deal with adult sexuality issues and homosexuality in the Christian context. The editors attempted to secure a study from Latin America, but without success. The strong Asian presence in the book serves to encourage and showcase Asia Spirit-empowered scholarship, and the editors are pleased with this end result, in spite of shortcomings.

In Conclusion

This book may be one of the first attempts to tackle this difficult issue from a distinctly Spirit-empowered perspective. Also, the three-stage approach to the theme at the Consultation (and of the book) is likely to serve as a theoretical framework for the future Consultations.

As the Scholars' Consultation program matures, its publications have found a new home: ORU Press. This new publishing program of Oral Roberts University signals the role of the university community to the global Empowered21 network as a community of learners. Indeed, two chapters of the book debuted in the theological journal of the university.[4]

May the Spirit continue empowering his church and people to bring a clear understanding of God's gracious intention, holy anger towards sin's devastating effects, and willing surrender to become change agents for the Spirit's restoration.

New Year, 2019
Editors

1.

God's Original Design for Human Sexuality and Spirit-Empowered Leaders in the Old Testament

Lian Mung

Abstract

This essay investigates God's design for human sexuality in creation and also probes the sexual behavior of selected Spirit-empowered leaders (Joseph, Samson, and David) in the Old Testament in light of that divine design. The first part reveals that human sexuality is part of God's good creation and his norm for marriage is heterosexual, monogamous, covenantal. Sexual union, therefore, is intended exclusively for husband and wife. The second part indicates that while the Spirit of God/Yahweh empowered leaders to carry out God's given tasks, only those who walked in the fear of Yahweh and submitted to his lordship could overcome sexual temptations. This finding has implications for modern Pentecostals and Charismatics: In order to live out God's original design for human sexuality, believers must continually submit ourselves to the leading of the Spirit who empowers us both to carry out God's given tasks and to walk in obedience to God and his ways.

Introduction

While recent decades have witnessed a growing scholarly interest in the relationship between the work of the Spirit and the moral failures of Spirit-empowered leaders,[1] little work has probed the Spirit-empowered leader's sexuality in light of God's design for human sexuality in the creation order. Thus, this study will explore the divine intention for human sexuality in creation and probe the sexuality of selected Spirit-empowered leaders in the OT in light of that divine design. This essay is organized into two parts. The first part will explore God's original design for human sexuality in the creation order in Genesis 1 and 2. In light of the findings of the first part, the second part will further examine the sexuality of three selected Spirit-empowered leaders. Joseph, Samson, and David are chosen in this study because they share commonalities:

(1) they all were empowered by the Spirit of God/Yahweh (2) they all played leadership roles in their respective contexts, and (3) the Hebrew Bible explicitly records how they all dealt with sexual temptations.

It is hoped that this essay may shed light on the moral standards that should govern one's practice of sexuality according to the divine design of sexuality in creation, and also on the role of the Spirit and human responsibility in relation to God's original design for human sexuality. Since there has been a general consensus that Genesis 1 and 2 serve as a foundational text for a theology of human sexuality and marriage,[2] we will begin our study by examining sexuality in Gen 1:26–31 and Gen 2:18–25. In this light, we will further examine selected passages in order to establish whether the aforementioned Spirit-empowered leaders lived out or distorted the original divine design for human sexuality. Then, implications for modern Pentecostals and Charismatics will be suggested.

God's Design for Human Sexuality in Creation

Sexuality in Genesis 1:26-31

In Gen 1:26–28, the narrator records that when Elohim created humankind in his own image, he created male *(zākār)* and female *(neqēbāh)* "to rule the earth under him."[3] Verse 26 reports "the initial decree of the creation of humanity in God's image," and vv. 27–28 records "the action God took to fulfill the proclamation in v. 26,"[4] where God said, "Let us make man in our image, according to our likeness." In v. 27, the poem is composed of three lines which repeatedly use the same verb *(bārā)* "create," linking the three lines together.

> v. 27a And God created *(bārā)* man *('ādām)* in his own image
> v. 27b in the image *of God* he created *(bārā)* him
> v. 27c male *(zākār)* and female *(neqēbāh)* he created *(bārā)* them

As highlighted above, the third line of the poem (v. 27c) explicates that the direct object "man" *('ādām)* in the first line (v. 27a) and another direct object ("him") in the second line (v. 27b) refer to both "male *(zākār)* and female *(neqēbāh)*" in the third colon ("them").[5] This implies that both male and female are equal bearers of "the divine likeness image,"[6] and "neither is more in the image of God than the other."[7] In the ancient Near East myths of creation, "copulation and procreation were mythically regarded as a divine event." In contrast, in Gen 1:26–28, the sexual distinction between male and female was "presented as a creation by God, not part of the divine realm,"[8] implying that human sexuality was God's gift to both man and woman whom he created in his image.

Mathews observes that God's creation of the sexual distinction between both male and female in v. 27 is also preparatory for understanding God's blessing of procreation in v. 28,[9] where both of them were given "the privileges to subdue the earth and to have dominion over animals."[10] Concerning the implication of v. 28, Groothuis argues, "Both [male and female] have been commanded equally and without distinction to take dominion, not one over the other, but both together over the rest of God's creation for the glory of the creator."[11] In v. 28 "God empowered humans with a special blessing in which he commanded them to be fruitful and increase in order that they might fill the earth and subdue (*kibbesh*) it."[12] When v. 28 is read in relationship with v. 27, which depicts God's creation of different sexes (male and female) who bear his image, it seems evident that heterosexuality (v. 27) is part of God's design for human and procreation, which is his mandate for humanity (v. 28; cf. 9:1).[13] Thus, as Dearman concludes, God's mandate for procreation in the creation account signifies that "marriage and family are the institutional setting for male and female in God's creation."[14] In Gen 1:31, when God saw all (*kol*) that he had made, he said, "behold, it was very good." Since the phrase "all (*kol*) that he had made" in v. 31 also refers to all of God's creation, including male and female whom he created in his image (vv. 26–30), it can be deduced that God's creation of human sexuality including sexual union between husband (male) and wife (female) is beautiful and good.[15]

Sexuality in Genesis 2:18–25

Whereas Gen 1:31 denotes that all that Elohim had made, including sexuality, was good, in Gen 2:18, Yahweh Elohim said, "It is not good for the man to alone." This signifies that "God, the Creator, knew that a man by himself could not experience the full dimensions of human existence,"[16] and thus made a helper suitable for him. While the word "helper" (*'ēzer*) in v. 18 "tends to suggest one who is an assistant, a subordinate," the frequent use of the word (*'ēzer*) to describe "God himself as the helper of Israel" in the Hebrew Bible suggests that the use of the word "helper" in this context neither implies a hierarchy of roles nor refers to a subordinate helper.[17] Donald G. Bloesch observes, "It is true that in Genesis 3:16 man is depicted as ruling over woman, but this describes the state of fallen humanity rather than the ideal state in which woman is a companion to man."[18] Allen P. Ross contends that the word "helper" in Gen 2:18 denotes, "one who provides what is lacking in the man, who can do what the man alone cannot do" because "human beings cannot fulfill their assistance except in mutual assistance."[19] Thus, in light of the above observations, the word "helper" in this context should be understood as "mutual assistance in the marriage relationship by one who corresponds (*kenegdô*) to man."[20]

Since there was no suitable helper for Adam among the animals (vv. 18–22), Yahweh Elohim made woman (*'iššâ*) from the rib that he had taken from the man and brought her to him. Adam's words, "This (*zō't*) is now bone of my bones and flesh of my flesh; she shall be called 'woman' (*'iššâ*) for she was taken out of man (*'îš*)" in v. 23 imply that "the woman is not a separate order of creation, but shares fully the nature of *adam*," and the man's need is met only with the woman who is a suitable helper for him.[21] The clause, "This is now bone of my bones and flesh of my flesh" denotes a kinship relationship, which suggests that the woman is a member of the man's family.[22] Instead of using a second person personal pronoun ("you are now bone of my bones," the man said, "This is bone of my bones," indicating his marital commitment and a covenant relationship, "I hereby invite you, God, to hold me accountable to treat this woman as part of my own body."[23] Thus, the narrator's account of the woman who was made to be a suitable helper for the man in vv. 18–23 denotes "the uniqueness of the woman and also the singular relationship shared by man and woman."[24] Further, it also serves as "'a powerful antidote to the problem with which the story begins' in v. 18: 'It is not good that the man should be alone.'"[25] The narrator further elaborates the relationship between the man and woman in v. 24.

> v. 24a Therefore a man (*'îš*) shall leave (*'āzab*) his father and his mother
> v. 24b and he shall hold fast (*dābaq*) to his wife (*'iššâ*)
> v. 24c and they shall become one flesh

While English translations (e.g., NAS, NIV, KJV, RSV, ESV) render the verb *'āzab* in the first colon of v. 24a as "leave," Gordon Wenham suggests that the verb *'āzab* in this context should be translated as "forsake" rather than "leave" because "the man continued to live in or near his parent's home even after he got married." This implies that "forsaking father and mother is to be understood in a relative sense, not an absolute sense" just as Jesus "remarks about hating father and mother, wife, and children in Luke 14:26."[26] Accordingly, Tarwater also writes, "To leave, therefore, while it may include a literal move from one house to another, does not necessitate it, but rather, figuratively refers to the establishment of a new family unity and loyalty to it. As a result, one assumes new responsibilities and obligations."[27] Thus, in this context, leaving or forsaking (*'āzab*) his father and mother in v. 24a implies that a man's priorities change on his marriage; while his first obligations are to his parents before his marriage, his priorities are toward his wife after his marriage.[28] The use of the verb *dābaq* in the second line (v. 24b), "and he shall hold fast (*dābaq*) to his wife," also affirms that "marriage requires a new priority by the marital partners where obligations to one's spouse supplant a person's parental loyalties."[29] Mathews aptly observes: "Marriage requires a new priority by the marital partners where obligations to one's spouse supplant a person's parental loyalties. Illustrative of this pledge is Ruth's earnest desire to remain with Naomi: "Ruth clung [*dābaq*] to her" (1:14) and "Don't urge me to leave [*'āzab*] you" (1:16)."[30] Thus, although the word "covenant" does not appear in v. 24, the use of the two verbs, *'āzab* and *dābaq* in the first line (v. 24a) and the second line (v. 24b), suggests that God's original design of marriage includes a covenant relationship between husband and wife.

Concerning the third line in v. 24c, "and they shall become one flesh," Tremper Longman III observes, "Becoming one flesh" is an idiom for sexual intercourse and thus reminds the reader that sexuality too is not a product of the rebellion, but rather a gift of God to his human creatures."[31] Whereas the phrase "one flesh" refers to sexual intercourse, the Hebrew word for "cling" (*dābaq*) in Gen 2:24c suggests that "the language of 'one flesh' is not simply a euphemistic way of speaking about sexual intercourse; it is a way of speaking about the kinship ties that are related to the union of man and woman in marriage, a union that includes sexual intercourse."[32] J. Andrew Dearman's observation is apt, "Becoming one flesh assumes both sexual union and a resulting bond."[33]

Concerning the implication of v. 24c, John Calvin argues that while there is no mention of "two" in Gen 2:24, just as what Jesus said in Matt 19:5, "They two will become into one flesh," God assigned only one way to Adam, and "the conjugal bond subsists between two persons only." Thus, in the light of Gen 2:24, Matt 19:1–12, and Malachi 2:15, "there is no doubt that polygamy is a corruption of legitimate marriage."[34] The above observations, therefore, signify that monogamy was God's intended design for marriage in the creation order because the one flesh union between a man and a woman was intended to be exclusive, implying that "no other should be involved" in that covenant marriage relationship.[35]

The last verse, Gen 2:25, "And the two of them were naked, the man and his wife, and they were not ashamed of themselves/before one another (*hithpolel*)," stands in contrast with Gen 3, where both the woman and women knew that they were naked (3:7) and hid themselves (3:10). This contrast, thus, signifies that "shameless sexuality was divinely ordered" but "shameful sexuality is the result of sin."[36] When Gen 2:25 is read in relationship with Gen 1:31, where everything God created was depicted as "very good," it is evident that before the fall, God's original design of creation was "wholesome, beautiful, and good."[37]

Summary of Findings

Our examination of God's intended designed for human sexuality in creation leads us to the following observations. First, God's creation of both male and female in both of the creation accounts (Gen 1 & 2) denotes that God's creation of human sexuality is his gift to human beings who are in a covenant marriage (2:4), and it is beautiful and good (1:31). Second, God designed a heterosexual relationship (male with female), not a homosexual relationship (man with man or woman with woman), to be a norm for marriage in creation. Third, a heterosexual marital form is further affirmed by God's mandate for procreation ("be fruitful and multiply" 1:28) through their sexual union ("They shall become one flesh" 2:24). Fourth, since both man and woman were created equally in the image of God (1:26–27) and they both were given authority to rule over the rest of creation, one gender should not dominate the other (1:28). Fifth, monogamy (a man and a woman), not polygamy, is clearly depicted as God's original design for marriage in creation, which is clearly taught by the Lord Jesus in Matt 19:4–6. Sixth, a monogamous marital relationship is intended to be a covenant marriage which involves a permanent commitment, an intimate relationship, and an exclusive sexual union between the two, husband and wife only. In the following, we will examine the sexuality of Spirit-empowered leaders in the Old Testament in light of the above findings.

Spirit-Empowered Leaders and Sexuality

Joseph

Joseph and the Spirit of God

In Gen 41, the role of the Spirit of God is associated with Joseph's wisdom and leadership skills. After Joseph had interpreted Pharaoh's dreams (41:25–32), he also suggested Pharaoh to appoint "a discerning and wise man" (v. 33) who would oversee the collection and keeping of the produce of the land of Egypt during the seven plentiful years before the seven years of famine to occur so that there would be enough food throughout the famine (vv. 33–36). Since Joseph's interpretation of the dreams and suggestions pleased Pharaoh, he [Pharaoh] said to his servants, "Can we find a man like this, in whom is the Spirit of God (*rûaḥ 'ĕlōhîm*)? (v. 38).

It has been suggested that since Pharaoh could have spoken from the perspective of polytheism, the phrase *rûaḥ 'ĕlōhîm* in Gen 41:38 can be translated as "the spirit of the gods" as NEB renders the phrase as "one who has the spirit of a god in him."[38] It is worth noting, however, that if Joseph's statement in v. 16 ["It would be God (*'ĕlōhîm*) who would "give" (*ya'ăneh*, third person masculine singular) Pharaoh an answer of peace,"] had influenced Pharaoh, then the phrase *rûaḥ 'ĕlōhîm* in v. 38 may be translated as "the Spirit of God."[39] This translation seems to be supported by the following verse (v. 39), where the same words ("discerning" and "wise") spoken by Joseph in v. 33 were repeated by Pharaoh who said to Joseph, "Since God (*'ĕlōhîm*) has shown you all this, there is no one so discerning and wise as you are" (v. 39; cf. v. 33). Since the Hebrew expression of *rûaḥ 'ĕlōhîm* in Gen 41:39 is identical with the phrase used in Gen 1:2, where *rûaḥ 'ĕlōhîm* was hovering over the surface of the waters, even if Pharaoh could have a polytheist in his mind, it is plausible that the narrator wanted his readers to see that the Spirit of God (*rûaḥ 'ĕlōhîm*) was the source of Joseph's wisdom and discernment.[40] Similarly, in Isa 11:2, the ideal ruler's wisdom and understanding were directly associated with the Spirit (*rûaḥ*) of Yahweh.[41] Thus, the above observations lead us to deduce that the Spirit of God was the source of Joseph's wisdom and leadership skills. Through the empowerment of the Spirit of God, Joseph was equipped with the charismatic gifts of wisdom and understanding

Joseph and Sexuality

In Gen 38–39, Judah's inappropriate sexual behavior toward Tamar (Gen 38) is contrasted with "the sexual purity of Joseph" who rejected and escaped the seduction of Potiphar's wife (Gen 39).[42] In Gen 39, Joseph's success was closely associated with the presence of Yahweh "who caused all that he did to succeed in his hands" (v. 3). In Gen 39:7, the narrator records that when Potiphar's wife asked Joseph to lie with her (v. 7), he gave "three reasons that the suggestion must be rejected: it is an abuse of the great trust placed in him (v. 6); it is an offense against her husband; and it is a great sin against God."[43] Joseph understood that adultery was "not just a crime on the human level but ultimately a sin against God."[44] Hamilton aptly observes, "Adultery is an offense against both spouse and deity. It is a sin against God because it is a violation of the boundaries he has placed on sexual expression."[45] Thus, seen in the light of the divine design of human sexuality in creation, Joseph's response to Potiphar's wife ("he has not withheld anything from me except you") in Gen 39:9b implies that Joseph viewed that sexual intercourse is exclusively for a husband and wife who were committed into a monogamous relationship, as designed by God (cf. 1:26–28; 2:18–25). The phrase, "this great evil" (*hārā'āh haggedōlāh hazzō't*) in Gen 39:9c also denotes that sexual union is beautiful and good (1:31) when exclusively practiced by a man and his wife (2:4), but it becomes evil and distorted when it is practiced outside of marriage. Hartley aptly observes that it is the fear of God that "guarded him [Joseph] against being caught by such a tempting offer."[46]

Thus, the clause in Gen 39:9c "How then could I do this great evil, and sin against God" signifies Joseph's fear of God, his submission to God's authority, and God's original design of sexuality. The narrator records that Joseph overcame the sexual temptation of Potiphar's wife (Gen 39), and in Gen 41, he was also depicted as a Spirit-empowered leader with one wife, Asenath, who bore two sons (Manasseh and Ephraim) to him (41:37–57). Thus, it can be deduced that Joseph's sexual practice is in harmony with the boundaries of God's original design for human sexuality that promotes a monogamous marital relationship.

In Gen 39, Joseph's success at Potiphar's house was attributed to Yahweh's presence and empowerment (Gen 39). Similarly, in Gen 41, the narrator associates Joseph's wisdom and the understanding, which he needed for interpreting Pharaoh's dream and carrying out his leadership tasks, with the work of the Spirit of God. It is worth noting, however, that Joseph's ability to overcome the sexual temptation of Potiphar's wife is associated with his fear of God and with his voluntary submission to God's authority and to God's norm for human sexuality in creation, where sexual union is confined exclusively within a marriage relationship.

Samson

Samson and the Spirit of Yahweh

It has been observed that Samson was a Spirit-empowered leader who frequently experienced the coming of Yahweh's Spirit (Judg 13:25; 14:6, 19; 15:14).[47] In Judg 13:7, the narrator records that Samson was to be a Nazirite for life; "for the boy shall be a Nazirite to God from birth to the day of his death" (v. 7). Samson's Nazirite vow was not a voluntary vow, but rather it was divinely imposed, signifying "Samson's role as a divinely appointed agent."[48]

When Samson grew up, Yahweh blessed him, and the Spirit began to stir (*pā'am*) him while he was in Mahaneh-dan, between Zorahan Eshtatol" (13:24–25). While the immediate result of the coming of Yahweh's Spirit upon Samson was not explicitly stated,[49] Ma argues that the verb "stir" (*pā'am*) in Judg 13:25 signifies "a more internal and personal nature of the Spirit's work" and "this experience is meant to remind Samson of his life calling and God's lordship.[50] Thus, it is probable that God intervened in Samson's life by stirring him through Yahweh's Spirit so that he would be able to start carrying out the plan, which was set for him (13:5–7).[51] In Judg 14:6, the coming of Yahweh's Spirit upon Samson resulted in physical empowerment which enabled him to tear the lion with his bare hands. In Judg 14:19, the narrator uses the same verb "rush" (*ṣālaḥ*) which he had used in 14:6 in order to depict how the Spirit of Yahweh empowered Samson. The same Spirit, who stirred him in Mahaneh-dan (13:25) and empowered him to kill the young lion (14:6), gave him supernatural strength to kill thirty of Ashkelon's elite leaders.[52] After killing these thirty men, he took their clothes and gave them to the thirty men to whom he owed thirty clothes.

The coming of the Spirit of Yahweh in 15:14 is significant in the

Samson narrative because he became the judge of Israel for twenty years after he defeated the Philistines. When the Philistines encamped in Judah to capture Samson, the three thousand men from Judah came to get Samson to deliver him to the Philistines because the Judeans were afraid of the Philistines and did not want any trouble from the Philistines.[53] After Samson was assured that his own people would not kill him, he let them bind himself with two new ropes. When Samson was about to be handed over to the Philistines near Lehi, the Spirit of Yahweh rushed (ṣālaḥ) upon him. "The ropes which were on his arms became as flax that has caught fire, and his bonds melted off his hands" (v. 14). Then he seized a fresh jawbone of a donkey and killed a thousand men of the Philistines (v. 15). Sasaki suggests that if the author did not mention "the Spirit of the Lord" in Samson's encountering with the Philistines, the account could be interpreted "merely as the story of Samson's revenge."[54] The narrator's statement ("the Spirit of Yahweh rushed upon him") in 15:14 indicates that Samson defeated the Philistines not by his human strength but by the power of Yahweh's Spirit. After his military victory, Samson judged Israel for twenty years in the days of the Philistines.[55] Despite his experience of the frequent coming of the Spirit of Yahweh upon him, Samson frequently violated his Nazirite vow by contacting with the lion's carcass and eating the honey which he took from the lion's carcass, taking part in the drinking feast which a Nazirite had to avoid, and also contacting with a dead body by using a fresh jawbone of a donkey as his weapon. Furthermore, Samson's life was driven by his lust which led him to his downfall (Judg 16).

Samson and Sexuality

The book of Judges records Samson's encounter with several women: His marriage with a Timnite woman (Judges 14), his relationship with a prostitute in Gaza (16:1–3), and also with Delilah (16:4–21). Samson's lust is most evident in chapter 16, where the narrator records that Samson went to a prostitute in Gaza (v. 1). Judges 16 begins with the narrator's statement, "And Samson went to Gaza, and saw there a prostitute (zônāh) and went into her" (16:1). Unlike his trip to Timnah ("His father and mother did not know that it was from Yahweh" 14:4), the narrator does not identify Samson's trip to Gaza in chapter 16:1–3 as a trip initiated or guided by Yahweh because Samson was driven by his lust. Younger's observation is apt: "Samson's going to a prostitute is once again indicative of his lack of regard for God's law. Moreover, he goes to Gaza, a Philistine city, which requires his traveling though the length of Philistia. This certainly speaks to intent. This is not a slip-up, a case of falling into sin. This is a deliberate rebellious act on Samson's part."[56]

In Gen 38:18, the clause, "and he went into her" (*wayyābō' 'ēleyhā*) is used to refer to Judah's sexual intercourse with Tamar, his daughter-in-law who pretended to be a prostitute (*zônāh*). After Judah gave his signet, cord, and staff to her, he went into her (*wayyābō' 'ēleyhā*), and she conceived by him (Gen 38:18). Seen in this light, the clause "and he went into her" in Judg 16:1 denotes that Samson had a sexual relationship with the prostitute (*zônāh*) in Gaza, and thus violated his Nazirite vows.[57] Samson's trip to Gaza where he had sexual intercourse with a prostitute was "a display of physical lust outside of marriage."[58] Samson both violated his Nazirite vows and distorted God's original design for sexuality by having sexual intercourse with a prostitute to satisfy his lustful appetites. As Block observes, the book of Judges records that "Samson wasted his life playing with the gifts God had given him and indulging in every sensual adventure he desired."[59] In Samson's story, "the role of women and their sexuality is a major governing characteristic of the Judge which leads to his death" (Judg 16:1–3; 4–31).[60] Thus, Samson's life driven by his lust illustrates "the failure of a charismatic leader, and divine powers wasted."[61]

David

David and the Spirit of Yahweh

In 1 Sam 16:13, the narrator records that Samuel's anointing of David was immediately followed by the coming of the Spirit of Yahweh; "Then Samuel took the horn of oil and anointed him in the midst of his brothers, and the Spirit of Yahweh came/rushed (*ṣālaḥ*) to David from that day forward. And Samuel arose and went to Ramah" (16:13). The simultaneity of David's anointing with oil and his receipt of Yahweh's Spirit in 1 Sam 16:13 signifies that David was Yahweh's chosen king who was "the man after God's own heart/mind" (cf. 1 Sam 13:14).[62] In the context of 1 Sam 16:13–14, the coming of Yahweh's Spirit upon David was followed by the departure of Yahweh's Spirit from Saul, implying that the Spirit of Yahweh that "bestows the gifts necessary for leadership cannot be given to two men, both supreme leaders, at the same time."[63] The coming of Yahweh's Spirit upon David in 1 Sam 16:13, according to Block, is "a most significant turning point in the history of Israel and her monarchy–the transfer of divine authority and support from Saul to David."[64]

The phrase "from that day forward" in 1 Sam 16:13c is particularly significant in this context because it signifies that unlike the judges and Saul on whom Yahweh's Spirit came "several different times, implying that it had left them in some way in the interim periods,"[65] the coming of Yahweh's Spirit upon David in 1 Sam 16:13 was to be permanent.[66] Concerning the role of the coming of Yahweh's Spirit, Hildebrand observes that Yahweh's Spirit equipped David with "military skills and charisma for his leadership skills," which are evident throughout his reign.[67] In 2 Sam 8:15, David is depicted as Israel's king who administered justice and righteousness to all his people. In 1 Sam 16:18, the narrator clarifies that David's success in all his undertaking was due to Yahweh's presence in his life; "And David was prospering [lit. "acting wisely"] in all his ways for Yahweh was with him."[68] In sum, the Spirit of Yahweh not only authenticated David as Yahweh's chosen king over Israel but also continually empowered him to carry out his tasks as the king of Israel who administered justice and righteousness in his kingdom. In the following, we will further explore the sexuality of David in light of God's norm for human sexuality in creation.

David and Sexuality

Despite experiencing the empowerment of Yahweh's Spirit, David fell "prey to the prevailing customs of bigamy, polygamy, or concubinage."[69] While David had a relationship with several women (e.g., Saul's daughter Michal, Abigal, Ahinoam of Jezreel, Bathsheba), because of the limited space, we will focus on David's sexual relationship with Bathsheba, the wife of Uriah, as described in 2 Sam 11. While some have portrayed Bathsheba as a seducer who secretly aimed to become queen, recent scholars view Bathsheba "not as an adulterer but as a victim of David's abuse of power."[70]

In 2 Sam 11:2, the narrator records that after David arose from his bed, he walked on the roof of the king's house and saw a very beautiful woman who was bathing. In v. 3, the beautiful woman was identified as the daughter of Eliam and the wife (*'iššâ*) of Uriah. In 2 Sam 23, both Eliam (23:34) and Uriah (23:39) were listed among David's loyal and heroic soldiers.[71] The messengers' statement that the beautiful woman whom David saw was the daughter of Eliam and the wife (*'iššâ*) of Uriah in v. 2 "should have picked David's conscience and restrained his lustful desires."[72] Yet, unlike Joseph who refused the seduction of Potiphar's wife because he considered having a sexual union with another man's wife was not only an offense against her husband but also a great sin against God (Gen 39:9),[73] David sent messengers and took Bathsheba, Uriah's wife, and when she came to him, he lay with her (2 Sam 11:4).

It has been suggested that the clause, "she came (*bô'*) to him" in 2 Sam 11:4 may denote that Bathsheba offered no resistance to David.[74] It is worth noting, however, that the narrator's similar statement that "And Uriah came (*bô'*) to him (David)" when David summoned him (vv. 6–7) indicates that Bathsheba's coming to David in v. 4 was in "obedient response to the explicit command of her king," just as Uriah's was.[75] This implies that she was a victim of David's abuse of power and sex. This is evident in the narrator's use of a "string of verbs in the narrative sequence ('saw...sent...inquired...sent... took her... lay with her')" in vv. 2–4.[76]

While God's original design for human sexuality in creation teaches that sexual intercourse is intended only within a covenantal marriage (Gen 2:24), 2 Sam 11:1–4 records that David, a Spirit-empowered leader, distorted the divine design by using his power to have sexual intercourse with Uriah's wife. Instead of submitting to Yahweh's lordship and living in the fear of Yahweh, David allowed himself to be controlled by his lustful desires. This led him to exploit Bathsheba to gain his own sexual satisfaction (vv. 1–5) and to murder Uriah, her husband (vv. 6–25). David tried to cover his sin with Bathsheba by taking her as his wife (*'iššâ*) after her mourning for her husband (Uriah) was over (vv. 26–27). However, the narrator explicitly records, "But the thing that David had done was evil (*rā'a'*) in the eyes of Yahweh" (2 Sam 11:27b). Thus, David's abuse of power and sex in 2 Sam 11 stands in contrast with Joseph who resisted the seduction of Potiphar's wife by saying, "How then could I do this great evil (*rā'āh*) and sin against God" (Gen 39:9c).

Conclusions and Implications

In the first part, our examination of the creation accounts in Genesis 1:26–31 and 2:18–25 reveals that human sexuality is part of God's good creation and his gift to husband and wife. Further, God's norm for marriage is heterosexual, monogamous, and covenantal. Sexual union, therefore, is intended exclusively for husband and wife.

In the second part, our examination of the sexual behavior of Spirit-empowered leaders in the light of the divine design for sexuality in creation leads us to the following conclusions. First, while the Spirit of God equipped Joseph with wisdom and understanding for his leadership task, his ability to overcome the sexual temptation of Potiphar's wife was directly attributed to the fear of Yahweh and his voluntary submission to his lordship. Second, although Yahweh's Spirit frequently empowered Samson to carry out the tasks set for him and to defeat his enemies, his life was driven by his lust and his sexual union with a prostitute to satisfy his lustful appetites signifies that he distorted the divine design for sexuality. Third, whereas David was authenticated as Yahweh's chosen king over Israel and was continually empowered by Yahweh's Spirit for his task as Israel's king, he committed adultery and murder. At those times, he was driven not by the fear of Yahweh but by his lustful desires (2 Sam 11).

The above findings have implications for modern Pentecostals and Charismatics who have received the Holy Spirit in their hearts as God's guarantee, seal, and down payment (2 Cor 1:22; Eph 1:13–14) and are also empowered by the Spirit to become effective witnesses of Jesus Christ (Acts 1:8). Although the Holy Spirit enables believers to carry out God's given task and also empowers them to walk in obedience to God, this fact does not negate the necessity of human responsibility. In Gal 5:16–18, Paul exhorts the believers in Galatia to keep on walking by the Spirit and to submit themselves to the will of the Spirit so that they will not gratify the desires of the flesh. In this context, Paul explicates that sexual immorality, impurity, and sensuality are the work of the flesh (v. 19), but faithfulness and self-control are the fruit of the Spirit (vv. 22–23). When vv. 16–18 are read in relationship with vv. 19–23, it is evident that only those who continue walking in the Spirit (v. 16) and those who are continually led by the Spirit (v. 18) can overcome the desires of the flesh, which include sexual immorality, impurity, and sensuality, (v. 19) and can also bear spiritual fruit, which includes faithfulness and self-control (v. 22–23).

Correspondingly, our study has shown that while the Spirit of God/Yahweh empowered Joseph, Samson, and David, to carry out God's given tasks, not all of them were able to live out the divine design for human sexuality. Samson distorted God's design for sexuality because he was driven by his lust throughout his entire life. Whereas David was known as a man after God's own heart, he also failed to live out the divine design for sexuality in creation when he was driven by his lustful desires. In contrast, Joseph was able to overcome the seduction of Potiphar's wife and lived out the divine design for sexuality because he walked in the fear of Yahweh and submitted himself to Yahweh's lordship. In sum, the above findings lead us to conclude that in order to overcome sexual temptations and to live out God's original design for sexuality in creation, we, modern Pentecostals and Charismatics, must continually submit ourselves to the leading of the Holy Spirit who empowers us both to carry out God's given tasks and to walk in obedience to God and his ways.

2.

A Historical and Hermeneutical Approach to the Vice-Lists: A Pauline Perspective Concerning Homosexuality and the Holy Spirit

Mark Hall

Abstract

The subject of homosexuality is controversial in the Church, even among Pentecostals; consequently, there has arisen a need for a historical and hermeneutical examination of the topic, especially in the Pauline corpus. The vice lists of ancient literature along with the ones in the Pauline epistles provide insight into the apostle's understanding of their purpose and function. Of the ones where Paul lists sexual sins, three specifically mention homosexuality: Romans 1:26–27, 1 Corinthians 6:9–10, and 1 Timothy 1:9–10. This article discusses Paul's understanding of the connection between homosexuality and idolatry and provides an in-depth analysis of the Greek words *malakoi* and *arsenokoitai*. It concludes by emphasizing the Pauline response to overcoming the vices he enumerates: follow the Spirit.

Setting the Stage: The Importance of the Subject

Paul Nathan Alexander, in his presidential address presented to the Society for Pentecostal Studies in 2013, entitled "Raced, Gendered, Faithed, and Sexed," discusses "constructions of race and white supremacy, diversities of religious faith, and constructions of genders and sexes together with the concomitant ongoing inequalities for females and limitations on discourse regarding LGBT+ realities."[1] Particularly, he points out the various views of the Pentecostal Churches concerning a Christian approach toward homosexuality and argues for inclusive understanding and dialog.[2] Alexander concludes, "I am hopeful we can thrive as a society even as we argue civilly and charitably about biblical, theological, ethical, historical, philosophical, practical, ecumenical, missional, and cultural perspectives regarding LGBT+ realities both within and beyond the pentecostalisms we experience and study."[3]

Certainly, dialog on any subject is to be welcomed. However, it is imperative that both doctrine and praxis emerge out of a proper historical and hermeneutical perspective. A valid and appropriate Pentecostal hermeneutic[4] is one that treasures Scripture and seeks a correct Spirit-inspired textual interpretation. To do anything else is to do violence to the Biblical text and to create a culture of scholarly eisegesis. What has been happening in recent scholarly pursuits is the placing of a filter over Scripture that ignores tried and true exegetical methodologies—ones that enlighten and enliven the text, that create space for revelation as inspired by the Holy Spirit, and that support interpretations grounded in Scripture. Gordon Fee, a premier Pentecostal scholar, and Douglas Stuart explain:

> The aim of good interpretation is simple: to get at the "plain meaning of the text." And the most important ingredient one brings to this task is enlightened common sense. The test of good interpretation is that it makes good sense of the text. Correct interpretation, therefore, brings relief to the mind as well as a prick or prod to the heart.[5]

Nowhere has this departure from truth and solid Biblical interpretation become more apparent than in the Church. Societal influences and the loud cacophony of voices advocating for special interests have replaced the reasoned and proven foundation of Scripture. Without rightly divided Scripture (2 Tim 2:15 NKJV), incorrect teaching and doctrine arise in the Church.

Paul's Vice Lists Compared to Other Ancient Literature

Paul's epistles advocate righteous living, and he promotes this specifically through his ethical catalogs. By presenting virtue[6] and vice[7] lists in his letters, Paul clearly demarcates the means by which the believer is to live a holy life—one pleasing to God—itemizing what is to be shunned and what is to be embraced. According to J. D. Charles, "vice and virtue lists in the N[ew] T[estament] function paraenetically [as moral exhortations] in different contexts. They may be used for the purpose of antithesis (e.g., Gal 5:19–23 and Jas 3:13–18), contrast (e.g., Titus 3:1–7), instruction (e.g., 2 Pet 1:5–7) or polemics (e.g., 1 Tim 1:9–10; 6:3–5; 2 Tim 3:2–5)."[8] "Common in ancient literature,"[9] vice lists are "a literary form widespread in secular moral writings as well as in the NT"[10]—including the twenty-one "vices" listed in Romans 1:29–31 and the twelve "vices" listed in 1 Clement 35:5 and "even longer lists in Philo and in other writings."[11] In the Pauline corpus, there are at least three of these passages that mention sexual sins, especially condemning homosexuality: Romans 1:26–27 (AD 57–58), 1 Corinthians 6:9–10 (AD 53–58), and 1 Timothy 1:9–10 (AD 61–66). As Paul delineates these iniquities and admonishes believers to reject them, he advocates they walk a Spirit-filled life.

Various vice lists exist outside of the New Testament, for example, in the Wisdom of Solomon, the Dead Sea Scrolls, 1 Clement, and the Didache. Similarities to the Pauline passages are apparent. In Wisdom of Solomon 14:23–26 (ca. 50 BC), the author mentions "unnatural lust" and "murder" (Rom 1:26–27, 29), "adultery" and "theft" (1 Cor 6:9–10), and "murder" and "perjury" (1 Tim 1:9–10):

> For while they practice either child sacrifices or occult mysteries, or frenzied carousing in exotic rites, they no longer respect either lives or purity of marriage; but they either waylay and kill each other, or aggrieve each other by adultery. And all is confusion—blood and *murder*, *theft* and guile, corruption, faithlessness, turmoil, *perjury*, disturbance of good people, neglect of gratitude, besmirching of souls, *unnatural lust*, disorder in marriage, *adultery* and shamelessness.[12]

The Dead Sea Scrolls also contain examples of vice lists as seen in "The Community Rule" (ca. 150 BC):

> But the ways of the spirit of falsehood are these: *greed*, and *slackness in the search for righteousness*, wickedness and lies, haughtiness and pride, falseness and deceit, cruelty and *abundant evil*, ill-temper and much folly and brazen insolence, *abominable deeds (committed) in a spirit of lust*, and ways of lewdness in the service of uncleanness, a blaspheming tongue, blindness of eye and dullness of ear, stiffness of neck and heaviness of heart, so that man walks in all the ways of darkness and guile. (1 QS 4:9–11)[13]

The vices mentioned in this DSS passage that are common to the Pauline corpus are "greed, and slackness in the search for righteousness," "abundant evil," and "abominable deeds (committed) in a spirit of lust." For example, Paul categorizes some of these sins as "being filled with all unrighteousness," "greed," "inventors of evil," and a description of unnatural lusts in Romans 1:26–32.[14] First Clement 35:5 (ca. AD 100) also incorporates vice lists, admonishing believers to cast off iniquities:

> But how shall this be, dearly beloved? If our mind be fixed through faith towards God; if we seek out those things which are well pleasing and acceptable unto Him; if we accomplish such things as beseem His faultless will, and follow the way of truth, casting off from ourselves *all unrighteousness* and iniquity, covetousness,

> strifes, malignities and deceits, whisperings and backbitings, hatred of God, pride and arrogance, vainglory and inhospitality.[15]

The vice lists in the Pauline corpus mention "all unrighteousness," "strife," "deceit," "haters of God," "arrogant," "gossips," and "slanderers" ("whisperings" and "backbitings," 1 Clement) (Rom 1:29–31). Of course, Clement is familiar with Romans since he quotes from the book.

Another detailed vice list occurs in the Didache 5:1 (AD 50–120):

> But the Way of Death is this: First of all, it is wicked and full of cursing, murders, adulteries, lusts, fornications, thefts, idolatries, witchcrafts, charms, robberies, false witness, hypocrisies, a double heart, fraud, pride, malice, stubbornness, covetousness, foul speech, jealousy, impudence, haughtiness, boastfulness.[16]

Some of the specific vices Paul notes in the lists above as well as general categories for others (e.g., lusts) are also reflected here in the Didache.

Paul's Vice Lists Mentioning Homosexuality (Especially Romans 1)

Paul's use of vice lists in Romans 1:29–31, Galatians 5:19–21, 1 Corinthians 6:9–10, and 2 Corinthians 12:21–21 hearkens back to a "moral tradition from the OT and Judaism especially from Deuteronomy," not just reflecting Greek or Hellenistic moral writings.[17] Anthony Thiselton notes, "[W]hat most scholars call 'the vice catalogue' is better interpreted in terms of the Deuteronomic covenant identity and convenient obligations."[18] He rightly observes,

> Evidence of similar patterns of style and parenetic catalogues within the NT…owe more to a common *catechetical Sitz im Leben* than to the hellenistic settings…. *If the background is catechetical, this transforms the significance of such a "list" into guidelines explicit for teaching on the nature of the Christian life.*[19]

In other words, Paul's epistolary vice lists reflect instructions the apostle gives to the Church, by which he establishes a moral framework based on the Old Testament upon which he commands believers to live righteously. In fact, Brian Rosner concludes that "the Scriptures were an indispensable and formative source for 1 Cor. 6:1–11." He asserts that Paul "showed himself to have Scriptural structures of thought, such as the notion that identity must inform behavior."[20]

In three of his vice lists, Romans 1:26–27, 1 Corinthians 6:9–10, and

1 Timothy 1:9–10, Paul condemns homosexuality. In Romans 1:26–27, Paul notes the effects of these "unnatural relations."

> For this reason God gave them over to degrading passions (disgraceful passions) (*pathē atimias*); for their women exchanged the natural function (*physikēn chrēsin*) for that which is unnatural (unnatural relations) (*tēn para physin*), and in the same way (*homoiōs*) also the men abandoned the natural function (*physikēn chrēsin*) of the woman and burned in their desire toward one another (they were inflamed in their lust for one another) (*exekauthēsan en tē orexei autōn eis allēlous*), men with men committing indecent acts (*tēn aschēmosynēn katergazomenoi*) and receiving in their own persons the due penalty of their error (the penalty...of their [idolatrous] perversion) (*tēn antimisthian...tēs planēs*).[21]

In the NASB, the Greek words *physikēn chrēsin* (from *chrēsis*) are translated "natural function" and *tēn para physin* (from *physis*) as "that which is unnatural."[22] The definition of *chrēsis* is the "state of intimate involvement w[ith] a pers[on], *relations, function*, esp[ecially] of sexual intercourse"[23] and *physis* means "the regular or established order of things, nature," with *tēn para physin* translated as "one contrary to nature"[24] or "what is against nature."[25] In order to move the understanding of this verse from the individual and his or her personal culpability to a broader, more palatable interpretation that encompasses the book of Romans as a whole, Eugene F. Rogers asserts that Paul is here discussing Gentiles. He connects this verse to Romans 11:24 where the same Greek words appear and asserts that "God is acting contrary to nature" because he is grafting the Gentiles to the Church. He maintains that "Paul's sex-talk is about something else: ethnic stereotype transformed into another proclamation of the gospel. It is our own Gentile salvation that we misunderstand, if we mis-hear how Paul reclaims the language of sexual stereotype for his purpose."[26] This lays the groundwork for Rogers' argument that Scripture does not forbid same-sex couples, and therefore the Church should embrace them.

A cursory examination of the text calls Rogers' view into question. Romans 1:27 is connected with the verse before it with the Greek word *homoiōs*, which can be translated "likewise' or "in the same way." Here Paul demonstrates that the "disgraceful passions" that cause women to participate in the "unnatural relations" of homosexuality are also responsible for "men committing indecent acts." Douglas Moo observes, "Homosexuality among 'males,' [*arsenes*, the same word used in the Septuagint when homosexuality is prohibited, Lev. 18:22; 20:13] like that among 'females,' is characterized as a departure from nature,... the natural order." Moo continues,

Paul uses strong language to characterize male homosexuality: "they burned [*exekauthēsan* from *ekkaiō*, a *hapax legomenon*, but has been used in writings apart from the NT to mean the "kindling" of sin] in their desire [*orexei*, another *hapax legomenon*] for one another, men with men doing that which is shameful [*tēn aschēmosynēn*, used here and in Revelation 16:15, with "closest parallels in intertestamental Judaism"] and receiving in themselves the just penalty [*antimisthian*, "a payment in place of," here meaning "penalty"] that was necessary for their error."[27]

Moo asserts that Paul believes this "penalty" "was necessary" because "God could not allow his created order to be so violated without there being a just punishment."[28]

In Romans 1:24, 26, and 28, Paul acknowledges God as being active in his response to those who decide to follow this path of immorality. The Greek words *paredōken autous ho theos* —can be translated "God gave them over,"[29] "God gave them up,"[30] or "God handed them over."[31] John Chrysostom, who according to C. E. B. Cranfield is "specially strong in exposition of the explicitly ethical sections" of Paul,[32] understands this Greek word as God withdrawing his presence from the idolaters, thus allowing them to keep committing wrong and to dive even deeper into sin. He writes:

> He "gave them up," here is, let them alone. For as he that hath the command in an army, if upon the battle lying heavy upon him he retreat and go away, gives up his soldiers to the enemies not by thrusting them himself, but by stripping them of his own assistance; thus too did God leave those that were not minded to receive what cometh from Him, but were the first to bound off from Him, though Himself having wholly fulfilled His own part.... They perverted to the opposite what they had received.[33]

For Chrysostom, the one committing the sin is responsible for its consequences, not God. Frederic Louis Godet presents the following analogy:

> The word *gave over* does not signify that God *impelled* them to evil, to punish the evil which they had already committed. The holiness of God is opposed to such a sense, and to *give over* is not to *impel*. On the other hand, it is impossible to stop short at the idea of a simple *permission*: "God let them give themselves over to evil." God was not purely passive in the terrible development of Gentile corruption. Wherein did His action consist? He positively withdrew His hand; He ceased to hold the boat as it was dragged by the current of the river.[34]

However, Douglas Moo argues that these explanations place God in too passive of a role; he believes the Greek word demands that God acts more intentionally: "God does not simply let the boat go—he gives it a push downstream. Like a judge who hands over a prisoner to the punishment his crime has earned, God hands over the sinner to the terrible cycle of ever-increasing sin."[35] As Everett F. Harrison and Donald A. Hagner observe concerning Romans 1:26–27: "'God gave them over' again to immorality, with emphasis on perversion in sexual relations. The sequence Paul follows—idolatry, then immorality—raises the connection between the two.... Sinning against God results in their sinning against their own nature."[36]

The Connection between Homosexuality and Idolatry

Earlier in Romans 1, Paul connects sexual sins to idolatry: "Professing to be wise, they became fools, and exchanged the glory of the incorruptible God for an image in the form of corruptible man and of birds and four-footed animals and crawling creatures. Therefore God gave them over in the lusts of their hearts to impurity, so that their bodies would be dishonored among them" (Rom. 1:22–24). Paul shows here that "sexual sin, specifically homosexuality, is the product of idolatry."[37] This connection between idolatry and fornication, a common one in Jewish literature, is also made in Wisdom of Solomon,[38] "For the idea of making idols was the beginning of fornication, and the invention of them was the corruption of life" (14:12 RSV), and "For the worship of idols not to be named is the beginning and cause and end of every evil" (14:27 RSV).[39] Idolatry inevitably leads to participation in the sin that it promotes: "In return for their foolish and wicked thoughts, which led them astray to worship irrational serpents and worthless animals, thou didst send upon them a multitude of irrational creatures to punish them, that they might learn that one is punished by the very things by which he sins" (Wisd 11:15–16 RSV).[40] These passages are reminiscent of the sin of the Israelites in worshipping the golden calf Aaron fashioned when Moses was in the presence of God receiving the Ten Commandments, an example of "idolatry [as] the source of immorality"[41]: "So the next day they rose early and offered burnt offerings [before the idol of the golden calf that Aaron made for them], and brought peace offerings; and the people sat down to eat and to drink, and rose up to play [participating in pagan orgies to celebrate their newfound god]" (Exod 32:6). Indeed, Paul believed that sexual immorality, especially homosexuality, displayed the highest rejection of God's moral order. According to Richard Longenecker

32 Human Sexuality and the Holy Spirit

> Likewise important for understanding Paul's rationale in highlighting homosexuality when explicating the connection between idolatry and immorality is the fact that Paul viewed homosexuality as the most obvious result of humanity's failure to respond appropriately to God's revelation in creation. For though it was often asserted by those who practiced it that homosexuality was "natural"—even, as argued both then and today, a legitimate feature of divine creation—Paul viewed such a claim as in direct opposition to the moral order established by God in creation, where only in marriage do a man and a woman "become one flesh" (Gen. 2:24).[42]

According to Paul, this sexual aberration is the direct result of worshipping some other god. J. A. Fitzmyer observes

> Thus pagan idolatry has become the "big lie," and pagans have no excuse; their godlessness and wickedness have made them objects of divine wrath. Second, the condition of pagan humanity results from the moral degradation to which their idolatry has brought them: to the craving of their hearts for impurity. Their idolatry has led to moral perversion: sexual excess (1:24, 26a) and homosexual activity (1:26b–27).[43]

In "The Testament of Naphtali, the Eighth Son of Jacob and Bilhah," the author discusses how both Sodom and the Watchers "changed the order of nature," which resulted in severe judgment from the Lord, a clear corollary to Romans 1.

> Be ye, therefore, not eager to corrupt your doings through covetousness or with vain words to beguile your souls; because if ye keep silence in purity of heart, ye shall understand how to hold fast the will of God, and to cast away the will of Beliar. Sun and moon and stars change not their order; so do ye also change not the law of God in the disorderliness of your doings. The Gentiles went astray, and forsook the Lord, and changed their order, and obeyed stocks and stones, spirits of deceit. But ye shall not be so, my children, recognizing in the firmament, in the earth, and in the sea, and in all created things, the Lord Who made all things, that ye become not as Sodom, which changed the order of nature. In like manner the Watchers also changed the order of their nature, whom the Lord cursed at the flood, on whose account He made the earth without inhabitant and fruitless (3:1–5).[44]

Anthony Thiselton also concludes, "What is clear from the connection between 1 Cor 6:9 and Rom 1:26–29 and their OT backgrounds is Paul's endorsement of the view that idolatry, i.e., placing human autonomy to construct one's values above covenant commitments to God, leads to a collapse of moral values in a kind of domino effect."[45] This emphasis would explain Paul's focus on homosexuality. Thomas Schreiner queries, "Why does Paul focus on homosexual relations, especially since it receives little attention elsewhere in his writings (1 Cor. 6:9; 1 Tim. 1:10)?" Schreiner sees both homosexuality and idolatry as unnatural:

> Idolatry is "unnatural" in the sense that it is contrary to God's intention for human beings. To worship corruptible animals and human beings instead of the incorruptible God is to turn the created order upside down. In the sexual sphere, the mirror image of this "unnatural" choice of idolatry is homosexuality.... Human beings were intended to have sexual relations with those of the opposite sex. Just as idolatry is a violation and perversion of what God indented, so too homosexual relations are contrary to what God planned when he created man and woman."[46]

For Paul, the connection between the two is axiomatic.

The Greek Words *malakoi* and *arsenokoitai*

Two other passages where Paul mentions homosexuality in his vice lists are 1 Corinthians 6:9–10 and 1 Timothy 1:9–10:

> Or do you not know that the unrighteous will not inherit the kingdom of God? Do not be deceived; neither fornicators, nor idolaters, nor adulterers, nor effeminate (*malakoi*), nor homosexuals (*arsenokoitai*), nor thieves, nor the covetous, nor drunkards, nor revilers, nor swindlers, will inherit the kingdom of God. (1 Cor 6:9–10)

> ...Law is not made for a righteous person, but for those who are lawless and rebellious, for the ungodly and sinners, for the unholy and profane, for those who kill their fathers or mothers, for murderers and immoral men and homosexuals (*arsenokoitais*) and kidnappers and liars and perjurers, and whatever else is contrary to sound teaching (1 Tim 1:9–10).

The Greek word *malakoi* has been translated variously as "effeminate" ("by perversion"), "homosexuals," "catamites," and "male prostitutes." Further analysis of the word reveals that the word can mean "males who are penetrated sexually by males"[47] or "being passive in a same-sex relationship, *effeminate* esp. of *catamites*, of men and boys who are sodomized by other males in such a relationship." The translation "male prostitutes" is considered by some scholars as "too narrow a rendering and 'sexual pervert'...is too broad."[48] The word *malakos* also has the connotation of softness, and for Philo means to change "the male nature to the female, becoming guilty of 'unmanliness'...and 'effeminacy'": "The male becomes 'womanish.'"[49] Philo writes that "another evil...has made its way among and been let loose upon cities, namely, the love of boys...which sin is a subject of boasting not only to those who practise it," but also to those who "are not ashamed to devote their constant study and endeavours to the task of changing their manly character into an effeminate one."[50] Gordon Fee asserts that *malakos* was "a pejorative epithet for men who were 'soft' or 'effeminate,' most likely referring to the younger, 'passive' partner in a pederastic relationship—the most common form of homosexuality in the Greco-Roman world" and believes the best translation of the word is "'male prostitute' (in the sense of 'effeminate call-boy')."[51]

The Greek word *arsenokoitai* that occurs in both 1 Corinthians 6:9 and 1 Timothy 1:10 "is a compound of 'male' and 'intercourse.'"[52] It can be translated as follows: "homosexuals," "abusers of themselves with mankind," "sodomites," "those who participate in homosexuality," "male homosexuals," "those who practice homosexuality," "males who sexually penetrate males,"[53] and "lying with men."[54] The word can be defined as "a male who engages in sexual activity w[ith] a pers[son] of his own sex, *pederast*"—"one who assumes the dominant role in the same-sex activity."[55] Paul's condemnation of same-sex conduct "cannot be satisfactorily explained on the basis of alleged temple prostitution...or limited to contract w[ith] boys for homoerotic service."[56] The word "does not refer...only to sex with young boys or to male homosexual prostitutes, but simply to homosexuality itself"[57]; "it denotes, unequivocally, the activity of male homosexuality."[58] Some translate *malakoi* and *arsenokoitai* together in 1 Corinthians 6:9 as "men who practice homosexuality," "men who have sex with men," and "sexual pervert(s)" because they believe the words refer to the "passive and active participants in homosexual acts."[59]

Some scholars have argued that homosexuality is not condemned by the New Testament. John Boswell asserts, "It is...quite clear that nothing in the Bible would have categorically precluded homosexual relations among early Christians.... The word 'homosexual' does not occur in the Bible."[60] He argues that *malakoi* has often been translated "masturbation" and that the proper translation of *arsenokoitai* is "male prostitute."[61] Robin Scroggs believes the former word should be understood as an "effeminate call-boy," and the latter as the one "who hires him on occasion to satisfy his sexual desires."[62] Dale Martin takes umbrage at *arsenokoitai* meaning homosexual "perversion" and asserts that *malakoi* should be translated as "effeminate," someone who attracts male and female lovers. He sees modern translations as purposefully reinterpreting the text, avoiding historical context and inserting cultural stereotypes that are biased against the gay community.[63] None of these authors believes that Paul forbids homosexuality in general. However, Robert Gagnon counters this understanding of the Pauline texts by translating *malakoi*, "literally...'the soft ones'" as "effeminate males who play the sexual role of females" and *arsenokoitai*, "literally...'male-bedders' as 'males who take other males to bed.'"[64] In his in-depth analysis of these Greek words, he demonstrates effectively their homosexual connotations.

Gordon Fee points out that this is the "first appearance [of *arsenokoitai*] in preserved literature, and subsequent authors are reluctant to use it, especially when describing the homosexual activity."[65] Since the Greek word does not appear before Paul's use, it seems likely that Paul has probably coined the term *arsenokoitai* from the LXX *arsenos koitēn* (Lev 20:13),[66] demonstrating his knowledge and acceptance of the condemnation of the act of homosexuality in the Mosaic writings. The passages in the Septuagint are Leviticus 18:22 and 20:13: "And thou shalt not lie (*koimēthēsē* —lit., 'go to bed'[67]) (*koitēn* —lit., 'in a marriage bed'[68]) with a man as with a woman, for it is an abomination" (Lev 18:22 LXX)[69]; "And whoever shall lie (*koimēthē* —lit., 'should have bedded') with a male (*arsenos koitēn* —lit., 'as the marriage bed') as with a woman, they have both wrought abomination; let them die the death, they are guilty" (Lev 20:13 LXX).[70] The Old Testament clearly indicates that "lying with a male is a general concept describing 'every kind of homosexual intercourse,' not simply male prostitution or sexual relations with youth."[71]

Even though certain types of homosexual behavior were acceptable in the Greek world of Paul's time, "Hellenistic Jewish texts are unanimous in condemning them and treat them and idolatry as the most obvious examples of Gentile moral depravity. Not surprisingly, Paul shares this Jewish aversion to idolatry and homosexual acts."[72] Paul's echoing of the Leviticus passages demonstrates that he views "homosexuality as a deviation from the Mosaic moral code."[73] Paul uses the Greek word *arsenokoitais* as "a broad term that cannot be confined to specific instances of homosexual activity such as male prostitution or pederasty." In the language of the Old Testament "lying with a 'male' (a very general term) is proscribed and relates to 'every kind of male-male intercourse.'" The Old Testament forbids "every type of homosexual intercourse (including a consensual one), not just male prostitution or intercourse with youths." While Paul's emphasis is "on homosexual *acts*, he would hardly have considered 'celibate' homosexual relationships as legitimate; for this would be to exchange a man's 'natural' function for what is 'unnatural.'"[74] This is in contrast to male friendships, which are legitimate. As Richard Longenecker observes, "Paul's attitude toward homosexual behavior could hardly be more adversely expressed. For he condemns it totally—as did also all Jews and all Jewish Christians of his day."[75]

The Pauline Response: Walking by the Spirit

Paul's desire is that Christians overcome the sins listed in his vice lists, not embrace them. Even so, believers are not expected to resist these vices on their own. After his vice list in Galatians 5:19–21, Paul asserts that Christ-followers are to leave sin behind: "Now those who belong to Jesus Christ have crucified the flesh with its passions and desires" (Gal 5:24), and he encourages them to live righteously through the power of the Holy Spirit: "If we live in the Spirit, let us also walk [*stoichōmen*] by the Spirit" (Gal 5:25). The Greek word *stoichōmen* (from *stoicheō*) means "to be in line with a pers[on] or thing considered as a standard for one's conduct, *hold to, agree with, follow, conform.*"[76] It can be translated to *"follow the Spirit."*[77]

Believers' bodies—temples inhabited by the Holy Spirit—are commanded to "flee immorality," for Paul, writing to the Christians in Corinth, teaches "that you are not your own," "for you have been bought with a price" (1 Cor 6:18–20). According to Anthony Thiselton, the basis for Paul's vice lists in 1 Corinthians 6:9–10, "is not Stoic or Jewish ethics, but Christian identity as temples of the Holy Spirit (6:19) redeemed at cost to belong to Christ as his (6:20). 'You are not your own' (6:19b) is as far from Stoic autonomy as can be imagined."[78] This forsaking of sin rather than its justification is a central Pauline doctrine, and as Robert Gagnon proclaims,

> [T]he good news is that God is on the side of believers in sparing no effort to transform them into the image of Jesus. God both empowers believers by means of the Spirit, and motivates them through God's unprecedented accomplishment of redemption in Christ and the hope of a magnificent salvation yet to be revealed. The God who once manifested wrath against those who turned to idols by handing them over to their shameful passions has now handed them over to the life-giving, transformative power of the Spirit of Christ.[79]

Paul commands that Christians are to "glorify God in [their] bod[ies]" (1 Cor 6:20). The Holy Spirit indwells and empowers the believer and provides for victory over iniquity and shows the way toward redemption.

3.

Leaving the Past Behind: A Historical Survey of the Church's Response to Homosexuality

Clayton Coombs

Abstract

It has been said that to fail to learn from history is to be condemned to repeat it. This chapter represents an endeavor to retrieve Godly wisdom for our present time from the history of the Church on the important issue/s of homosexuality. It arises from four fundamental convictions. First, that all humans alike are sinners in the eyes of God before they encounter his transformative power. Second, the gospel is good news to all. Third, that the *modus operandi* of the Church is love. And fourth, that the Bible is the eternal inerrant Word of God containing the answers in every culture and every generation to every issue humans face. For us, particularly as Spirit-empowered believers, the discourse must be about compassion rather than judgment, wholeness rather than hatred, faithfulness rather than a phobia.

From this foundation, this chapter surveys four ways that the Church has traditionally responded to the reality of homosexuality—to treat it as an 'Abomination,' as an 'Aberration,' as an 'Illness,' and more recently as an 'Injury'—and discusses the relative merits (and consequences) of these responses. The approach is necessarily representative rather than exhaustive. While each of these arguably arises from Scripture, a fifth and more basic approach ultimately commends itself, namely to see homosexuality as part of the (Fallen) human experience. To acknowledge this has the effect of humanizing homosexuality and thus, on the one hand, providing the basis for a response of compassion rather than judgment, while on the other eliciting the hope of transformation by the power of the Spirit.

Introduction

Needless to say, the stakes of the discussion are incredibly high, since how we view homosexuality will tend to dictate how we deal with people. Ideas have consequences and theology can never be divorced from pastoral care. On the one hand, those who identify as gay (queer, etc.) may be constantly reminded by some teachings of the Church that because God does not approve of the homosexual lifestyle, a greater and eternal torment awaits when they escape the torment of this life. When they insist that they did not choose to feel this way, they are often met with lectures or with being ignored or dismissed. This has the effect of dehumanizing rather than offering hope. On the other hand, when those who identify as Christians, politely (or otherwise) insist on their right to hold to the truth of the Bible on this issue,[1] they are denounced as motivated by fear (homophobic) and preaching hate. While Christians would argue that they are motivated by love rather than fear, it is ironically the fear of offense and ridicule which has largely silenced the voices of those who claim to have experienced a change in 'orientation' due to an encounter with the Spirit of God. For Pentecostal Christians, who believe passionately in the transformative power of the Holy Spirit, this is surely a gap in the literature that needs to be courageously and compassionately addressed. And yet there is another gap in the literature that should be of concern to Pentecostals. Voices from the Early Church are conspicuous by their absence. There are as yet few if any scholarly treatments of Early Church voices on this issue. There is, of course, much that is said about the Church and its attitude to gay people. This includes various references to some of the more hostile things that the ancient Church has said, usually quoted out of context and calculated for maximum shock value. Given the 'journey' motif of many who have written from their own experience on this issue, references to the Past are typically only produced to support the case, presumed self-evident, that we should leave it behind where it belongs and move on to more enlightened attitudes. Much less common is a sympathetic reading of the Church Fathers with sustained engagement regarding their treatment of Scripture.

The present chapter attempts (at least to begin) to address this gap by presenting a reception history of 1 Corinthians 6:11 from the Patristic period.[2] This period has been chosen for two main reasons. First, some of the most important theologians in the history of the Church lived and wrote in this period. Second, it is broadly acknowledged that outside of the first century Church itself, the Church of this period had the greatest regard for and expectation of the supernatural involvement of the Holy Spirit. 1 Corinthians 6:11 has been chosen as a source text for this study because it names homosexual practices specifically,[3] and it also mentions the agency of the Holy Spirit in bringing about transformation. In other words, for those seeking a distinctly Pentecostal response to homosexuality, 1 Cor 6:11 is a natural choice. Beginning with Irenaeus, the following proceeds with an author by author presentation of the Church Fathers who cited this passage which includes a discussion of how each interpreted the verse.[4] Of special interest for this publication is how each author understands the agency of the Holy Spirit. The chapter concludes with a summary and synthesis.

As it primarily takes a historical focus, this study will not engage the modern debate over this issue except to recommend where we might learn from the ancient one.

The Power of the Holy Spirit in Evidence: A Reception History of 1 Cor 6:11

Irenaeus

Irenaeus of Lyon discusses 1 Corinthians 6:11 and the passage within which it is contained several times in his extant corpus. Three of these occur in his *Against Heresies*, an important qualification to begin with, since his express purpose throughout this work is to refute the various heresies that were, in his day, attempting to make inroads into mainstream Christian teaching. In the 27th section of Book 4 of this work, he is refuting the heresy that the God of the Old Testament is somehow different from the God revealed in Christ in the New Testament. Of the proponents of this heresy, Irenaeus says:

> [A]ll these men are found to be unlearned and presumptuous, nay, even destitute of common sense, who, because of the transgressions of them of old time, and because of the disobedience of a vast number of them, do allege that there was indeed one God of these men, and that He was the maker of the world, and existed in a state of degeneracy; but that there was another Father declared by Christ, and that this Being is He who has been conceived by the mind of each of them; not understanding that as, in the former case, God showed himself not well pleased in many instances towards those who sinned, so also in the latter, "many are called, but few are chosen."[5]

In a withering pastiche of New Testament judgment passages including Ephesians 5:3–7, 1 Corinthians 5:9–11, and (importantly for the present study) Romans 1:18, Irenaeus demonstrates that while the gospel does deal with sin, it by no means changes its definition. It is in this context that he brings in 1 Corinthians 6:9–11:

> ...and the apostle says, "Know ye not that the unrighteous shall not inherit the

kingdom of God? Be not deceived: neither fornicators, nor idolaters, nor adulterers, nor[6] effeminate, nor abusers of themselves with mankind,[7] nor thieves, nor covetous, nor drunkards, nor revilers, nor extortioners, shall inherit the kingdom of God.[8]

The point here is not so much the judgment though, as it is to demonstrate the continuity between the Old Testament and the New. God's attitude towards sin has not changed. Lest his readers think that judgment for sin applies only to those outside, Irenaeus reminds them of the Apostle's words from 1 Corinthians 6:11, "And that is what some of you were. But you were washed, you were sanctified in the name of the Lord Jesus Christ and by the Spirit of our God." Because of that sanctifying activity of the Spirit, the standard, if anything, is higher. For just as under the Old Covenant "those who led vicious lives, and put other people astray, were condemned and cast out, so also even now the offending eye is plucked out, and the foot and the hand, lest the rest of the body perish in like manner."[9]

Several sections later in the same book, Irenaeus, having established that God's will for purity in his people has not changed, insists that it is within the power of the believer to achieve God's will in this regard. Beginning from Paul's premise that "everything is permissible for me but not everything is beneficial" (1 Cor 10:23), he continues thus:

> ...referring both to the liberty of man, in which respect "all things are lawful," God exercising no compulsion in regard to him; and [by the expression] "not expedient" pointing out that we "should not use our liberty as a cloak of maliciousness," for this is not expedient. And again he says, "Speak ye every man truth with his neighbour." And, "Let no corrupt communication proceed out of your mouth, neither filthiness, nor foolish talking, or scurrility, which are not convenient, but rather giving of thanks." And, "For ye were sometimes darkness, but now are ye light in the Lord; walk honestly as children of the light, not in rioting and drunkenness, not in chambering and wantonness, not in anger and jealousy. And such were some of you; but ye have been washed, but ye have been sanctified in the name of our Lord" (1 Cor 6:11). If then it were not in our power to do or not to do these things, what reason had the apostle, and much more the Lord Himself, to give us counsel to do some things, and to abstain from others? But because man is possessed of free will from the beginning, and God is possessed of free will, in whose likeness man was created, advice is always given to him to keep fast the good, which thing is done by means of obedience to God.[10]

What is clear from Irenaeus' references to 1 Corinthians 6:11 is that he does not single out the sin(/s) of homosexuality for special treatment. It is condemned along with 'foolish talk,' 'rioting,' 'drunkenness,' 'jealousy,' and the rest. Any and all of these things may characterize a believer before conversion, but should not after. Believers are expected, reasonably in Irenaeus' view, to live without the former sins, because human beings have been created in the image of God with free will. What is implicit here is that this free will is clearly damaged in unbelievers. However, the change that the "washing" of baptism and the sanctification of the Holy Spirit achieves in the name of the Lord Jesus Christ, restores the believer's God-created free will to enable him/her to live in obedience to God. And so in book 5, Irenaeus, foreseeing the objection of those that would twist Paul's meaning, draws together the several New Testament passages along with 1 Cor. 6:9–10 that delineate the things that will preclude a person "receiving the kingdom." From Galatians 5:22–23 Irenaeus suggests that, just as it is actions (of the flesh) which bring death, it is also actions (of the Spirit) that bring life, namely actions of love, joy, peace, patience, kindness etc. But these actions, the "things which save" all boil down to "the name of our Lord Jesus Christ, and the Spirit of our God."[11] He then proceeds to explain how the image of God (and thus the free will necessary to refuse sin) is renewed by the power of the Holy Spirit:

> Now this which he says, "as we have borne the image of him who is of the earth," is analogous to what has been declared, "And such indeed ye were; but ye have been washed, but ye have been sanctified, but ye have been justified in the name of our Lord Jesus Christ, and in the Spirit of our God." When, therefore, did we bear the image of him who is of the earth? Doubtless it was when those actions spoken of as "works of the flesh" used to be wrought in us. And then, again, when [do we bear] the image of the heavenly? Doubtless when he says, "Ye have been washed," believing in the name of the Lord, and receiving His Spirit. Now we have washed away, not the substance of our body, nor the image of our [primary] formation, but the former vain conversation.[12] In these members, therefore, in which we were going to destruction by working the works of corruption, in these very members are we made alive by working the works of the Spirit.[13]

Tertullian

For Tertullian, mention is made of 1 Corinthians 6:11 in section 21 of his treatise *On the Soul* where he is exposing the heresy that the soul is not subject to change. If that is so, Tertullian argues, then it follows that,

> God will not be able any longer to raise up from the stones children unto Abraham, nor to make a generation of vipers bring forth fruits of repentance. And if so, the apostle too was in error when he said in his epistle, "Ye were at one time darkness, (but now are ye light in the Lord)" (Eph 5:8) and, "We also were by nature children of wrath;" (Eph 2:3), "Such were some of you, but ye are washed" (1 Cor 6:11).

> The statements, however, of holy Scripture will never be discordant with truth. A corrupt tree will never yield good fruit unless the better nature be grafted into it; nor will a good tree produce evil fruit, except by the same process of cultivation. Stones also will become children of Abraham, if educated in Abraham's faith; and a generation of vipers will bring forth the fruits of penitence if they reject the poison of their malignant nature.[14]

In contrast to Irenaeus' high view of Free Will, Tertullian here sees the agency of God's grace as overriding our free will, albeit through the transformation of the new birth:

> This will be the power of the grace of God, more potent indeed than nature, exercising its sway over the faculty that underlies itself within us—even the freedom of our will, which is described as αὐτεξούσιος (of independent authority); and inasmuch as this faculty is itself also natural and mutable, in whatsoever direction it turns, it inclines of its own nature.... Now that which has received its constitution by being made or by being born is by nature capable of being changed, for it can be both born again and re-made...[15]

It is worth noting that Tertullian, though his high view of the power and grace of God to transform a human life is clearly in evidence in the quote above, also has a high view of baptism which, while common among the Fathers, is not perhaps shared to its fullest extent among Protestant Christians today. In the following quote from *De Pudicitia*, he again cites 1 Corinthians 6:11, but makes (perhaps a little too) much of the past tense:

> "But such indeed ye *have been*; but ye *have received* ablution, but ye *have been sanctified*, in the Name of the Lord Jesus Christ, and in the Spirit of our God;" in as far as he puts on the paid side of the account such sins before baptism, in so far after baptism he determines them irremissible, if it is true, (as it is), that they are not allowed to "receive ablution" anew.[16]

Tertullian then, clearly considers the 'washing' of baptism to be absolute and any sins committed after baptism to be unforgivable. He makes no special mention in either passage of any of the sins mentioned in 1 Cor 6:9–10. He merely takes it for granted that all can be forgiven and cleansed, and that Christians can and must avoid such sins after baptism.

Origen

Origen is well known as being the master allegorist. It is not surprising then, when we find him in full allegorical flight in the 15th of his

Homilies on Joshua, drawing the inevitable parallel between Joshua, the Jesus of the Old Testament,[17] and the Jesus of the New Testament. Here he is talking about the victories of Joshua over the various inhabitants of the land of promise. Citing Joshua 11:19–20 Origen notes that Joshua took

> ...all into his possession by war, it says, "because it happened that their heart was strengthened by the Lord and they hastened into battle against Israel." It did not say that by war Jesus [that is, Joshua] took some and did not take others, but that he took all into his possession, that is, he captured and destroyed all. And, indeed, the Lord Jesus has purged every kind of sin and destroyed all." For we all "were irrational, unbelieving, errant, serving various desires, acting in malice and envy, hateful, and hating one another," and (we possessed) every type of sin that is found in persons before they believe. Therefore, it is well said that Jesus [again, Joshua] kills all who have gone to war. For Jesus—who is the word and the "wisdom of God"—is greater than any kind of sin, no matter how terrible. For he overcomes and conquers all sins. Or do we not believe this, that every kind of sin is carried away when we come to the saving bath? For the apostle Paul also alludes to this, who, when he had enumerated the whole class of sins, adds something after them all and says, "And indeed you were these; but you were washed, you were sanctified, you were justified in the name of our Lord, Jesus Christ." Therefore, in this way, Jesus is said to have seized all in battle and to have destroyed all.[18]

Origen does not distinguish between the various sins in the sin list. Indeed, he evidently considers the list in Titus 3:3 an adequate substitute for the rather longer list in 1 Cor 6:9–10. Certainly, the parallel is a good one. In Titus 3 the solution is expressed in much the same terms as in 1 Cor 6, namely, "not by works of righteousness which we have done, but according to his mercy he saved us, through the washing of regeneration and renewing of the Holy Spirit, whom he poured out on us abundantly through Jesus Christ our Savior" (Titus 3:5–6).[19] He makes the same association in his fourth homily on Leviticus.[20] Clearly, it is not the nature of the sins that he is concerned to highlight but the completeness of the solution. For him, sin arises from demonic temptation anyway, since "for almost every human there are several spirits stirring up diverse kinds of sins in them."[21] Sexual sin for Origen—for it seems clear that at least here, he is happy to subsume the several different types of sexual sin enumerated in 1 Cor 6:9 into the broader category of 'fornication'—is part of the old human nature which is defeated by the battle of the New Testament Jesus. In other words, it is a normal human problem that can be overcome by God's power experienced through conversion.

The transformation to purity is, for Origen, absolute, as he makes clear in Homily 6 on Joshua. Here again, we see the master allegorist at work, this time, paralleling Rahab the prostitute with the life of the Church (on account of her having been joined to the house of Israel and found in the genealogy of Christ). The one who was once a prostitute has become the pure bride of 1 Corinthians 11:2:

> But now let us neither recall nor impute to her the old fault. Once she was a prostitute, but now "a pure virgin, to one man" she has been united, "to Christ." Hear the Apostle speaking of her: "But I have determined this itself, to present you to Christ, a pure virgin to one husband." It was also surely of her that someone said, "For once we ourselves were also foolish, unbelieving, wandering, serving desires and various forms of pleasures." Do you still wish to learn more about how the prostitute is no longer a prostitute? Hear Paul saying in addition, "And this surely you have been; but you have been washed, you have been sanctified in the name of our Lord Jesus Christ, and in the Spirit of our God."[22]

And of course, the allegory is incomplete without making the connection between the scarlet cord by which Rahab was saved and the blood of Christ through which we are saved.

Cyril of Jerusalem

1 Corinthians 6:11 is a fitting verse in the context of Cyril of Jerusalem's *Catechesis*, in which he is preparing the newly converted for baptism. In the tradition of Origen he makes a passing reference to Song of Solomon 5:3, "I have taken off my robe, how am I then to put it back on?" For Cyril, this is a fitting picture of the Christian convert who 'takes off' the old self (Col 3:9) in repentance. He amplifies this repentance as follows:

> What must be done, then, and what are the fruits of repentance? "Let him who has two tunics share with him who has none".... While aspiring to the grace of the Holy Spirit for yourself, will you deny bodily food to the poor? Do you seek great things, but share not the small?

> Though you be a publican or fornicator, yet hope for salvation. "The publicans and harlots are entering the kingdom of God before you." Paul testifies to this when he says: "Neither fornicators nor idolaters," nor the rest, "will possess the kingdom of God. And such were some of you, but you have been washed, and you have been sanctified." He did not say, some of you "are," but some of you "were." The sin committed in ignorance is pardoned, but persistent wickedness is condemned.[23]

As with Tertullian, Cyril takes a high view of baptism, considering it quite rightly to be a definitive break from the past. No sin is excepted from its cleansing; the solution to all is the same. Repentance. Indeed, he makes it clear that in his view nobody, save only martyrs, attains salvation without baptism.[24] This makes all the more significant his commentary on the superiority of the baptism of the Holy Spirit to water baptism which directly follows the material quoted above:

> "You have for the glorification of baptism the Only-begotten Son of God Himself. Why should I speak any further of man? John was great, but what was he compared to the Lord? Loud was his voice, but what compared with the Word? Noble was the herald, but what he to the King? Glorious was he who baptized with water, but what in comparison to Him who baptizes "with the Holy Spirit and with fire"? The Savior baptized with the Holy Spirit and with fire when: "suddenly there was a sound from heaven as of a violent wind coming, and it filled the whole house where they were sitting. And there appeared to them parted tongues as of fire, which settled upon each of them. And they were all filled with the Holy Spirit."[25]

This association between Pentecost and the agency of the Holy Spirit in 1 Cor 6:11 is an important one for Pentecostal readers of the Fathers, and is reminiscent of the earlier holiness theology of the baptism of the Spirit which once pervaded the movement.

John Chrysostom

John Chrysostom is known as being one of the greatest preachers of all time. His use of 1 Cor 6:11 is important because it involves several important cross-references and accompanies an extensive discussion of 1 Cor 6:9–10 including several examples of homosexual sin in its various forms. The citation is found in a collection of homilies on the pastoral epistles. The text with which he begins the fifth of these homilies is Titus 2:11–14, the theme of which is clearly parallel to 1 Cor 6:9–11:

> For the grace of God has been revealed, bringing salvation to all people. And we are instructed to turn from godless living and sinful pleasures. We should live in this evil world with wisdom, righteousness, and devotion to God, while we look forward with hope to that wonderful day when the glory of our great God and Savior, Jesus Christ, will be revealed. He gave his life to free us from every kind of sin, to cleanse us, and to make us his very own people, totally committed to doing good deeds (NLT).

Following a discussion on the nature of sin and in particular of lust, Chrysostom speaks of the comprehensiveness of the *new birth*; an entirely fresh start:

> Strange! How were we drowned in wickedness, so that we could not be purified,

but needed a new birth? For this is implied by *Regeneration*. For as when a house is in a ruinous state no one places props under it, nor makes any addition to the old building, but pulls it down to its foundations, and rebuilds it anew; so in our case, God has not repaired us, but made us anew. For this is *the renewing of the Holy Ghost*. He has made us new men. How? *By His Spirit...* (emphasis original to the translation).[26]

Chrysostom then launches into a description of human depravity before Christ which he derives mainly from Greek drama and Plato's *Republic*. He mentions the ancient practice of pederasty along with various other perversions as proof that "...every species of wickedness prevailed."[27] Making it clear that in addition to Titus 3:4–7 he has in mind Romans 1:26–27, Chrysostom says:

> O ye subverters of all decency, who use men, as if they were women, and lead out women to war as if they were men! This is the work of the devil, to subvert and confound all things, to overlap the boundaries that have been appointed from the beginning, and remove those which God has set to nature.[28]

For Chrysostom, as for the other Fathers discussed, the solution to this, however, is the same as the solution to all other sins, regardless of how perverse they may be—the new birth which is entered into by repentance and faith and affected by the power of the Holy Spirit. That this was a live issue for Chrysostom's own congregation at Constantinople in the fourth century, and not merely some detached theological speculation, is made clear by his pastoral advice, contained towards the end of the sermon on how to approach the people of the world thus afflicted:

> Let us then give thanks to God, and not revile them; nor accuse them, but rather let us beseech them, pray for them, counsel and advise them, though they should insult and spurn us. For such is the nature of those who are diseased. But for those who are concerned for the health of such persons do all things and bear all things, though it may not avail, that they may not have themselves to accuse of negligence.

He urges Christians to "at least imitate" the loved ones of sick people suffering in the hospital who will spare no expense, do all in their power, and implore the attending physician to effect the healing of the person.[29] Though his advice may sound insensitive to modern ears which have been calibrated to the modern commentary on this issue, it must be said that he is motivated by pastoral concern and a stubbornly passionate belief that God's grace can forgive any sin, his power transform any sinner.

There are also hints, in a sermon from another series, in which

Chrysostom likewise cites 1 Cor 6:11, that he was aware of this issue in the present struggle of some of his congregants, not merely in their pre-Christian experience. First highlighting the multiple benefits of the new birth found in 1 Cor 6:11, he urges Christians to continue in their New Birth identity enduring to the end:

> "He hath not limited his redemption to mere deliverance, but hath greatly extended the benefit: for He also hath made thee clean. Was this then all? Nay: but he hath also *sanctified*. Nor even is this all: He hath also *justified*. Yet even bare deliverance from our sins were a great gift: but now He hath filled thee also with countless blessings. And this He hath done, *In the name of our Lord Jesus Christ:* not in this name or in that: yea also, *In the Spirit of our God.*
>
> Knowing therefore these things, beloved, and bearing in mind the greatness of the blessing which hath been wrought, let us both continue to live soberly, being pure from all things that have been enumerated... and the noble birth which God hath freely given us, the same let us preserve to the end."[30]

If his solution to sin in general and the sins associated with homosexuality, in particular, is the new birth, the remedy for persistent homosexual temptation after conversion is the engagement of the renewed will to persist in the purity of the New Birth identity.[31]

Ambrosiaster

Ambrosiaster (literally "would-be Ambrose") is the name given to the anonymous author of a commentary on Romans and 1 and 2 Corinthians that had been falsely attributed to Ambrose of Milan.[32] The work is attested in Latin and is from the same period in which Chrysostom (and indeed Ambrose himself, discussed next) writes. In a strikingly similar treatment of 1 Cor 6:9–11 to Chrysostom's, the author of the commentary may be interpreted as acknowledging the presence of ongoing homosexual temptation among converted Christians. At the very least, he is acknowledging the presence of ongoing temptation in general of the sorts of sins listed in 1 Cor 6:9–10 when he suggests quite strongly that the New Birth is not just a past event to be celebrated by Christians but an ongoing process that needs to be appropriated in faith.

> *Do you not know that the unrighteous will not inherit the kingdom of God? Do not be deceived; neither the immoral, nor idolaters, nor adulterers, nor sexual perverts,*[33] Paul indicates that they are not sinning unknowingly, and so it is that much harder to excuse them.... *And such were some of you. But you were washed, you were sanctified, you were justified in the name of the Lord Jesus Christ and*

> *in the Spirit of our God*.... The Corinthians had received all the benefits of purity in their baptism, which is the foundation of the truth of the gospel. In baptism the believer is washed clean from all sins and is made righteous in the name of the Lord, and through the Spirit of God he is adopted as God's child. With these words, Paul is reminding them how great and how special is the grace which they have received in the true tradition. But afterward, by thinking which is contrary to this rule of faith, they had stripped themselves of these benefits. For this reason he is trying to bring them back to their original way of thinking, so that they can recover what they had once received.[34]

As the commentator explains if cleansing from sin and sanctification is effected by the name of the Lord Jesus Christ, adoption as God's children is made possible through the Holy Spirit. And yet, even for those who have been thus adopted, the grace once received can be forfeited, and its benefits stripped by a reversion in the thinking of a converted Christian to their pre-Christian way.

The Ambrosiaster material is a commentary, and not a sermon; however, it is easy to imagine that the commentator's pastoral experience forms the backdrop of his interpretation of Paul at this point. Viewed in this way, 'Ambrosiaster' is urging his own readers (in much the same way as Chrysostom exhorted his congregation) to persist in the "great" and "special" grace that they had received, by continuing to think of themselves in their renewed identity as they did when first converted.

Augustine

This investigation would not be complete without a discussion of the great preacher and theologian, Augustine of Hippo, the last of the period under investigation to make a significant citation of 1 Cor 6:11. Though much of his teaching in his 161st sermon is on 1 Cor. 6:15 specifically,[35] the passage for his sermon is 1 Cor 6:9–15. What is fascinating for the present discussion is that for Augustine, it all comes down to is *identity*. In the third part of his sermon Augustine explicitly addresses those in his audience that are identified by the behaviors listed in 1 Cor 6:9–10:

> "*Make no mistake; neither fornicators, nor idol-worshippers, nor adulterers, nor the effeminate, nor men who lie with men, nor thieves, nor the grasping, nor the drunken, nor the scurrilous shall possess the kingdom of God* (1 Cor 6:9–10)....Many people, you see, who commit such sins nurse fond hopes for themselves. It's because of people who live abandoned lives, and nurse fond hopes of the kingdom of heaven, where they are not going to get to.... Any of you like that should choose now where you would like to dwell, while there is still the chance for you to change."[36]

He is similarly uncompromising in section 11, as he begins to make his conclusion: "So let's have no more fornications. *You are God's temple, and the Spirit of God dwells in you. If anyone reduces God's temple to ruins, God will ruin him* (1 Cor 3:16–17)."[37] And yet the tone of his sermon is not merely blunt denunciation, but rather a pastoral invitation to live into the truth of the identity that Scripture declares. Sexual sin, Augustine declares, devalues the sinner because God has chosen to make us; our very bodies; part of his holy temple:

> "[You] are despising Christ in yourselves, and not recognizing your Lord, or giving a thought to your price, your true value....Has such great worth, such tremendous dignity, really grown so cheap? If it hadn't been bestowed, it would be desired; because it has been bestowed, is it to be despised?
>
> 2. But these bodies of ours, which the apostle says are members of Christ thanks to Christ's body, which he took to himself of the same nature as our bodies; so these bodies of ours the apostle also says are the temple of the Holy Spirit in us, whom we have received from God. Because of Christ's body, our bodies are members of Christ; because of Christ's Spirit dwelling in us, our bodies are the temple of the Holy Spirit. *Which of these two within you are you prepared to despise? Christ whose member you are, or the Holy Spirit whose temple you are?*" (emphases mine).[38]

To emphasize the importance of identity, Augustine continues:

> Wherever you go, after all, Jesus can see you; the one who made you and when you were lost redeemed you, and when you were dead died for you. *You don't know who you really are* but he never takes his eyes off you... (emphases mine).

In the subsequent sermon in his series, Augustine speaks in particular of sins classed as fornication. For Augustine, fornication 'in general' counts for cleaving to anything other than God.[39]

Discussion and Conclusions

What then may we learn for the present day from the wisdom of the Fathers? How in particular did they view homosexuality? What was their response? And can we see evidence of the Holy Spirit's activity through the way that they discuss the topic? A few observations are appropriate.

First, from the evidence presented, the Fathers are united in considering homosexual acts to be sinful, and in violation of God's plan. There is no qualification. There is no equivocation. There is no lengthy examination in the Ancient Church that Paul must have meant something other than what he apparently said. Perhaps this should go without saying, but apparently, it doesn't always. And yet its significance should not be missed. Surely the ancient interpreters, closer in time, culture and language to the New Testament are no *less* qualified than interpreters in our own day to correctly apprehend the intent of Scripture. Seen from the perspective of history, and the united voice of the Church throughout the ages, it is interpreters in our own day that are out of step. To ignore the wisdom of the ancient Church on this issue because of modern concerns over so-called 'pre-critical exegesis' amounts to little more than what C.S. Lewis called chronological snobbery. Similarly, to dismiss the witness of the Patristic Church because it is somehow a betrayal of the Protestant Reformation is a naiveté that should no longer be tolerated amongst Pentecostals.

Of course, modern voices like to object at this point that the conversation concerning homosexuality is less nuanced in the ancient Church because they did not possess the construct of sexual orientation that was only 'discovered' relatively recently (chronological snobbery again). Yet there is ample evidence that sexual preference was known and discussed in ancient times, indeed well before the First century.

In the discussion above, Chrysostom seems to allude to a passage in Plato's *Symposium*, in which a satirical creation narrative is offered by Aristophanes. In this narrative humanity was originally created in inseparable pairs, but because of sin were split down the middle such that each half spends its life looking for its 'other half.' Some of these were male-female pairs, but others were female-female pairs and still others male-male pairs, a point which Aristophanes uses to explain the sexual preference for men which was common in his all-male circle of friends. This preference he held to be superior to the preference of weaker men for women. The presence of this alternative creation narrative—satirical or otherwise—serves to demonstrate that what we believe about humanity comes back to what we believe about its origin. In the biblical creation story, rather than creating one and splitting it into two, God creates male and female and unites them as one in marriage.

What is clear from the Church Fathers is that they *did* acknowledge an orientation. It is called the sin nature and predisposes a person to sin in any number of ways. What they *did not* acknowledge was any notion of an 'identity' that survived conversion and baptism. Temptations persist beyond conversion, but sin should not, since the will necessary to resist temptation has been restored. And while conversion does change the state of a person, it is seen as a reversion from what is unnatural (the fallen human condition) to what is original and natural (the redeemed condition).

Beyond this, however, the sin of homosexuality is largely unremarkable. Ambrosiaster does make the point that sexual sin is worse than other sins, but here he simply echoes the judgment of the apostle Paul. We have no reason to suppose that he sees homosexual sins as worse than heterosexual sins, since both fall under the more general term *fornicatio* and both, as sexual sins, are sins against the body. It is true that mention is made, particularly in Chrysostom's evidence above,[40] of homosexual sins being 'against nature.' However, as Origen noted, since the devil himself is ultimately the origin of these sins, and the desires that lead to them, no human sin is too monstrous to be forgiven.

The Fathers have an extremely high view of Christian baptism, and while at many other points their convictions seem to resonate with Pentecostals, in respect of water baptism we are furthest from their belief and practice. Having said that, the Pentecostal emphasis on the baptism of the Holy Spirit, which, in its fullest historical Pentecostal understanding brings with it both cleansing and empowerment, ensures that while we may resist the notion of 'sacramental efficacy' in baptism, we nevertheless contend for the real spiritual transformation that the Fathers talk about. For them, baptism releases the power of God in the presence of the Holy Spirit to bring about total transformation, regardless of the magnitude of the sin, which results in a change in identity *back* to God's created intent. God gives, with this new (restored original) identity, the power to resist the temptation to slip back into pre-baptism patterns of thought and behavior.

Rather they saw it as a human problem, specifically, as one of many symptoms of the fallen human nature. And this is an insight that is worth restoring to the present discussion, for to acknowledge it as part of the human condition prevents us from dehumanizing responses, but to acknowledge that it is a symptom of the fallen nature is to offer the hope of a true transformation, *back* to God's original intent, and hence *forward* to true and full humanity. If we truly believe in the unique authority of the name of the Lord Jesus Christ, the transformative power of God and the empowering presence of the Holy Spirit, we would do well to emulate the judgment of the Fathers to pursue, particularly as Pentecostal Christians, a theology of encounter.

And so perhaps instead of 'leaving the past behind' in the sense of ruling out of court the views of the Ancient Church, we should rather retrieve from our forefathers their simple and uncompromising belief that the old nature itself can truly be left behind, for "that is what some of you *were*. But you were washed. You were sanctified, you were justified in the name of our Lord Jesus Christ and by the Spirit of our God."

4.

Querying Queer Theory: Gender Expression and Transgender Identity in Manifold Perspective

Michael McClymond

Abstract

This essay summarizes and evaluates some of the recent literature on transgender identity—from social, medical-empirical, theoretical, autobiographical, political, and theological perspectives. It first considers some definitional questions pertaining to key terms, such as "sex," "gender," "queer," and "transgender." It then considers some of the empirical and clinical data on the phenomenon of transgenderism; and turns to the theoretical aspects of queer theory (Judith Butler) along with some anti-theoretical challenges coming from within the transgender community (Viviane Namaste). The next section surveys a number of first-person or autobiographical narratives, from North America and from Thailand, including accounts of detransitioned as well as transitioned transgender persons. The final sections of the essay examine transgenderism from the perspective of politics, of queer exegesis and queer theology, and of mainstream Christian thinking—including both Roman Catholic and evangelical viewpoints, which in recent years have tended to converge on the broad themes of marriage and family. The overall argument of the essay drives toward two general conclusions: first, that Christian believers should "love their transgender neighbors as themselves," bearing in mind the traumatic life-histories of many persons who experience gender dysphoria and who self-identify as transgender; and, second, that Christian believers should reject some of the common claims of transgender ideology, e.g., that the correct (or only possible) interpretation of gender dysphoria is that males are "trapped in women's bodies," while females are "trapped in men's bodies."

Introduction: Swimming in a Sea of Fluidity

Each year the academic editors of the *Oxford English Dictionary*—the largest and most impressive dictionary ever produced in any language—announce the new words that are to be added to their monumental word-shrine. Katy Steinmetz notes that "the editors at the *Oxford English Dictionary* typically wait and watch for years before giving new words a chance to be included in their hallowed pages." So when those editors decide to add new words, "you know there is nothing willy-nilly (or shilly-shally) about it." The words have been "weighed, measured and determined to be a notable event in the history of the English language, silly as it may sound." Steinmetz finds "notable" the 2016 addition of *"gender-fluid*, a term describing someone who doesn't necessarily identify as male or female — or who might feel rather female one day and rather male the next. Of all the evolutions going on in the English language, [*OED* editor Katherine] Martin sees the 'speed at which the English language is expanding' to accommodate identities like this to be…thrilling."[1]

Think of the mental image associated with the word "fluid." A bottle containing water, or coffee, or orange juice, can be poured into any other container and the fluid will immediately adopt the shape of that new container. Fluidity implies a complete lack of fixity, permanence, or continuity in shape or form. One might line up a dozen containers, pouring liquid from one to another in sequence and so displaying the liquid in a dozen shapes. *Is this how human life is?* Can I myself, like a liquid, be poured into a new shape? And if I am the one pouring the liquid—as well as the liquid being poured—can I choose at will the shape I will assume? *Are we all shape-shifters?* And does this apply in a special way to our sexual desires and experiences, and/or to our gendered identity?

Ryan T. Anderson's book, *When Harry Became Sally* (2018), notes that the culture of the USA since 2015 has been in the midst of what some have called a "transgender moment." "Within the space of a year, it [i.e., transgenderism] became a cause claiming the mantle of civil rights…and therefore any failure to accept and support a transgender identity amounts to bigotry."[2] In 2014, Facebook began allowing its users to pick from among 58 different gender options.[3] Who would have imagined this in 1980, or even as recently as 1990, or 2000? The letter "P" (for polyamory) might be another letter to be added to the ever-lengthening "LG…etc." acronym. In the aftermath of the *Fifty Shades of Grey* book and film series, those involved in domination/submission or sadism/masochism may soon insist on adding the letters "S" and "M" to all the rest.[4]

A new theory or ideology of gender is currently establishing itself in popular opinion and in the legal systems of various nations. In Quebec, Canada, the civil code has removed references to "father" and "mother" and replaced these with the vague term "purveyor of genetic forces."

In Spain today, the words "progenitor 1" and "progenitor 2" are used in place of "father" and "mother." Consider the case of the Canadian parents, who concealed from their friends the sex of their child at birth, whom they named "Storm." Their intent is to allow the child later on to choose his/her/its own gender.[5] In the USA, the Obama Administration in May 2016 reinterpreted the decades-old ban on "sex discrimination" to include "gender identity discrimination." This decision meant that all health-care plans regulated under the Affordable Care Act (or Obamacare) would be required to cover the costs of sex-reassignment procedures and to provide physicians to perform the procedures. Yet there was a problem. A month later, the Centers for Medicare and Medicaid Services released a report indicating that they would not mandate coverage of sex reassignment surgery because medical and clinical evidence did not demonstrate it to be beneficial. The report stated: "Based on a thorough review...there is not enough evidence to determine whether gender reassignment surgery improves health outcomes for...beneficiaries with gender dysphoria."[6] The Obama Administration was endorsing and seeking to fund a medical procedure—involving surgery—that had no convincing empirical evidence to support its efficacy.[7]

There is presently a struggle in certain circles in regard to the use of pronouns such as "he" and "she" or "him" and "her." In some school districts in the USA, teachers are being told to avoid the expression "boys and girls" when addressing their pupils. Even more radical is the proposal to use—or to require the use of—wholly new gender-neutral pronouns, such as "ne," "ve," "ze," or "spivak."[8] The New York City Commission on Human Rights in 2016 prescribed a fine of $250,000 for anyone who knowingly and repeatedly refers to someone by a non-preferred pronoun.[9] This legal guidance is almost certainly unconstitutional—in light of the right to free speech guaranteed in the United States Bill of Rights. Yet, remarkably, it was proposed as policy in America's largest city.

Activists who claim to speak for the transgender community sometimes show a hair-trigger sensitivity regarding the various verbal "trans-gressions" that one is supposed to avoid. Television host Katie Couric evoked widespread criticism when she inadvertently used the term "transgenders" as a plural for "transgender persons" or "trans persons"—the phrases accepted by activists. In another incident, a liberal gay man who had worked on behalf of LGBTQ+ people slipped up by speaking of someone as "transgendered" rather than "transgender," was called out for it, and chided himself for his own insensitivity.[10] What made the term "transgendered" offensive was the implication of a *process undergone,* contradicting the activists' dogma that "trans persons" have always been "trans." Such persons never *changed* their gender identity but simply *recognized* the gender identity they had always been. Along these lines, transgender activists have increasingly come to reject the previously accepted phraseology of "gender transition" or "sex reassignment." This is because the language of "transition" is said to be "inaccurate to describe the process a transgender person is going through from that person's perspective." From the outside, there may appear to be a change, but those who identify as transgender see this as a process of "settling in" or coming home" to what they always were on the inside. Activists now prefer to speak of "gender-affirming therapies" rather than "sex-reassignment therapies."[11]

These transgender rules regarding pronouns seem to be binding even if the reference is to someone's prior life, i.e., prior to "transition." To be politically correct, then, we must now refer to the 1976 Olympic Decathlon winner Bruce Jenner as "she," since "Bruce" was even then ontologically female and was already "Caitlyn"—even though Jenner did not then use this name or self-present as a woman. One wonders: Should the International Olympic Committee revise its official records to show "Caitlyn Jenner" as the Gold Medalist? To apply the principle consistently, one would need to rewrite the entire personal histories of transgender persons, and, in this particular case, rewrite a little bit of Olympic history too. To use the phraseology of George Orwell's novel, *Nineteen Eight-Four,* the name "Bruce Jenner" must disappear into the "memory-hole."[12]

There are not only points of tension between LGBTQ+ persons and the heterosexual majority but also within the LGBTQ+ world.[13] In various global cities, the annual Pride Fest or Pride March sometimes engenders conflict. The conflicts are generally rooted in distinctions within the community. Even the letter "T" means not one thing but several different things. Included under the banner of transgender are at least four distinct groups, including: "transsexuals" who have made a full transition (sometimes involving hormonal treatment and surgery) to living in a new gender identity; the "crossdressers" who are mostly heterosexual males who sometimes dress as women (and usually find sexual arousal and fulfillment in doing so); the "drag queens" who are generally gay men who perform as ultra-feminized women in highly theatrical, staged, and campy performances; and the "drag kings," who are generally lesbians who perform theatrically as men.[14] In connection with the Pride Event in Glasgow, Scotland, a conflict broke out when transgender women or transsexuals objected to participating in the same event alongside of cis-gender, cross-dressing males, or gay male drag queens. Male-to-female impersonation, argued the transsexuals, was *merely an act or a performance* for these others, whereas for them it was far more serious since it *defined their core identity*. Things seem later to have been partially patched up between the various Scottish "T" groups, when an Alternative Pride Event decided to allow drag queens to participate.[15]

Another dispute arose, once again in connection with the annual Pride March in London. Some lesbians, along with some heterosexual feminists, contend that no men—including those undergoing male-to-female transition—could ever understand the full experience of being a woman—e.g., experiencing discrimination as a girl, having to worry about getting pregnant, sexual harassment in the workplace, the fear of rape, the experience of giving birth, etc. A man who decides when he is thirty, forty, or fifty years old, to transition to being a woman, will never have the history that makes him part of the feminist sisterhood. Those who hold this position are sometimes impolitely referred to as "TERFS," for "trans-exclusionary radical feminists."[16] On 7 July 2018, as London prepared for its annual Pride March, and a group of lesbians arrived, with banners and placards stating, "Lesbian, not Queer," and "Transactivism Erases Lesbians." A furor erupted, and when the lesbians were told that they would not be allowed to march, they responded by lying down in the road, and blocking the march. When they were allowed to march, and walked at the front of the pack, this upset some participants and onlookers, as implying that the trans-exclusionary lesbians were leading the whole march. London Mayor Sadiq Khan condemned what he called an "anti-transgender group" for "hijacking" the event.[17]

Unresolved Questions in Transgender Theory and Thinking

In his book *When Harry Became Sally,* Ryan Anderson points out some of the unresolved tensions or contradictions in transgender ideology. First, "it holds that the real self is fundamentally separate from the material body, yet insists that transforming the body is crucial for personal wholeness." We might ask: If the true self is not tied to biological sex, or to a particular body-type, then why should persons bother to change their body-type?[18] Second, transgender ideology "attaches a notion of authentic gender identity to stereotypical activities and dispositions, yet it grows from a philosophy holding that gender is an artificial construct." Some observers have commented on the 2015 *Vanity Fair* cover image of Caitlyn Jenner, there portrayed not just as a woman but as a glamorously feminine woman. How could this possibly be helpful to biological women who look in the mirror and realize that they will never look like any of the glamorous women on magazine covers? And why should a sex change require anyone to become a stereotypical female sex-object? The optics of the cover shoot seem not to be *progressive* but *conservative*—not an overcoming but a reaffirmation of gender norms.

Third, transgender ideology "promises a radical subjectivity in which individuals should be free to do whatever they wish and to define the truth as they choose, yet it calls for enforced conformity of belief in transgender dogma." If the new gender theory embraces the principle of individual freedom, then individuals should be free not only to change genders but also to believe or disbelieve in transgender ideology. Otherwise, the trans activists are in effect promoting freedom-for-me-but-not-for-thee. To Anderson's three points, we might add a fourth: Transgender ideology holds that gender is fluid rather than fixed, and yet it accepts *changes in one direction only*—from one's so-called "assigned sex" at birth to a different gender identity. It seems incoherent though to argue that "gender is fluid" and then to denounce "detransitioners" (i.e., those who underwent sex reassignment or "transition" and changed back) as though they are somehow traitors to the cause of transgenderism. A consistent belief in "fluidity" would welcome those who transition in as many ways, or as many times, as they might wish. Anderson believes that "we should…call on transgender activists to stop trying to silence detransitioners." Their voices and views should receive a hearing, no less than those who have transitioned and who remain happy with their transition.[19]

This essay will first consider some definitional questions pertaining to key terms, such as "sex," "gender," "queer," and "transgender." It will then summarize empirical and clinical data on the phenomenon of transgenderism and turn to the theoretical aspects of queer theory (Judith Butler), along with some anti-theoretical challenges coming from within the transgender community (Viviane Namaste). The next section will survey a number of first-person or autobiographical narratives, from North America and from Thailand, including accounts of detransitioned as well as transitioned transgender persons.[20] The final sections of the essay will examine transgenderism from the perspective of politics, of queer exegesis and queer theology, and of mainstream Christian thinking—including both Roman Catholic and evangelical viewpoints, which in recent years are surprisingly alike on the themes of marriage and family. The overall argument of the essay drives toward two broad conclusions: first, that Christian believers should "love their transgender neighbors as themselves," bearing in mind the traumatic life-histories of many persons who self-identify as trans-gender; and, second, that Christian believers should question some of the common claims of transgender ideology, e.g., that "men" may be "trapped in women's bodies," while "women" may be "trapped in men's bodies."

The scientific evidence summarized in this essay does not support the claim that gender dysphoria (i.e., the feeling of belonging to something other than one's sex at birth) is due to biological causes. Moreover, clinical evidence does not definitely indicate that sex reassignment—by the usual means of hormonal treatment and/or surgery—leads in general to positive mental health outcomes. The life-stories of many gender transitioners (see below, the accounts from Thailand) as well as gender detransitioners (see below, the accounts from the USA) suggest that gender dysphoria is often rooted in traumatic early life experiences. Transgenderism may be more a matter of *disidentification* than of *identification*. That is, many transgender persons had specific reasons to reject their birth sex and the gender traits that they associated with it. The path to healing for such persons will likely involve a revisiting of early-life trauma, so that these difficult experiences can be integrated into a present sense of selfhood, thus addressing both a painful past and the resulting experiences of gender dysphoria.

Questions of Definition: "Sex," "Gender," and "Queer"

Until the late twentieth century, the terms "sex" and "gender" were often used interchangeably. The introduction of the term "gender" in distinction from "sex," in something like its contemporary use, may be traced to the New-Zealand-born psychologist, John Money (1921–2006).[21] Money was an early promoter of the theory of sexual or gender fluidity.[22] Heterosexuality, for Money, was socially constructed and so he regarded it as essentially superficial. In Money's work, "sex" refers to biological identity at birth, and "gender" to behavior or personal identity.

The British sociologist and feminist, Ann Oakley (b. 1944), published a monograph, *Sex, Gender, and Society* (1972), that further enforced the distinction between "sex" and "gender." For Oakley, "sex" was a biological given, while "gender" was socially constructed from a mix of family environment, cultural context, and personal choices. "Gender" was no more fixed than culture is fixed, and for this reason "gender" can and does evolve. "Gender" simply designates the sexual identity constructed by each individual as a function of subjective perceptions. The study of transgender persons has played a role in evolving theories of sex and gender. The American psychiatrist Robert Jesse Stoller (1924–1991) found that the imagined or visualized gender identity among transgender persons displaced the reality of their biological sexual identity. Stoller developed his ideas in his works, *Sex and Gender: On the Development of Masculinity and Femininity* (1968), *Splitting: A Case of Female Masculinity* (1973), and *Pain & Passion. A Psychoanalyst Explores the World of S & M* (1991).[23]

The long-term agenda of gender ideology, writes Joseph-Marie Verlinde, is "to reject entirely the idea of conditioning by nature," and so "progressively to replace the word 'sex' with the word 'gender,' freely defined by the and individual and always revisable." Verlinde explains that "Sexual identity, disconnected from the biologically sexed body, may be freely constructed by individuals, and may equally change in accord with the fluctuations of one's individual tendencies."[24] Within this outlook, any presumption of a natural or normal attraction of men to women and women to men—now called "heterosexism"—becomes an odious form of prejudice, comparable to racial discrimination by white persons against people of color. Some LGBTQ+ advocates insist that children from their earliest ages need to be exposed to a whole variety of sexual proclivities, so that they are not subjected to a distorting, "heterosexist" prejudice in early life.

One term in the contemporary discourse on sexuality and gender is the word "queer." In older English, this was often a derogatory term for a homosexual person, and yet the term has acquired new significance in the last twenty-five years. In her book, *Tendencies* (1993), gender theorist Eve Kosofsky Sedgwick first publicly embraced the word "queer," defining it as "the open mesh of possibilities, gaps, overlaps, dissonances and resonances, lapses and excesses of meaning when the constituent elements of anyone's gender, of anyone's sexuality aren't made (or *can't be* made) to signify monolithically."[25] The term "queer" here suggests a rejection of fixed categories.

Taking the term in this sense, the "queers" are the self-conscious barrier-breakers and nonconformists of the LGBTQ+ world. For just this reason, some on the "queer" side of the sex-and-gender spectrum were not particularly interested in the more mainstream political effort to secure the right to same-sex marriage in the USA. The Russian political exile and human rights activist Masha Gessen spoke candidly of her views regarding monogamy. "It's a no-brainer that [homosexuals] should have the right to marry, but I also think equally that it's a no-brainer that the institutional of marriage should not exist.... Fighting for gay marriage generally involves lying about what we are going to do with marriage when we get there—because we lie that the institution of marriage is not going to change, and that is a lie." She adds: "The institution of marriage is going to change, and it should change. And again, I don't think it should exist.... I have three kids who have five parents, more or less, and I don't see why they shouldn't have five parents legally."[26]

Empirical Perspectives on Same-Sex Desire and Transgenderism

The earlier history of the transgender movement from the 1950s and 1960s is little known in today's post-Obergefell context—i.e., since the legalization of same-sex marriage by the United States Supreme Court in 2015. Harry Benjamin was an endocrinologist and sexologist who first coined the term "transsexual" in 1954. The later transgender "Standards of Care" were named in Benjamin's honor. A colleague of Benjamin's, Charles Ihlenfeld, who administered hormone therapy at Benjamin's clinic to some five hundred transgender persons over a six-year period, told an audience in 1979 that 80% of those who had been treated would have been better off without having received treatment. Ihlenfeld also spoke of the pervasive unhappiness and frequent suicides occurring among those who had undergone gender reassignment.

Another early advocate of medically-assisted gender reassignment was John Money, who was the key medical professional involved in a tragic case of twin boys, from the Reimer family, one of whose male organs (following botched attempt at circumcision) were removed after birth. In Money's well-documented gender experiment, one of the boys was raised as a girl, without being told (at Money's insistence) that he had been born as a boy. The boy in question lapsed into depression in late childhood, refused to meet with Money, and at that point was told he had been born a boy. From that point onward, David Reimer identified himself as male. In 2004, when Reimer was thirty-eight-years old, he committed suicide. His brother had died two years earlier from a drug overdose. Money publicly presented this as a successful case of gender reassignment, though the facts of the case in no way supported this claim.[27]

The representation of LGBT issues in the mainstream media in recent years generally conveys the impression that same-sex desires are fixed and invariant, essentially programmed into an individual's biological makeup from birth. Somewhat paradoxically, the opposite is thought to be the case with regard to those with a perceived disparity between their biological sex at birth and their inward sense of gender identity. If *biology is destiny* for those experiencing same-sex attraction, then for transgender persons the opposite claim is made that *biology is not destiny*.

Yet empirical evidence challenges the now culturally accepted narrative that *sexual desires are fixed while gender identities are fluid*. The truth might be the reverse of the accepted notion—i.e., that *sexual desires are fluid for many persons, while gender identities are fixed biologically and from birth*. The fluidity of sexual desire is supported by some surprising data recently assembled by Lawrence Mayer of the Mayo Clinic, and Paul McHugh—the latter author a former Psychiatrist-in-Chief at Johns Hopkins University Hospital, and one of the most important American psychiatrists of the last half century. Their report released in 2016 "shows that some of the most frequently heard claims about sexuality and gender are not supported by scientific evidence."[28] As a result of their review of around two hundred peer-reviewed scientific research studies on sexuality and gender, they came to the following conclusions regarding sexual desire and sexual orientation:

- "The understanding of sexual orientation as an innate, biologically fixed property of human beings—the idea that people are 'born that way'—is not supported by scientific evidence."

- "There are no compelling causal biological explanations for human sexual orientation."

- "Longitudinal studies of adolescents suggest that sexual orientation may be quite fluid over the life course for some people, with one study estimating that as many as 80% of male adolescents who report same-sex attractions no longer do so as adults."

- "Compared with heterosexuals, non-heterosexuals are about two to three times as likely to have experienced childhood sexual abuse."[29]

The best studies of gender dysphoria in children indicate that between 80% and 95% of those who at one point report gender dysphoria will come in time to identify with their birth sex if their natural development is allowed to proceed. The data thus cast grave doubts on the wisdom of giving hormones as "puberty blockers" to gender dysphoric children, following the procedures pioneered at Boston Children's Hospital. Puberty, as Paul McHugh has said, is not a "disease" requiring medical treatment. Some have asserted that "puberty blockers" are safe and reversible, but in fact these drugs carry long-term health risks. Moreover, people who have *already transitioned* with a full surgical procedure are *nineteen times more likely* than the average person to die by suicide.[30] The statistics suggest that "transition" through hormonal treatment and surgery does not address the underlying psychological disorders experienced by self-identified transgender persons.

One of the surprising lines of evidence in showing the fluidity of sexual desire among today's adolescents and young adults in the USA lies in the pregnancy rate of self-identified lesbian women, as well as the number of children fathered by self-identified gay males. On the basis of a study done in Minnesota, Allie Shah in 2015 wrote that "gay teens...are far more likely than their straight peers to become pregnant or have gotten someone pregnant." Gay or "questioning" males were four times more likely than straight males to report getting someone pregnant—the obvious implication being that many self-identified gay males were significantly involved in heterosexual sex as well as gay sex. Bisexual females in this study were five times more likely than heterosexual females to have become pregnant. Erin Wilkins, of the Family Tree Clinic—a community sexual health clinic in St. Paul, Minnesota—comments that "people's sense of sexuality tends to be black or white, gay or straight," and that "there isn't as much of an understanding of the middle ground, where many people live."[31] This data supports the conclusions of Mayer and McHugh regarding the fluidity rather than fixity of sexual desires and practices in the LGBTQ+ community, at least within the younger age cohort today.

Scholars in the field of sexuality have recently raised questions about female sexual orientation, with some even asking whether a fixed female sexual orientation actually exists. Lisa Diamond's *Sexual Fluidity* (2008) argues against the assumption that female lesbianism is comparable to male homosexuality. She asserts that the belief that "L" is like "G" may be due to gay-normativity and male prejudice in research. She is hopeful that attitudes are beginning to change, revealing a picture of male and female sexual orientation as "distinct phenomena instead of two sides of the same coin." Diamond suggests that "one of the fundamental, defining features of female sexual orientation is its fluidity," meaning "situation-dependent flexibility in women's sexual responsiveness." This flexibility in desire makes it possible for some women to desire either men or women, depending on the circumstances, and regardless of their self-assigned sexual orientation. Diamond writes: "This is why a woman like Anne Heche can suddenly find herself falling madly in love with Ellen DeGeneres after an exclusively heterosexual past, and why a longtime lesbian can experience her very first other-sex attraction in her forties." Diamond's work suggests that lesbianism is not a "sexual orientation," as this term is generally understood, and might better be interpreted as a situation-specific sexual activity of some females.[32] Gay males, in contrast, are more likely to "stay in one lane" over time—although, as noted above, the evidence from Mayer and McHugh regarding same-sex attraction may indicate that males who experience such attraction in adolescence often later cease to do so.

In reviewing the scientific literature on gender and transgender identity, Mayer and McHugh presented a further set of conclusions, as follows:

- "Studies comparing the brain structures of transgender and non-transgender individuals have demonstrated weak correlations between brain structure and cross-gender identification. These correlations do not provide any evidence for a neurobiological basis for cross-gender identification."

- "The hypothesis that gender identity is an innate, fixed property of human beings that is independent of biological sex—that a person might be 'a man trapped in a woman's body' or 'a woman trapped in a man's body'—is not supported by scientific evidence."

- "According to a recent estimate, about 0.6% of U.S. adults identify as a gender that does not correspond to their biological sex."

- "Members of the transgender population are…at higher risk

of a variety of mental health problems. Especially alarmingly, the rate of lifetime suicide attempts across all ages of transgender individuals is estimated at 41%, compared with 5% in the overall U.S. population."

- "Compared to the general population, adults who have undergone sex-reassignment surgery continue to have a higher risk of experiencing poor mental health outcomes. One study found that, compared to controls, sex-reassigned individuals were about 5 times more likely to attempt suicide and about 19 times more likely to die by suicide."

- "Only a minority of children who experience cross-gender identification will continue to do so into adolescence or adulthood."

- "There is little scientific evidence for the therapeutic value of interventions that delay puberty or modify the secondary sex characteristics of adolescents.... There is no evidence that all children who express gender-atypical thoughts or behavior should be encouraged to become transgender."[33]

Studies have shown that people with gender dysphoria have other psychological issues some 63% of the time.[34] When the underlying psychological issue or issues receive treatment, then the individual experiencing gender dysphoria often may find that the desire to change gender abates over time and may become content to live in accordance with his or her birth sex. A 2004 headline in the left-leaning British periodical, *The Guardian*, reported that "Sex Changes are Not Effective, Say Researchers." The author, David Batty, summarized these results based on a thorough analysis of published scientific literature: "There is no conclusive evidence that sex change operations improve the lives of transsexuals, with many people remaining severely distressed and even suicidal after the operation....The review of more than 100 international medical studies of post-operative transsexuals by the University of Birmingham's aggressive research intelligence facility (Arif) found no robust scientific evidence that gender reassignment surgery is clinically effective."[35]

In an online editorial, Paul McHugh summarizes his decades of medical research and experience in sexuality and gender as follows: "The idea that one's sex is a feeling, not a fact, has permeated our culture and is leaving casualties in its wake. Gender dysphoria should be treated with psychotherapy, not surgery.... At Johns Hopkins, after pioneering sex-change surgery, we demonstrated that the practice brought no important benefits. As a result, we stopped offering that form of treatment in the 1970s." He continues:

> The most thorough follow-up of sex-reassigned people—extending over thirty years and conducted in Sweden, where the culture is strongly supportive of the transgendered—documents their lifelong mental unrest. Ten to fifteen years after surgical reassignment, the suicide rate of those who had undergone sex-reassignment surgery rose to twenty times that of comparable peers.... Although much is made of a rare "intersex" individual, no evidence supports the claim that people such as Bruce Jenner have a biological source for their transgender assumptions. Plenty of evidence demonstrates that with him and most others, transgendering is a psychological rather than a biological matter.

McHugh came to this conclusion:

> Gender dysphoria—the official psychiatric term for feeling oneself to be of the opposite sex—belongs in the family of similarly disordered assumptions about the body, such as anorexia nervosa and body dysmorphic disorder. Its treatment should not be directed at the body as with surgery and hormones any more than one treats obesity-fearing anorexic patients with liposuction. The treatment should strive to correct the false, problematic nature of the assumption and to resolve the psychosocial conflicts provoking it. With youngsters, this is best done in family therapy.[36]

Yet in medical practice as well as in law, transgenderism increasingly is being treated as a right to be defended, and not a condition needing treatment. Paul McHugh notes that in several states in the USA "a doctor who would look in the psychological history of a transgendered boy or girl in search of a resolvable conflict could lose his or her license to practice medicine."[37]

Perhaps the issues of gender dysphoria and transgenderism are now coming near to a tipping point, or at least with regard to the fraught issue of dysphoria in children and teenagers. The recent essay by Jess Singal in *The Atlantic*, "When Children Say They Are Trans," is open-ended in tone, proposing that this topic leads us to difficult questions, and not to any quick fix: "Hormones? Surgery? The choices are fraught—and there are no easy answers."[38]

Theoretical and Anti-Theoretical Perspectives on Gender

Alongside the medical and clinical approaches to transgenderism is the development, especially since the 1990s, of so-called "gender theory." At most of the major research universities today, "gender theory" and "gender studies" have established themselves as part of the academic curriculum. This development in academe is directly pertinent to recent changes in social attitudes on sexuality and gender, and to feminist, gender, and transgender advocacy in the political sphere. From its origins, gender theory has been strongly tied to poststructuralist and postmodernist thought. Perhaps the most influential literary or non-scientific gender theorist today is Judith Butler (b. 1956), who teaches at the University of California, Berkeley, where she is now Maxine Elliot Professor in the Department of Comparative Literature and the Program of Critical Theory. She is also the Hannah Arendt Chair at the European Graduate School. Her Yale University Ph.D. dissertation in 1984 focused on French interpretations of Hegel's philosophy.[39] In her breakthrough book, *Gender Trouble* (1990), Butler argued that masculine gender and heterosexual desire in male bodies, and the correspondence of feminine gender with heterosexual desire in female bodies, is not "natural" as such. Instead, this correspondence of body type with desires and practices is culturally constructed through the repetition of stylized acts. Repeated acts thus create an appearance of "ontological" gender. But gender, along with sex and sexuality, is *performative*—i.e., akin to a theatrical performance. Butler has been politically active and served, for a period of time, as the chair of the board of the International Gay and Lesbian Human Rights Commission.[40]

Butler explicitly challenges biological accounts of binary (male and female) sexual identity. The supposed naturalness of binary sexual identity shows that its "discursive production" is well hidden. Subjected to "regulative discourse," human beings are forced into supposedly natural, ontological, and inevitable gender identities. Butler's gender theory has a liberative or emancipatory aspect, seeking to empower persons to break free of the misleading and confining gender binary of heterosexual maleness or femaleness.

Butler's aim is to confound, destabilize, and deconstruct the gender binary.[41] Her discussion in *Gender Trouble* begins from the question: "What [is the] best way to trouble the gender categories that support gender hierarchy and compulsory heterosexuality?"[42] Butler's position is that the "fictive" categories of sexual identity are "constructed" through language so that a change in language is key to the deconstruction of the gender order. Butler's aim is the "subversive confusion and multiplication of gender identities." Her technical language may conceal the extent to which her claims conflict with empirical reality: "'Sex' is an ideal construct which is forcibly materialized through time. It is not a simple fact or a static condition of the body, but a process whereby regulatory norms…achieve this materialization through a forcible reiteration of those norms."[43] As a practitioner of "queer theory," Butler not only rejects the "binary" of male-female but also the "binary" of heterosexual-homosexual, which for her are confining categories. The term "queer" is more open-ended since it can refer to anything other than heterosexuality.

For Butler, gender identity is fluid and flexible, and there is neither male nor female, but only a certain kind of behavior that can change at any time. One of her central claims is that "there need not be a 'doer behind the deed,' but…the 'doer' is variably constructed in and through the deed."[44] She asserts that the incest taboo is the cause of the "phantasm" of binary gender identity as well as the traditional prohibition of homosexuality. For this reason, the incest taboo must be abolished.[45] Butler recognizes that the dissolution of fixed male and female identities might be bad news for the cause of feminism, but she asks "whether feminist politics could do without a 'subject' in the category of women."[46] As German sociologist Gabrielle Kuby points out: if "women" do not actually exist, then it stands to reason that "women" cannot be oppressed. (In this way, the real-world problem of women's oppression around the world finds resolution on a strictly theoretical plane!) Butler sees families as formed by arbitrary acts of momentary belonging, rather than by a stable and perhaps lifelong marital bond between a man and a woman. In the world she envisages, children would not be "conceived" in the traditional way, but rather "designed" with the aid of sperm donation, egg donation, surrogate motherhood, artificial wombs, and gene manipulation.[47]

One of the more important and intriguing critiques of Judith Butler—and of gender theory generally—comes from the transgender scholar Viviane K. Namaste, in the book *Invisible Lives: The Erasure of Transsexual and Transgendered People* (2000).[48] The author describes her basic reason for writing this book as follows: "Very few of the monographs, articles, and books written about us deal with the nitty-gritty realities of our lives, our bodies and our experience of the everyday world." She adds that "our lives and our bodies are…more than a theory that justifies our very existence, more than mere performance, more than the interesting remark that we expose how gender works."[49] The central problem with gender theory is that it "neglects the everyday social world," while French poststructuralism in particular "voids the possibility of...transsexual bodies." Namaste argues that "transsexuals are...perpetually *erased* in the cultural and institutional world." Academic authors have written extensively on the cultural meanings implied in transgenderism, but this does not mean that they have understood the lived experiences of the people themselves, Namaste observes. "Critics in queer theory write page after page on the inherent liberation of transgressing normative sex/gender codes, but they have nothing to say about the precarious position of the transsexual woman who is battered and who is unable to access a woman's shelter because she was not born a biological woman."[50]

Namaste admits the importance of Butler's work in aiding the advancement of queer theory and gender studies. Yet she takes issue with Butler's understanding of drag queens and drag performance. Butler writes, "Drag implicitly reveals the imitative structure of gender itself—as well as its contingency. Indeed, part of the pleasure, the giddiness of the performance is in the recognition of a radical contingency in the relation between sex and gender in the face of cultural configurations of causal unities that are regularly assumed to be natural and necessary."[51] In her analysis of drag, Butler "fails to account for the context in which these gender performances occur. The drag queens Butler discusses perform in spaces created and defined by gay male culture." These spaces involve many paradoxes. Namaste points out that drag queens are tolerated in the gay bars, and yet the queens must remain on stage and cannot descend from the stage to interact with the clientele. Gay bars that have drag queens on stage often deny entrance to all (non-transsexual) women. Some gay bars admit women, but then set up segregated areas based on sex/gender distinctions.[52] There is thus a complicated set of inclusions and exclusions occurring in the physical space of the gay bar that Butler omits from her discussion. These exclusionary practices show that the drag performance may not challenge or overturn sex-gender distinctions and hierarchies, and may serve instead to reinforce them. Butler's Francophonic theoretical fixation on "discursive formation" makes these concrete social conditions all but invisible within her cultural analysis.

Namaste explains, "That gay men can accommodate the presence of drag queens on stage does not mean that gender liberation has arrived. Indeed, relegating such gender performances to the stage implies that gay men do not 'perform' their identities: they just *are*." The inference from the embodied practice is that "drag is about performance, while the homoerotic is about identity." The "performance," in other words, is contained within the space of the stage, while spectators viewing the stage are not themselves seen as "performers." Thus the physical arrangements and exclusions within the typical gay bar do not support but rather *militate against* Butler's performative theory of gender. "Drag queens are reduced to entertainment, coifed personalities whose only purpose is to titillate the gay male viewer." This means that "the relegation of drag queens to the stage…excludes transgendered people even as it includes us."[53] Butler's gender-as-performance theory allows and encourages her to ignore evidence that does not fit in her preconceived theory. Her theory "laud[s] drag practices over transsexual identities."[54]

Namaste finds an even more problematic passage in Butler's *Bodies That Matter* (1993), where she offers an interpretation of the transsexual prostitute, Venus Extravaganza, based on the film *Paris is Burning*.[55] Rather than dealing with the situation of the transsexual prostitute in New York City, Butler argues that Venus enacts an imaginary relationship to the category "woman" in order to escape the cruel realities of her class (i.e., poor) and her ethnicity (Latina). When Venus is found murdered—presumably by one of her clients—Butler writes that her death represents "a tragic misreading of the social map of power."[56] Namaste comments, "In this interpretation, Butler elides both Extravaganza's transsexual status and her work as a prostitute. Here is the point: *Venus was killed because she was a transsexual prostitute*." Yet this is something that "Butler chooses to ignore." "Since Butler has reduced Extravaganza's transsexuality to allegory, she cannot conceptualize the specificity of violence with which transsexuals, especially transsexual prostitutes, are faced. This, to my mind, is the most tragic misreading of all." Butler is not interested in "transsexuality" but wants instead to "speak about race and class."[57]

Namaste argues that the French poststructuralists—such as Michel Foucault and Jacques Derrida—characteristically refused to accept the idea that individual human beings can be viewed as "masters" of their own lives and identities. "Queer theory" therefore emerged as an "academic inquiry that is contemptuous and dismissive of the social world." By aiming "to demonstrate the textual production of sexual and gender identities," queer theory offers only a "limited frame of reference," so that the theory itself "determines the selection and presentation of evidence."[58] Butler's own interpretation of the drag performance, for example, could have been written by a theoretically conversant scholar who had never set foot in a gay bar, but who had seen a video version of the performance. Butler's mode of scholarship does not *observe* but instead *infers* social reality from the cultural products she has chosen to discuss. The interpretation is deracinated. Foucault was concerned with "questions about how discourse produces its own object." In this way, "by privileging literary and cultural objects, and by ignoring the social and institutional relations in which these objects are located and embedded, queer theory enacts a restricted use of the notion of 'text.'" Namaste then concludes that "queer theory as it is currently practiced must be challenged because it exhibits a remarkable insensitivity to the substantive issues of transgendered people's everyday lives." More than this, it "authorize[s] a political agenda that robs transgendered people of dignity and integrity." Despite its elaborate exhibition of theoretical finesse, "queer theory is blind to its own institutional workings," as some other scholars have argued as well.[59]

From the preceding section, it would seem that the empirical or medical claims of transgender activists regarding the efficacy of hormonal treatment and surgical procedures for dealing with gender dysphoria should not be taken at face value. From the present section, it should be clear that gender theory—at least in the form presented by Judith Butler—does not fare much better. Neither the public claims nor the academic literature does a very good job at capturing the lived reality of transgender persons. We turn in the next two sections to consider what transgender people have to say about themselves and their own experiences.

Autobiographical Perspectives I: Detransitioners from North America

The term "detransitioners" refers to those who underwent the hormonal and/or surgical process to begin life with a new gender identity, but later changed their minds, and returned to their birth sex/gender. Here we will consider what a representative group of detransitioners have to say about their life-experiences.

Cari Stella is a twenty-two-year-old detransitioned woman, who resides in the "trans-friendly" region of Portland, Oregon. She sums up her present-day experience in this way: "I'm a real live 22-year old woman with a scarred chest and a broken voice and a 5 o'clock shadow because I couldn't face the idea of growing up to be a woman. That's my reality."[60] She comments, "I detransitioned because I knew I could not continue running from myself, dissociating from myself, because acknowledging my reality as a woman is vital to my mental health." Cari writes that "a lot of women don't feel like they have options. There isn't a whole lot of place in society for women who look like this, women who don't fit, women who don't comply." The therapists do not say that "it's okay to be butch, to be gender nonconforming, to not like men, to not like the way men treat you." The therapists "don't tell you that there are other women who feel like they don't belong," but instead "they tell you about testosterone." She adds:

> I think that prospect of completely changing your body, your life, your identity, is very compelling to a teenager, who is just learning to cope with mental health issues....The current rhetoric around transition really discourages any kind of questioning; it really frames transitioning or trans identity as the solution to any kind of gender issues or gender confusion. And I think it's really important for therapists not to frame transition as the only solution.[61]

Cari asks: "How many other medical conditions are there where you can walk into a doctor's office, tell them you have a certain condition, which has no objective test, which can be caused by trauma or mental health issues or societal factors, and receive life-altering medication on your say-so?" She speaks of how the process of transition turned out to be unsatisfying. "Transition didn't really make my dysphoria better, it just kind of kept moving the goalposts." She adds, "I never got any closer to where I wanted to be," and so "I could keep going and changing my body in search of this finishing point." On Cari's view, therapists should "encourage people not to take their feelings and urges entirely at face value, to be critical, to really think about where those thoughts are coming from." "I know women who were on testosterone three, four, five, even ten years before they were able to recognize that it was f**king them over. It can be damn hard to figure out that the treatment you're being told is to help you is actually making your mental health worse. Testosterone made me even more dissociated than I already was." To those who would wish to dismiss the detransitioners, Cari comments that "you may not agree with us, but the fact is that we exist, we're going to continue to exist, and our numbers are growing."[62]

Another female-to-male transitioner and detransitioner is named "Max." "I felt that I had no choice but transition for a long time, and the reason I felt that way was because other choices were not offered to me." Today Max is critical of trans activists who "see advice for coping with distress that doesn't involve medication or surgery as inherently invalidating." She adds that "a lot of detransition, for me, has been about listening to myself, and learning to take the pain I experienced as a result of transition seriously. Paying [my physician] to cut away healthy tissue from my body, being seen as a man when I'm not one, effects from testosterone...how the medical-industrial complex fails women and girls in pain."[63]

Another female-to-male transitioner and detransitioner is named "Crash." Her experience taught her that "being supported in my trans identity didn't help me, letting go of it and accepting myself as a woman did. Changing my body didn't help me find lasting peace." Crash has reflected on the reasons for her desire to transition: "I realized that my dysphoria and trans identity were rooted in trauma and internalized misogyny. I was severely bullied and harassed starting when I was a young girl and continuing throughout my teenage years." Another factor pertained to Crash's fraught relationship with her mother. "I also see a connection between my decision to transition and my mom's suicide. She killed herself when I was 20 and I started hormones about three months after she killed herself. We greatly resembled each other and I think one of my motivations for changing my body is I wanted to differentiate myself from her." In summary, she says, "I transitioned because I was severely harassed for being a lesbian and traumatized by my mom's suicide." Crash still struggles to understand that her physician "treated us [trans persons] with understanding and respect," and yet "she hurt me" and "helped me hurt myself. That definitely wasn't her intention but that's still what happened. This contradiction is difficult to face and understand." She adds, "When I look back, I'm horrified and creeped out. There's something disturbing about doing something you think is good for yourself but that turns out to be really self-destructive and it's even worse when so many other people were helping you." Crash says that in detransition, "we have to learn to live in a modified body and this usually involves grieving. All of us who took [testosterone]...have altered voices. There is a very deep, painful symbolism behind losing your original voice and having no way of getting it back."[64]

Crash offers some thought-provoking reflections on her experience and that of other transitioners and/or detransitioners:

> We transitioned for a lot of different reasons. We lived through event(s) terrible enough that it damaged our sense of self and so we created a new self to cope and survive. That self was our trans or male or genderqueer identity....Whatever trauma we lived through typically had something to do with being a woman....I had

traits like an Adam's apple, body hair, an angular face, and so on, leading many to speculate on what sex I was. Eventually, other people's judgments got inside my head and infected how I saw myself until I started questioning whether I was really female too.... I rejected and betrayed myself.... I took other people's hatred into my own body. My body is now marked forever by that hatred, and that can be a lot to carry.... Detransitioning is as much about facing trauma as it is about figuring out how to live in an altered body. Transitioning was all about trying to get away from what hurt us, and detransitioning is finally facing that and overcoming it.... It's about remembering terrible, scary, upsetting memories and integrating them.[65]

Many of those who have gone public about their detransition experiences are women, but there are some cases of men who transitioned to female and then back to being men again. One such case is "TWT," who transitioned when he was nineteen and detransitioned at age thirty-nine. TWT sees the recent spike in the numbers of persons who are transitioning as due to a more accepting culture and a kind of "social contagion," which encourages people to transition when they might be better off not doing so. Now pursuing a Ph.D. degree in psychology, TWT comments, "One of the things I learned in my clinical training...is just in general how little you know about someone when you see them once or twice or three times. There's so much we don't know."[66]

TWT's desire to become a girl was intimately connected to some of his early-life experiences. "When I was young, I was physically the slowest boy but also very intellectually advanced like a child prodigy. By fourth grade, I was going to the high school...[but] I was the weakest.... So I suffered a lot of bullying and violence. It peaked in middle school where every day I would have some sort of violence directed at me. When I was a child, I started to have this fantasy of being a girl, because it meant I could be safe and not suffer from this violence due to being at the bottom of the male hierarchy. I could also be softer." During college, TWT went for counseling and this led to him being prescribed "a high dose of estrogen" and this "created a kind of euphoria and emotional intensity," that "was considered to be a confirmation that I had found my true self." Once he succeeded in passing as a woman, "I got quite a bit of attention from men, many of them the same sort of men that used to bully me as a teenager. This attention validated my then fragile sense of self-worth."[67]

The twenty years of living as a woman did not resolve TWT's dysphoria. "It just made me uncomfortable with different parts of my body that weren't feminine.... I had really big hands and a big jaw and so I still had the same problem of hating parts of my body."[68] Eventually, TWT started to see a regular therapist rather than a gender therapist, and this helped him to understand the deeper reasons that he felt disconnected from his own body:

> I wasn't working on my gender, but on why I couldn't have relationships and why my body was so tense.... I eventually became aware I was really disconnected to my body.... I...came to understand the roots of this with the bullying and feeling unsafe about being myself and a man in the world. I didn't see things in this way in an intellectual sense, but in a visceral [way].... It was also a big revelation because I thought my gender identity of being female was fundamental. It seemed like an absolute truth and an absolute axiom, and then it turned out not to be that at all. It turned out to be something that could be changed.[69]

TWT now finds "no...consistency in the whole ideology" of gender theory, since the assumption is that gender identity is "permanent but it also can be fluid and it can also change but it doesn't change."[70]

Walt Heyer was born male, underwent sex reassignment surgery, detransitioned in his forties, and is now in his seventies. He traces his gender dysphoria to the event in early childhood, when his grandmother would dress him up as a girl.

> My grandmother withheld affirmations of me as a boy, but she lavished delighted praise upon me when I was dressed as a girl. Feelings of euphoria swept over me with her praise, followed later by depression and insecurity about being a boy. Her actions planted the idea in me that I was born in the wrong body. She nourished and encouraged the idea that over time it took on a life of its own.[71]

As a consequence of this, Heyer's uncle began mocking him and sexually abused him, and Heyer's parents did not believe him when he told them. He eventually married and had children but could not shake the persistent feeling that he was actually a woman inside a male body. "Unbeknownst to my wife, I began to act on my desire to be a woman. I was cross-dressing in public and enjoying it. I even started taking female hormones to feminize my appearance."[72]

Heyer says that his male-to-female transition brought him a measure of relief, and yet the relief was only transient. "Hidden deep underneath the make-up and female clothing was the little boy carrying the hurts from traumatic childhood events.... Being a female turned out to be only a cover-up, not healing." He writes that

> I felt peace for the first four or five years after I transitioned. Then I realized the high cost of that tenuous peace. Being transgender required destroying the identity of Walt so that my female persona, Laura, would feel unshackled from Walt's past, with all of its hurt, shame, and abuse...it's a marvelous distraction for a while, but...the underlying issues remain unaddressed.[73]

After speaking with a medical doctor, Heyer came to the "maddening" realization that he had "developed a dissociative disorder in childhood to escape the trauma of the repeated cross-dressing by my grandmother and the sexual abuse by my uncle." Now Heyer regards the cross-dressing at the hands of his grandmother to have been a form of child abuse. He has started a mutual-support network of detransitioners. "Every single one of them," writes Heyer, "had unwanted pain caused by sexual abuse, deep trauma, mental disorders, horrible loss, or terrible family circumstances in early life." Heyer writes, "The world of regretters that I see and support is vastly different from the world of the transition advocates, those in a relentless pursuit to convince the world that being transgender is the ultimate of all genders." He notes that many of those who detransition "live in secret and hide the shame and disappointment of falling for the fraud of gender change."[74]

Something generally missing from the transgender success stories appearing in the popular press in recent years is the impact that gender reassignment has on family members. In her essay, "When My Father Told Me He Wanted to Be a Woman," Denise Shick tells of her memory of being nine years old and having her father tell her that he wished to become a woman. She kept this secret over many years, even though by age eleven she began to suffer emotional and sexual abuse from her father. "As his desires intensified, he began to borrow my clothing. Many times I discovered my underclothes and tops....in places I had not been." Whenever she discovered a piece of her clothing that he had worn, she resolved never again to wear it herself. Her father's fixation on becoming a woman caused Shick to begin to reject her own emerging womanhood: "When I began to wear makeup, I had to block out the images I had of him applying makeup or eye shadow or lipstick. He was destroying my desire to become a woman." Fortunately, Shick was able to overcome these early difficulties and to come to love a man who later became her husband. Yet, on her wedding day, as she waited for her father to walk her down the aisle, she says that "he looked me in the eye and said, 'I wish it were me in that dress.'" Shick's heart-wrenching story of her experiences as the daughter of a gender-dysphoric father might not be comparable to the stories of other such children, but her account shows clearly some of the ways that transgenderism may affect families as well as individuals.[75]

Autobiographical Perspectives II: *Kathoey* Transitioners from Thailand

An expression of transgender identity that differs culturally from that of the USA and other Western nations is found among the *kathoey* (or *katoey*) of Thailand. This term refers to transgender, transsexual, or effeminate gay males.[76] Many Thais perceive and speak of the *kathoeys* as belonging to a third gender. Though born as males, they take on a woman's look and habits but are nonetheless not socially regarded simply as women, but as something neither strictly male nor strictly female. Fourteen first-person accounts of *kathoey* experience are included in LeeRay Costa's and Andrew Matzner's *Male Bodies, Women's Souls: Personal Narratives of Thailand's Transgendered Youth* (2007).[77] There is some fluidity in Thai references to transgender persons, with such phrases as "third gender," "transvestite," "transsexuals," "lady boy," and *kathoey* used to refer to the same group of persons.[78] The *kathoey* are generally very clear that they themselves are "not gay," and many of them have a low view of what they regard as the promiscuous way of life among most gay males in Thailand. The life aspiration of most *kathoey* is not to have a variety of sexual partners.[79] The goal instead is fully to embody the female role in Thai culture (i.e., soft, quiet, meek, nurturing), to attract and hold onto a "real man" (i.e., a strict heterosexual), and then to remain in a long-term and monogamous relationship with him.

One of the striking features in *kathoey* narratives is the inherently interpersonal dimension of their transgender identities. Unlike many Western transgender persons, the *kathoey* are not on a quest to find their own true gender identity as individuals, but instead to inhabit the role of the Thai woman in relation to those around them. Those who have met *kathoey* in Thailand or elsewhere are often astonished at the degree to which they are indistinguishable to those who are born as women. The *kathoey* are not sexually attracted to other *kathoey*. They instead are attracted to men regarded as heterosexual, and they seek to make themselves attractive to such "real men."[80] Costa and Matzner note that the *kathoey* are generally more socially acceptable in Thai culture than are gay men. Arguably this is the reverse of the contemporary situation in most Western countries, inasmuch as transgender identity is considered to be further away from heterosexual norms than same-sex relationships. A certain Western liberal romanticization of Thai culture exists today outside of Thailand, whereby their culture is regarded as open to the whole gamut of sexual and gender identities, while Western cultures are only partially so. Thai attitudes are not as accepting as is commonly believed.[81] Costa and Matzner note that the *kathoey* by feminine appearance and deportment replicate and reinforce the strong gender binary in Thai culture, while gay men—by having sex with one another—are seen as violating the gender binary.

University students who were interviewed displayed positive attitudes toward kathoey who "behaved themselves" in public, while they reacted negatively to those who "drew attention to themselves through loud voices, sexy clothes, or aggressive behavior"—all of which were seen as inappropriate for women in Thai culture. Moreover, "the sexual partners of *kathoey* identify as heterosexual, and therefore *kathoey* are rationalized as women, not homosexual men."[82] Though it might seem ironic or strange in a Western context, many *kathoey* express anti-gay attitudes, saying that gay sex between males is a purely physical affair that lacks the all-important elements of "understanding and caring." The *kathoey* seek not only to act as women, but as women who are *riabroi*—a Thai word for "polite" or "well-mannered."[83]

Religious ideas play a role in the interpretation of the *kathoey* phenomenon. An informant named Dini says that being *kathoey* was "my karma and they [i.e., my parents] couldn't change it." Dini went on to say that "I must do good so that in my next life I can be born either as a regular woman or man who does not have anything wrong with them." Another *kathoey*, named Tammy, said that her gender identity "came from a deep part of my soul," and "I still sometimes think that it might be because of sins from a past life."[84] In Thai folk religion, most spirit mediums are female, but those who are male are often *kathoey*. As Costa and Matzner explain, the Thais believe that in "becoming possessed by *jao* [i.e., spirits]...this 'forces' them to become spirit mediums," and "having entered into the role of medium, *kathoey* may more freely adopt and perform the feminine role in terms of clothing and behavior."[85]

Beyond these religious explanations, Costa and Matzner note that the narratives they recorded suggest social or psychological explanations: "[*Kathoey*] frequently view women as positive role models and men as negative.... Thai men are commonly described as irresponsible, selfish, abusive, promiscuous, and alcoholic." As a result, "these expressions of masculinity are devalued...and, as a result, they [i.e., kathoey] want to avoid any association with masculinity in constructing their own subjectivities."[86] This pattern is repeated time and again in the fourteen narratives contained in the collection.

Growing up as a boy, Ek speaks of having been beaten by his father, especially whenever Ek displayed feminine traits. At the same time, Ek was being teased by his sisters and forced to wear a dress and put on makeup, and Ek felt that he was "beginning to absorb this femininity." Along with other *kathoey*, Ek speaks of taking birth control pills—a form of self-administered hormone therapy.[87] Ping comments, "I grew up in the midst of a family of women," and "I was treated like a girl by my grandmother." "There was no warmth in my family at all," says Ping, and "every time my father came home, he would argue with my mother." So "I...vowed not to take him as a role model." "One reason that caused me to behave in the way I did...[is] because I admired my mother very much. She...was much more responsible than my father."[88] Satree Lek remembers, "I was born into a family that had more women than men.... I was dressing as a woman and playing with paper dolls," and "my father did not often come home."[89]

Waranat speaks of how his father drank often and constantly quarreled with his mother. "I could only sit and cry." While Waranat was a teenager, his father became drunk and would not allow him to leave the house. He was so angry at his father that he kicked the bed that his father was sleeping on—a sign of great disrespect. Waranat believes that "the hormones in my body are abnormal," and comments that, "if I were given a choice, I would like to be born as a man with a man's soul. But seeing as I was born the way I was, I have no choice but to live my life the best I can." Though his "father and mother still hope that I will eventually become a real man, like other men," Waranat says that "I don't think that will be possible."[90] Like the other *kathoey*, Wanchaya writes that "it was difficult for me to be close with my father." "My childhood was spent largely around women. I guess it isn't strange that I ended up having some feminine behaviors." In school, Wanchaya spent time with *kathoey* and came to like this group.[91] Like others who became *kathoey*, Phi was dressed up as a girl by another family member.[92]

Thai Silk's narrative follows the common pattern. As a boy he was "much more attached to my mother than to my father," and in general was "very spoiled" as a child. "As a child, all of my heroes were women, and I always imitated them. They were able to stand up to men. At that time I thought that women were the better sex...because men only picked on women who didn't have a way to fight back." The father provoked an opposite reaction: "I was beaten by my father very many times, so much so that it made me hate and fear him very much; I didn't want to think that this man was my father." Thai Silk writes:

"Sometimes I saw my father speak abusively to my mother, but she would never answer back. This made me hate men like my dad who bullied women...it made me want to be a woman who was enduring and patient, like my mom."[93] Diamond notes that as a boy he was closer to my mother than to my father, who "went out...almost every night," and spent his time with "a number of mistresses over the years." As a result, "this situation made me idolize my mother...[and] I didn't have any respect or love for my father at all." So "I began to think that I mustn't be like my father, and instead took up the fighting spirit from my mother." While in university, Diamond began to "think more deeply about the causes of my problems."[94]

The stories of Dini and Go fit in with the general pattern of the narratives. Dini writes:

> What I remember most about my childhood is the image of my father and mother arguing. My father liked to drink until he got drunk and passed out.... My mother played a big role at home...she had the last word in the house." "I really admired her and felt in my heart that she was a hero. At the same time, my father never showed me any love. It's possible that I needed love from the same sex. Besides that, all the relatives I grew up with and ran around and played with were girls.[95]

Go's story—narrated in the third-person by Aom—is as follows:

> Go became a *kathoey* because of her father. When she was a child Go saw her father verbally and physically abuse her mother every day. She saw her mother cry out in pain. Go was not able to help at all. Seeing this happen every day, she began to hate her father more and more. In hating her father so much, she also turned to hating men as well—Go did not want to be a man. So she completely changed herself—her outward manner, appearance, and spirit all became just like a woman's.[96]

The stories of *kathoey* just surveyed suggest that the phenomenon of Thai boys' *identification* with femaleness and femininity has much to do with their *disidentification* from maleness and masculinity. This disidentification, in turn, is linked to experiences of trauma and abuse in early life. Costa and Matzner comment, "Morality in the Thai context is intimately bound up with appearance and conformity."[97] Becoming *kathoey* means conforming to Thai notions of femaleness and femininity in connection with a correlative rejection of the perceived negativism of Thai maleness and masculinity.

Political and Sexual Revolutions: The Marxist and Leftist Connections

Sexuality and gender may be, in the first instance, a "personal" matter, but recent developments disclose an inescapable "political" dimension. Ryan Anderson notes, "Most people with a discordant gender identity are not activists of any sort. But there are activists pushing a transgender ideology...and their views have greatly influenced how our society responds to gender dysphoria."[98] A 1960s and 1970s slogan held that "the personal is the political." This became a rallying cry of radical student movements and of second-wave feminism, underscoring the connections between personal experience and the larger social and political structures. Applied to the current context, the saying might mean something like this: the *personal* sex-and-gender identity that people claim for themselves has inescapable *political* repercussions. In particular, the LGBTQ+ quest for "dignity" involves not merely the decriminalization of homosexual acts, or even the legal sanctioning of same-sex marriage, but a much more wide-ranging (and perhaps elusive) quest for public respect from everyone else in society.[99]

To cite one relatively recent legislative issue in the USA, in the State of California a bill passed in the lower chamber of the state legislature that bans "conversion therapy" in all forms, i.e., therapeutic efforts to aid someone in changing their sexual orientation from same-sex attraction to opposite-sex attraction. Yet critics point out that the state law is so loosely worded that it might, in fact, outlaw the publishing of books or articles, the dissemination of audio and video content, and perhaps even sales of the Bible—in short, any commercially-transacted communication that might be construed as unfavorable toward the idea that LGBTQ+ identities are fixed in stone and can never be changed.[100] Assembly Bill 2943 did not pass in the upper chamber of the California legislature—and it was thought that it might not do so, since this bill would certainly be subjected to a legal challenge, and might be in conflict with the First Amendment of the U. S. Constitution that guarantees freedom of speech. The fact that the bill was introduced, and won such strong support, shows that the idea of a live-and-let-live between the LGBTQ+ community, and its critics or opponents, has given way to a much more socially and politically contentious situation.

Current transgender activism raises issues regarding parental rights. The literature of PFLAG (Parents, Families, and Friends of Lesbians and Gays) says that it is "most important" that parents take at face value "what our children are telling us."[101] Some experts apply this to preschoolers. (Of course, preschoolers may claim not only to have changed sex, but also to have become mermaids, dragons, or lions!) PFLAG also affirms that school officials may know better than parents how to do what is in the child's best interest: "Schools officials interact with the student on a daily basis and focus on supporting the student's growth and development, which gives school personnel unique insight into the student's needs without the biases parent can or are perceived to have."[102]

Recent developments in social attitudes, culture, media, and politics with regard to transgenderism cannot be fully understood without considering the history of efforts to revise, reform, or replace the traditional, heterosexual, male-headed household. Such efforts were underway for more than a century prior to the 1960s and 1970s Sexual Revolution. One of the first modern attempts to theorize a rejection of the traditional family occurred in connection with the French utopian thinker Charles Fourier (1772–1837). He was one of the few authors of the early nineteenth century to advocate something like "free love" in contrast to male-female monogamy.[103] Another was the Robert Owen (1771–1858), founder of a small-scale community, who in his "Declaration of Mental Independence" (1826) wrote, "Man up to this hour has been in all parts of the earth a slave to a trinity of the most monstrous evils…[of] private property, absurd and irrational systems of religion[,] and marriage."[104] Owen declared war on marriage, the family, and private property.

Sociologist Gabrielle Kuby judges that "all sexual revolutionaries in the twentieth century have their spiritual roots in Marxism."[105] The sexual revolution has always been linked with political revolution. In *The Communist Manifesto* (1848), Karl Marx (1818–1883) and Friedrich Engels (1820–1895) stated: "[Communists] openly declare that their ends can be attained only by the forcible overthrow of all existing social conditions." The Marxist plan for "forcible overthrow" included not only the economic sphere, but also what Marx and Engels called the "bourgeois family." Because of pervasive adultery, Marx wrote that "bourgeois marriage is, in reality, a system of wives in common." It was a "dirty existence" of "domestic slavery" and "general hypocrisy." Marx expected that "the bourgeois family will vanish as a matter of course"—in the same way, that supposed eternal truths, morality, and religion would also pass away. The abolition of private property and the rise of socialism would lead to the disappearance of the traditional family. In Richard Weikart's words, Marx and Engels "never masked their contempt for present family relationships and their hope for radically new social relations in communist society."[106] Many of the key Marxist ideas on the family appeared first in the first work jointly written by Marx and Engels, *The German Ideology*, which was not published during their lifetimes. Marx and Engels had almost nothing to say about the relations between parents and children—except for the insistence that they would not be allowed to live together.[107]

Friedrich Engels, in *The Origin of the Family, Private Property and the State* (1884), proposed that "The first class-antagonism appearing in history coincides with the development of the antagonism of man and wife in monogamy, and the first class-oppression with that of the female by the male sex." For Marx and Engels, the integration of women into economic production was one and the same with their "liberation." From the beginnings of the Communist movement, "bourgeois morality" was thought to impede the achievement of a classless society.[108] Engels allowed for marriages easily to be dissolved, and rather cynically appealed to the feeling of love as the only justification for the continuance of any marriage: "Only a union based on love is moral; hence the union should last only as long as love lasts. When love ceases to exist, or when it is succeeded by a new passion, divorce becomes a benefit."[109] Engels's influence has continued up to the present. One researcher found that Betty Friedan, while writing her best-selling and widely influential book, *The Feminine Mystique* (1963) had scribbled into her notes various lines from Engels's 1884 book.

Engels called for women to be channeled into factories, and for private housework to be nationalized by the state. Housework would become a public industry, with communal cleaning, cooking, and childcare. Engels said that he wanted "to bring about the gradual growth of unconstrained sexual intercourse and with it a more tolerant public opinion."[110] In this book and in other writings, Engels prescribed that marriage would not be a legal relationship at all but would become purely a private affair. This is ironic because matrimony was one of the few areas in which Marx and Engels actually favored privatization. Divorce in Communist Russia was made easy in 1918—involving nothing more than the mailing of a postcard—and abortion was legalized in 1920.[111] Divorce increased during the Soviet era, and by the late 1960s, there were some Russians who had been married and divorced as many as fifteen times. During the 1960s there were also women who had had as many as twenty abortions. In Communist China, the one-child policy led to vast numbers of forced abortions, and one of the most severe infringements on family life that was ever inflicted by any government on its people.[112]

In the aftermath of the Russian Revolution, Alexandra Kollontai (1872–1952) was the first woman to serve on the St. Petersburg Revolutionary Council, and she functioned as the commissar for public welfare under Vladimir Lenin. She also established communal houses and promoted free love as a way of liberating women from what she called the "choice between marriage and prostitution." Kollontai's "Communism and the Family" (1920) declared, "There is no escaping the fact: the old type of family has had its day. The family is withering away not because it is being forcibly destroyed by the state, but because the family is ceasing to be a necessity." She claimed that "Communist society will take upon itself all the duties in the education of the child." The new Soviet woman would no longer have any sense of possession regarding her children: "The worker-mother must learn not to differentiate between yours and mine."[113] Just as there would be no "private possessions," there would be no "private children" either. The private life was dead—long live the Communist collective! The Bolsheviks wanted to be entirely in charge of childrearing, so that the Soviet children would all grow up to be obedient Communists. Women were to become economically productive and were no longer to remain with their husbands and children in the home.[114] The Soviet opposition to the traditional family has found expression in the declaration of the Thirteenth Congress of the Communist Party of the Soviet Union that the family was a "formidable stronghold of all the turpitudes of the old regime." Another early Bolshevik decree declared that all women ages seventeen to thirty-two were "property of the state," with the "rights of husbands" to consider them as wives "abolished."[115]

The so-called New Left of the 1960s took up in Western Europe and in North American the anti-family cause that the Soviets, the Chinese, and other Communist regimes had already championed. The radical West German youth of the 1960s embraced slogans such as the these: "Destroy what is destroying you!" "Battle the bourgeois nuclear family!" "If you sleep with the same one twice, you're a slave of bourgeois vice!"[116] Herbert Marcuse's widely read book, *Eros and Civilization* (1955), might be described as the "Bible" of the New Left and the student radicals. It argued that the deepest cause of dictatorial power relationships in the world was the widespread repression of eros. This repression resulted in a socio-pathological dynamic in which certain people came to dominate other people, eventually resulting in war and mass murder. Marcuse called for the elimination of "the achievement principle" and its replacement with "the pleasure principle." No longer were sexual desires to be "sublimated," as Sigmund Freud suggested, but they were henceforth to find full expression in all their glorious variety and vagary. Living in the here-and-now, and seeking pleasure, was now defined as a revolutionary act. Absurd as it may sound, Marcuse argued that the unbridled indulgence of one's sexual urges would produce a virtuous society purged of all domination and bring a permanent end to war and genocide. Marcuse's theories help to explain the hippy slogan: "Make Love, Not War." Marcuse promoted intolerance toward those who disagreed with his program, and in a rather Orwellian fashion, he inverted the meanings of words so that "tolerance" of differing views was a form of "repression," while "intolerance" was a form of "liberation."[117]

At a 1969 gathering in New York City, feminist author Kate Millett led the group in attendance in a chant: "How do we destroy the family?" she called out. "By destroying the American Patriarch," they shouted back. "How do we do that?" "By destroying monogamy." "How can we destroy monogamy?" "By promoting promiscuity, eroticism, prostitution, and homosexuality!" they resounded.[118] Just as Marcuse might have suggested—a glorious new society would arise once the traditional family had been abolished. The student radical group of the 1960s, The Weathermen, had as one of their major slogans: "Smash Monogamy!" The "Smash Monogamy" campaign was intended to destroy bourgeois sexual inhibitions in the same way that street fighting would "smash" inhibitions against engaging in violence. Student radicals in this group were required to embrace non-monogamy by sharing with others their spouses, boyfriends, or girlfriends. They also engaged in group sex and tried unsuccessfully—in the name of political radicalism—to convince heterosexual male members to overcome their inhibitions and pursue gay sex with one another.[119]

Excursus: Queer Biblical Interpretation and Queer Theology in Brief

For queer interpreters of the Bible, the Christian scriptures as traditionally interpreted have been an *oppressive object* that has fallen upon and crushed its vulnerable readers. Gender theorist Mary Ann Tolbert calls for "strategies of reading for disarming the Bible's potential for 'clobbering'...marginalized or oppressed groups."[120] To the extent the biblical text is monolithic (or is interpreted monolithically), queer interpreters insist that it must be *broken into pieces*. Once the text has been broken apart, among the fragments one may pick up pieces that serve a liberative function. Yet queer interpreters of the Bible share no common methodology, and indeed the notion of a single, dominant, hermeneutical method would be incompatible with the sometimes whimsically playful, sometimes deadly serious, queer commitment to anti-form and anti-structure. Tolbert explains that "queer readers of the Bible reclaim...its texts by destabilizing them, playing with them, laughing at them, tricking them—all wonderfully inventive strategies."[121]

Among the more common strategies of queer interpretation is the construction of a *counternarrative* to undermine or displace existing biblical narratives. For Tolbert, the counternarratives come into existence as readers become textual "co-creators." She writes that "all texts, including the biblical texts, are generally ambiguous and indeterminate, thus requiring readers to refine and complete their meanings.... Readers of texts literally become the co-creators of their meanings."[122] For Robert Goss and Mona West, the biblical interpreter ought to function as a "trickster." They assert, "To read as a trickster [is] to recover our voices within the biblical tradition...transgressing boundaries is a rebellious act that breaks conceptual categories."[123] "Tricksters," says Virginia Ramey Mollenkott, "incorporate a spirit of disorder."[124]

Goss and West in their edited collection—*Take Back the Word: A Queer Reading of the Bible* (2001)—praise Christopher King's essay on the biblical Song of Songs for "loosening the reading of the Song from exclusive heterosexuality" and "envision[ing] queer love...identifying with...the outsider."[125] Readers might be wondering how it is that the Song of Songs breaks free from "exclusive heterosexuality."[126] The answer lies in what I will here term the *associative-assimilative* aspect of queer biblical interpretation. Queer readings are often based on homology, in which two or more persons, objects, or elements, by sharing one particular trait in common, are understood as connected or interchangeable. The young woman who debuts in the first chapter of the Song of Songs—as "black and lovely" (Song 1:5)—is an outsider to the royal court.[127] The erotic love in this text occurs between an insider (i.e., royal) and an outsider (i.e., commoner). So the implied argument runs thus: queers are outsiders in today's culture. The young woman in the ancient text is an outsider, and so she is queer, and thus the Song of Songs includes the theme of queer love and may offer a vindication of today's queer love.

As in other instances of queer exegesis, the implied argument breaks down on examination. If two queers love one another (as might generally be the case today), then *two outsiders* would be involved, not an outsider and an insider, as in the first chapter of the Song of Songs. Even according to the loose logic of association-assimilation, one would need to find biblical instances of *outsider-outsider* and not *insider-outsider* romance if one wanted to find in scripture some foreshadowing of contemporary queer, outsider-outsider love. What makes the queer interpretation even more problematic here is that the Song's portrayal of the ruler who picks a lovely yet lowly girl as his companion comes across as patriarchal and perhaps as oppressive. What could be more hierarchical than a king picking out for himself a village maiden as concubine or wife? (Does this woman have any *choice*? Is she a royal sex slave?) One must thus employ a good deal of *eisegesis* (i.e., reading into the text) to find "queer love" in any sense in the biblical Song.

What, in the end, is the point of queer interpretation? The answer seems to be: the aim of today's queer interpretation is not *liberation* as much as *subversion*. The subversive hermeneutics of queer reading seeks to destabilize, disrupt, undermine, and collapse systems of meaning or assertions of truth that might be made on the basis of the biblical text. Queer reading not only rejects hetero-normative sexuality, but other forms of normativity as well. There is a focus on themes of death, pain, suffering, violation, suffering, and transgression. So we find here a remarkable series of inversions: death not life, pain not wellness, sickness not health, violation not innocence, and unhappiness not happiness.

Lee Edelman's *No Future: Queer Theory and the Death Drive* (2004) is summarized by the publisher in this way:

> In this searing polemic, Lee Edelman outlines a radically uncompromising new ethics of queer theory. His main target is the all-pervasive figure of the child, which he reads as the linchpin of our universal politics of "reproductive futurism." Edelman argues that the child, understood as innocence in need of protection, represents the possibility of the future against which the queer is positioned as the embodiment of a relentlessly narcissistic, antisocial, and future-negating drive. He boldly insists that the efficacy of queerness lies in its very willingness to embrace this refusal of the social and political order. In *No Future*, Edelman urges queers to abandon the stance of accommodation and accede to their status as figures for the

force of a negativity that he links with irony, *jouissance*, and, ultimately, the death drive itself.[128]

Edelman's book offers a form of queer nihilism—antisocial, misanthropic, and death-devoted. The rejection of sexual reproduction reminds one of the so-called voluntary extinction movement that regards *homo sapiens* as a pestiferous species that ought to be collectively euthanized.[129] Seemingly, the only affirmative principle in Edelman's *No Future* lies in what the author calls "raw sex"—a sheer, physical act performed for the sake of momentary pleasure, and without regard for future consequences, well-being, or posterity. Perhaps the assumption here is that civilization is doomed. The barbarians are at the gates, the partygoers bolt themselves inside, and revel on until the door is kicked in, and death arrives for one and all. As in Edgar Allen Poe's story, "The Masque of the Red Death," there is festivity among those locked in the castle, but destruction stands near.

Queer theologian Marcella Althaus-Reid is less nihilistic than queer theorist Lee Edelman, yet she is equally transgressive. In *Indecent Theology* (2001) she writes:

> Indecent Sexual Theologies...may be effective as long as they represent the resurrection of the excessive in our contexts, and a passion for organizing the lusty transgressions of theological and political thought. The excessiveness of our hungry lives: our hunger for food, hunger for the touch of other bodies, for love and for God.... Only in the longing for a world of economic and sexual justice together, and not subordinated to one another, can the encounter with the divine take place. But this is an encounter to be found at the crossroads of desire, when one dares to leave the ideological order of the heterosexual pervasive normative. This is an encounter with indecency and with the indecency of God and Christianity.[130]

In *The Queer God* (2003), Althaus-Reid reflects on the holiness of the gay club, and the intersection of vibrant faith with total sexual self-indulgence. Inverting the traditional interpretation of Jeremiah 2:23–25, she takes this text not as a critique but as an affirmation of uncontrolled lust: "A young camel deviating from her path: a wild she-ass accustomed to the wilderness, sniffing the wind in her lust. Who can repel her desire? And you said, No! I love strangers, the different, the unknown, the Other, and will follow them."[131] Both Edelman and Althaus-Reid show us how the queer themes of rejection, subversion, and transgression have largely displaced such earlier queer motifs as social acceptance, inclusiveness of queers with non-queers, and liberation from hurtful or harmful narratives in scripture.

Roman Catholic and Evangelical Perspectives on Sex, Family, and Gender

The Roman Catholic Church from the nineteenth century onward came to oppose Socialism and Communism for their rejection of traditional marriage and family life. Pope Leo XIII's 1878 encyclical *Quod Apostolici muneris* ("On Socialism") declared, "They debase the natural union of man and woman, which is held sacred even among barbarous peoples; and its bond, by which the family is chiefly held together, they weaken, or even deliver up to lust." He wrote that "Family life…redounds to the right ordering and preservation of every State and kingdom." Yet "the doctrines of socialism strive almost completely to dissolve this union; since that stability which is imparted to it by religious wedlock being lost, it follows that the power of the father over his own children, and the duties of the children toward their parents, must be greatly weakened."[132]

Recent pontiffs—including Pope John Paul II, Pope Benedict XVI, and Pope Francis—have all sounded many of the same themes that one finds in nineteenth- and early-twentieth-century papal declarations. In his address on 21 December 2012, Pope Benedict XVI spoke of the profound challenges to Christian ideas and ideals of marriage and family in our era:

> While up to now we regarded a false understanding of human freedom as one cause of the crisis of the family, it is now becoming clear that the very notion of being—of what human really means—is being called into question.… The profound falsehood of this theory…is obvious. People dispute the idea that they have a nature, given by their bodily identity, that serves as a defining element of the human being. They deny their nature and decide that it is not something previously given to them, but that they make it for themselves. According to the biblical creation account, being created by God as male and female pertains to the essence of the human creature. This duality is an essential aspect of what being human is all about, as ordained by God.…
>
> Now we decide for ourselves. Man and woman as created realities, as the nature of the human being, no longer exist. Man calls his nature into question. From now on he is merely spirit and will.… If there is no pre-ordained duality of man and woman in creation, then neither is the family any longer a reality established by creation. Likewise, the child has lost the place he had occupied hitherto and the dignity pertaining to him.… From being a subject of rights, the child has become an object to which people have a right.… When the freedom to be creative becomes the freedom to create oneself, then necessarily the Maker himself is denied and ultimately man too is stripped of his dignity as a creature of God, as the image of

God at the core of his being. The defense of the family is about man himself. And it becomes clear that when God is denied, human dignity also disappears. Whoever defends God is defending man.[133]

The French Catholic Joseph-Marie Verlinde authored a small but thought-provoking book, *L'ideologie du gender* (2012).[134] The book's subtitle poses a key question: "Is sexual or gender identity received, or else chosen?" In his exposition, Father Verlinde cites statements on sexuality and gender from Pope John Paul II and by Pope Emeritus Benedict XVI. Authoritative Catholic assertions on this topic are recent and brief, yet clear and pointed. Pope Francis—though more progressive in certain respects than Pope John Paul II or Pope Benedict XVI—spoke out strongly in October 2016 on the dangers posed by "gender theory." Pope Francis commented: "A great enemy of marriage today is the theory of gender.... Today, there is a global war trying to destroy marriage...they don't destroy it with weapons, but with ideas. It's certain ideological ways of thinking that are destroying it...we have to defend ourselves from ideological colonization."[135]

The Greek Catholic Church, centered in the Ukrainian city of Kiev, produced a 2016 encyclical, "Concerning the Danger of Gender Ideology."[136] Archbishop Sviatoslav Shevchuk authored this encyclical on behalf of the Synod of Bishops of the Major Archeparchy of Kiev–Galicia. Their country was in the midst of a civil war, and yet the bishops there found it important to address this topic at this time. The subheadings in the text are "Human Dignity in God's Plan," "The Concept of Gender," "Destructive Outcomes of Gender Ideology," and "Proclaiming the Truth of Christ in the Context of an Expanding Gender Ideology." The bishops warn that gender ideology is not accompanied by "open and bloody persecution," like twentieth-century Communism, and yet it uses "hidden" and often "covert" means that nevertheless has the similar result of "destroying Christian faith and morality, as well as universal human values."[137]

It is perhaps not surprising then that the Christian church in formerly Communist countries has shown itself most astute in recognizing the dangerous tendencies of the new gender ideology. Archbishop Sviatoslav of the Greek Catholic Church states that gender ideology "denies the most obvious anthropological reality." For "people are born male and female, and the natural complementarity of the gifts of the two sexes is an extraordinary richness for all of humanity, which gives hope for progress. Promoting vague and undefined ideas of 'gender identity' creates a dangerous psychological instability that leads to absurd conflicts between bodily and psychological sexuality, which naturally stems from the physical." The archbishop adds that gender theory not only "destroy[s] the concept of family as a community of husband and wife in which children are born and brought up," but it "promotes many forms of sexual identity and behavior that do not at all correspond to human nature." As a result of this, "gender theories lead to promiscuity and further demoralization of society. Such a situation leads to disappointment, anger, and the self-destruction of the human race, because its natural foundations and principles are undermined." Properly understood, "human sexuality...is a natural gift of God and precisely through it we discover the joy of being co-creators."

Gabrielle Kuby, in *The Global Sexual Revolution* (2015), speaks of contemporary Western culture as engaged in a mistaken battle against the "tyranny of nature":

> The goal is absolute freedom, unfettered by any natural or moral limitations. It sees the human being as merely a 'naked' individual. For such absolute freedom...any natural precept is an obstacle that must be removed.... The concrete weapons in this war include deconstruction of male-female sexuality, alteration of the population's social norms and attitudes (especially among youth), complete legal equivalency of homosexual partnership with marriage, and even social ostracism and legal criminalization of any opposition to these new 'norms'....
>
> A person sexualized from childhood is taught: 'It is *right* to live out all of your instincts without reflection. It is *wrong* for you to set boundaries for them.' He uses his own body, and the bodies of other people, for satisfying his sex drive, instead of for expressing personal love.... A person driven in this way loses his freedom. He no longer hears the voice of his conscience. He loses the ability to love and the ability to bond. He loses the desire to give children the gift of life. He becomes incapable of cultural achievement. He becomes mentally and physically sick. He loses his desire and ability to maintain his own culture, thereby setting it up for domination by a more energetic one.[138]

In a foreword to Kuby's book, Robert Spaemann speaks of the present danger of mistaken notions of freedom. "The word 'emancipation' once meant something like liberation," and yet "emancipation from our nature can only mean liberation from ourselves."[139] Such freedom-from-oneself would take shape as a self-negating act borne of delusion or an *emancipative self-destruction*. We might picture a fish that wants to be free of the water, and so jumps from the pond and perishes. Alternatively, we might think of a person so sick of the house he inhabits that he decides to burn it down—while he is still inside it.

To a remarkable extent, there has been a recent convergence of views on sex and gender issues among biblically- and traditionally-oriented Catholic and Protestant Christians. In reading some of the major critiques of the current sex-and-gender ideology, one would not be able to identify to what tradition or confession the Christian author belongs.

In their recent book on maleness and femaleness in biblical perspective, *The Grand Design* (2016), Owen Strachan and Gavin Peacock comment on global crisis regarding gender identity. From Paris to London, Hong Kong, Mexico City, Sydney, and Capetown,

> a gender-neutral world convinces us that manhood and womanhood aren't important. Complementarity is a fiction. It's no big deal to be a man or a woman. Many people today believe secularism. They pursue androgyny. As a result, boys want to be girls today and girls want to be boys. Many men embrace the traits and attitudes traditionally associated with womanhood. Many women do the same thing with manhood. Both sides avoid at all costs hard-and-fast stereotypes. The ultimate transgression today is to fit into past conceptions of the sexes. Nobody wants to be some sort of manly man's mountain man or a Victorian-era tea-sipping countess. Men have grown increasingly passive, effeminate, and unsure of themselves. Women have grown increasingly manly, aggressive, and unsure of their future. These are hard words today, but they sum up the drift of a secularizing world.
>
> In 2016, the sexes have lost the script for their lives, and so many don't know what role to play in life. Try asking a male friend at a coffee shop, "What is your manhood *for*? What's the purpose of being a man?" Or try querying a young woman at the local university, "What meaning does womanhood have? Does it matter at all?" A good number of folks would, in being asked these kinds of questions, look at us like we had just invited them on a lunar cruise in a tugboat. Outside of affirming feminism, transgender identity, and shape-shifting sexual orientation, it's taboo today to speak of manhood and womanhood in any fixed way.
>
> This is true in secular circles, and it's increasingly true even in Christian circles. The confusion extends to sex. When it comes to this perennial hot topic, we are told that fluidity trumps biology. There is no specific meaning of manhood and womanhood, and thus there is no structure or plan for sex. You just be who you choose to be, and you experiment with whoever strikes your fancy. You don't need to wait, you don't need to restrain your natural desires, you don't need to commit yourself. You need only to act on your impulses. When you're doing so, in fact, you find out who you really are. You're then happy, alive, liberated, and *human*.[140]

Strachan and Peacock devote the rest of their slender volume to unpacking these statements and showing what is wrong with the current secular recipe for personal and sexual fulfillment. In the words of the authors, "Christians have something better to offer—something incomparably better," in acknowledging the created complementarity of man and woman.[141]

Conclusions: On Balancing the Personal and the Political

The argument of this essay has gradually built toward two conclusions that might be summed up in terms of two (slightly modified) biblical imperatives. The first of these is "love your [transgender] neighbor as yourself" (Mk. 12:31). The second is "do not believe every [ideological] spirit, but test the spirits to see whether they are from God" (1 Jn. 4:1). The first is the *personal application,* and the second the *political application.* Some Christians, on coming personally to know transgender persons, have become acutely attuned to the personal aspects of transgender experience, and may be prone to turn a blind eye to its political dimension. In light of the material presented above, the situation and status of transgender persons are clearly linked to the legacy of Sexual Revolution of the 1960s and 1970s, and this, in turn, must be understood in light of a larger struggle in Western society between secular and Christian conceptions of the human life, the nature of the human person, sexuality, marriage, family, and child-rearing. One would be naïve to ignore this political dimension. On the other hand, a fitting Christian response must flow from a recognition of transgender persons as human beings created in God's image (Gen. 1:26-27). As image-bearers, transgender persons possess an essential dignity that must be acknowledged and respected. As the autobiographical excerpts above might suggest, each trans person's story is inescapably individual and idiosyncratic, and for this reason, those engaging the transgender community will need to do a great deal of attentive listening to understand the persons whom they are encountering.

An effective engagement with transgender ideology on the political level must be based on an awareness of its philosophical underpinnings. Gender ideology, as presented by Judith Butler and others, rests in fact on an atheistic presupposition that *there is no Creator* and that *human beings are not creatures.* Since, on this view, each human being is but wisp of smoke that briefly appears and then vanishes forever, then why should we not, as Butler's theories might suggest, *put on a good performance in the meanwhile*? In Butler's worldview, each person's life is like a separate stage and each of us gets to be the playwright, director, and acting cast for our own theatrical production. It is telling that Butler's early work focused on the philosophy of Jean-Paul Sartre—a militant atheist, who from his youth denied God's existence, and insisted that each person is called to self-fashioning or self-creating. The famous summation of Sartre's atheistic existentialism is that "existence precedes essence." This meant that there is no essential human nature that shapes individual lives, and that each of us is therefore radically free. What Butler has done since the 1980s is to apply Sartre's atheistic philosophy of self-creation to the field of gender studies. Butler's gender theory is thus founded on *a presumption of atheism*, and Christian leaders engaging it ought to keep this in mind. And medical science is starting to mimic the philosophical changes in Western society. Among physicians today, as Paul McHugh writes, "there is a deep prejudice in favor of the idea that nature is totally malleable." A postmodern worldview is shifting medicine from being a profession that restores health and wholeness, to a set of techniques that provide customers with whatever it is that they desire. "Without any fixed position on what is given in human nature, any manipulation of it can be defended as legitimate. A practice that appears to give people what they want…turns out to be difficult to combat with ordinary professional experience and wisdom."[142]

Since the Bolshevik Revolution of 1917, the international Communist movement bears sobering witness to the political dangers of an atheistic philosophy of human self-creation. The emerging gender ideology, writes Archbishop Sviatoslav of Ukraine, is not merely being proposed but is being forcibly imposed, with no toleration for dissent:

> Therefore, at its present stage of development, gender theory begins to acquire the characteristics of totalitarian ideology and is similar to those utopian ideologies that in the twentieth century not only promised to create paradise on earth, supposedly building true equality between people, but also tried to forcibly introduce their own way of thinking, eradicating any alternative point of view. The tragic history of the twentieth century has shown us what such ideologies that promise 'happiness to all humanity' turn into.

The denial of human nature and natural moral law by gender ideology, writes the archbishop, will inevitably lead to the destruction of the "concept of human identity." For this reason, "one can say with conviction that gender theory is destructive and anti-human."[143] The freedom promised by the Sexual Revolution of the 1960s and 1970s is increasingly coming to resemble a *coercive freedom*—i.e., a supposed liberty that is wholly intolerant of those who believe that there are ethical norms in sexuality and a natural order for the family.

In balancing political awareness with personal compassion, Christian believers should remember that transgender activists may be hard at work, and yet the transgender neighbor is not necessarily a part of any sort of plot against monogamy or calculated effort to take down traditional marriage. Each transgender person must be approached on his or her (or, its, zer, spivak, etc.) terms, and not prejudged in advance as a member of a particular, gender-identity grouping. The research summarized above by Paul McHugh—as well as the University of Birmingham (UK), and by Swedish researchers—shows that it would be a mistake for Christians, in the name of empathy and compassion, to support methods of treatment that have not proven their effectiveness in combatting gender dysphoria. Ryan Anderson summarizes:

> There is no solid scientific evidence that transgender identities are innate or biologically determined, and there is some evidence that other factors are most likely involved. But, in truth, very little is understood about the causes of discordant gender identities. Many psychologists and psychiatrists think of gender dysphoria as being much like other kinds of dysphoria, or serious discomfort with one's body, such as anorexia. These feelings can lead to mistaken and harmful beliefs. The most helpful therapies do not try to remake the body to conform with thoughts and feelings—which is impossible—but rather to help people find healthy ways to manage this tension and move toward accepting the reality of their bodily selves.... An effective therapy looks into the reasons for the child's mistaken beliefs about gender, and addresses the problems that the child believes will be solved if the body is altered...so they understand that real boys and real girls don't all conform to narrow stereotypes.... We need to respect the dignity of people who identify as transgender, but without encouraging children to undergo experimental transition treatments.[144]

Some comments from two of the female detransitioners are worth recalling. Crash wrote that *"transitioning was all about trying to get away from what hurt us and detransitioning is finally facing that and overcoming it."* For Christian believers, to engage the transgender community is to encounter those who have been deeply hurt by life, and to direct them to God's healing power in Christ. Those who profess to believe in Jesus, but who are doubtful regarding the depth and power of divine healing, should probably not involve themselves in this way. Consider Cari's statements as well: *"There isn't a whole lot of place in society for women who look like this, women who don't fit, women who don't comply."* The therapists do not say that *"it's okay to be butch, to be gender nonconforming."* A common theme throughout the stories of transgender persons is that of self-hatred and self-rejection. As the above accounts suggest, the process of self-rejection typically begins with bullying and mockery from family members, friends, and the surrounding community. Girls and young women who have masculine traits *need acceptance as they are*—as God created them, and not as measured by a cultural construct of femininity. Boys and young men who have feminine traits also *need acceptance as they are*—as God created them, and not according to equally artificial standards of masculinity. If the church does not practice and model the acceptance of persons—as God has created them—then where will and how will acceptance be found?

Postscript (May 2019). A researcher at Brown University, Lisa Littman, reported in an August 2018 article that gender dysphoria seemed often to appear in clusters of adolescent females who were already acquainted with one another and were together influenced by social media.[145] This led to a new concept, known as "rapid onset gender dysphoria" (ROGB). Littman wrote: "In on-line forums, parents have reported that their children seemed to experience a sudden or rapid onset of gender dysphoria, appearing for the first time during puberty…[and] in the context of belonging to a peer group where, one, multiple, or even all of the friends have become gender dysphoric and transgender-identified during the same timeframe. Parents also report that their children exhibited an increase in social media/internet use prior to disclosure of a transgender identity." Littman proposed that "social influences" as well as "maladaptive coping mechanisms" among adolescents can "contribute to the development of gender dysphoria." The publication of this study evoked such strong and immediate protests that the Dean of the Brown University School of Public Health issued an apology, commenting that the study might be used to "invalidate the perspectives of members of the transgender community." The journal featuring Littman's paper undertook a reassessment of the article, leading to the publication of a "Correction" from the author. This "Correction" noted that "this is a study of parent report[ing] and consideration of what information parents may or may not have access to is an important element of the findings." In response to these developments, the former Dean of Harvard University Medical School, Jeffrey Flier, claimed that objections from "unnamed parties" in terms of "some vaguely defined harm to other third parties is a spurious basis for the university's actions." University of Texas sex researcher, Mark Regnerus, suggested that the additional scrutiny of Littman's work was politically and not scientifically motivated. "The obvious problem," for Littman's opponents, was that "the evidence doesn't fit an immutability narrative, or even the 'I felt it as a child' explanation. On the contrary, ROGD appears to be 'infectious' in some post pubertal social groups." Regnerus asks: "Just how common is this? We don't know." Regnerus called for additional studies of ROGD, but noted that the present climate of opinion surrounding trangenderism might be an obstacle to new research in this field.

II

Learning from Real Life

5.

Sexuality, Gender, and Marriage: Pentecostal Theology of Sexuality and Empowering the Girl-Child in India

Brainerd Prince and Atula Walling

The focus of the article arises from a case study of an Indian woman and her adopted child, Sunita and Komal. There are three key issues that can be abstracted from the story of Sunita and Komal. The abandoned "girl-child" Komal raises the question of sex—what am I? What does it mean to be biologically female? What consequences are there for being born female? Sunita's and Komal's rejection from their families has led them to ask the question about their gender—who am I? What does it mean to be a girl or woman in a predominantly Hindu society? How is my female identity constrained and constructed by my society? Finally, Sunita, as a young wife and in light of her miscarriages, recasts the question of marriage itself—how am I supposed to live as a woman in society, particularly in the context of family? What role and functions are expected of me as a woman? Thus, the three issues raised are sexuality, gender, and marriage of the Hindu girl-child. This article seeks to explore, in response, a Pentecostal theology of human sexuality along these lines.

Introduction

Five-and-one-half-year-old Komal is one of the children whom we serve at Shiksha Rath. Komal's mother, Sunita, got married at the very young age of fourteen. She faced a lot of problems as she was unable to manage the household chores she had to perform in her husband's house. Furthermore, being very young, she had two miscarriages. The doctor had already warned the family that she would not be able to bear children in the future if pregnancies continued, as her body was not ready to bear children. Meanwhile, the villagers found an abandoned premature girl baby (born in the seventh month) in the forest.

The doctor diagnosed that the baby would not survive for long. Sunita's in-laws, thinking that the baby would die soon, forced Sunita to take the baby and look after her. They thought this would be a distraction for Sunita and ease the pain of her two miscarriages. They believed that the baby would surely die, so there was no question about adopting it. Unwillingly Sunita took the baby, but soon found herself genuinely taking care of her. By the time the baby Komal reached two months of age, she got healthier, and Sunita had developed a great attachment to her. Seeing the baby getting healthier and growing, Sunita's husband and family got worried and told her to give away the baby as it was not their own. But Sunita was not willing to abandon Komal again. Sunita was physically abused for not listening to them and was told to leave the house. In addition to her husband's family, all the villagers started taunting her. She left her husband and in-laws and came to her parents' home with Komal. But even her own family was not supportive of her decisions. Sunita brought Komal to Delhi to begin a new life in the Outram Lines slum. She is working as a maid to support both Komal and herself. In addition to her work, Sunita is taking tuition classes to complete the tenth grade so that she can get a better job.

Shiksha Rath

Shiksha Rath ("chariot of education") is an after-school holistic educational program for the slum children living in Outram Lines, North Delhi. There are eighty children between the ages of five and fourteen from sixty-eight households who regularly attend our daily classes. Shiksha Rath aims to help these underprivileged children in their studies and give them opportunities to develop their skills and talents and most of all gives them an environment of love and acceptance and a place to learn the principles and teachings of Jesus. This is done in a non-conventional way of evangelism. We do not talk or teach about religion directly, but mostly demonstrate it through our lifestyle and deeds. We work very closely with the parents and the community as a whole. Our approach is to be a true light and salt in this community and to allow our good deeds amongst them to speak about the love of Jesus that motivates our work.

Most of the children and the families we serve belong to different kinds of Hindu traditions. They may be Shaivites or Vaishnavites and would worship many gods and goddesses and broadly live out the Hindu life, even if they are not consciously indoctrinated in it. Even as we have served these children for over seven years, we have gotten close to their families and have been able to observe the deeper issues and challenges they face—particularly the girl-children and their mothers. Komal's and Sunita's story is an example. It is well documented that the Hindu traditions predominantly have a low view of women and female sexuality, particularly with respect to the girl-child, at least in the practical sense of their role and function in society. Hence, wonderful stories in the tradition that honor women seem exceptional, although revisionist historians have built the argument that the marginal notion of women has not always been the case. However, in the context of our work, the girl-child and often their mothers are disrespected as they are seen as a dowry curse. Furthermore, the anticipation of their early marriage and going away alienates the girl-child from her own family from a very young age, as she is perceived as belonging to the other. The practice of female child marriage also translates into a lack of present care of the girl-child as well as fuels a disinterest in her welfare through education or other means. These issues are not only seen as emerging in the Sunita-Komal story but are also generally well documented within the larger Hindu society. In the Indian social world, these oppressive and abusive structures continue to persist, fed by unchallenged social customs that are often termed religious.

There are three key issues that can be abstracted from this story. The abandoned girl-child Komal raises the question of sex—what am I? What does it mean to be biologically female? What consequences are there for being born female? Komal's and Sunita's rejection from their families has led them to ask the question about their gender—who am I? What does it mean to be a girl or woman in predominantly Hindu society? How is my female identity constrained and constructed by my society? Finally, Sunita, as a young wife and in light of her miscarriages, recasts the question of marriage itself—how am I supposed to live as a woman in society, particularly in the context of family? What role and functions are expected of me as a woman? Thus, the three issues raised by the above vignette are sexuality, gender, and marriage of the Hindu girl-child. This article seeks to explore a Pentecostal theology of human sexuality along these lines.

The methodology followed is the method of correlation with the following structure. First, after an initial description of these issues—sexuality, gender, marriage—problems are identified by the survey research done with the girls and mothers in Shiksha Rath. Second, the issues are explored and engaged from the Hindu point of view within whose horizons the Shiksha Rath women experience their lives. Finally, building on what Shiksha Rath is doing practically, we will offer a theological reflection from a Pentecostal perspective. Through this case study on the work of Shiksha Rath, it will be argued that a Spirit-empowered ministry intervention can go a long way in engaging these issues and reforming the cultural and religious practices, particularly related to the dignity of the Hindu girl-child in India.

However, before we get to the main sections, three preliminary points will be addressed: a) the method of correlation used in this article; b) the status of Pentecostal studies on human sexuality; and c) the three-part conceptual structure of Ricoeur's narrative identity, which will provide the theoretical scaffolding for this work.

Method of Correlation

In a general sense, this work lies within the theology, and particularly contextual Pentecostal theology, of human sexuality. However, it is not a mere review of theological material that concerns us here: rather this is an attempt to make a contribution to a Pentecostal theology of human sexuality from the ground up, in a sense, from the problems faced in a particular context in which theology is asked to respond and seek for an answer. Paul Tillich called it "dialectic" or "answering" theology, which he developed in his *Systematic Theology Volume 1* as the method of correlation. Tillich states that "the method of correlation explains the contents of the Christian faith through existential questions and theological answers in mutual interdependence[1] In other words, the questions are raised in "real life," as in the case of the project of Shiksha Rath, which depicts the human condition, and an attempt is made to seek theological answers. It is in this correlation that the contents of the Christian faith are revealed. However, for Tillich, the entire process possesses a circularity within which God has a predominant place. He writes,

> God answers man's [sic] questions, and under the impact of God's answers, man [sic] asks them. This formulates the questions implied in human existence, and theology formulates the answers implied in divine self-manifestation under the guidance of the questions implied in human existence.[2]

Thus, in a sense, there is a predominance of theology in the method of correlation. Adrian Thatcher provides a helpful insight in his introduction to *The Oxford Handbook of Theology, Sexuality, and Gender*. While this method of correlation has been heavily critiqued, he argues, "Tillich was right on several counts" and that "he was right to insist that for revelation to occur at all, it must first be received in human context." Thatcher affirms that "Tillich was right to demand 'answering theology.'" He also claims that the *Handbook*, published in 2015, attempted "to provide 'answers' to very modern and pressing questions arising from the experience and study of sexuality and gender, within and beyond the Christian faith."[3] This article seeks to follow in the lineage of such an inquiry, attempting to articulate a Christian response to issues of gender, sexual identity, and marriage in a Hindu context, with a view to contributing to a Pentecostal theology of human sexuality.

Pentecostal Perspective on Human Sexuality

It has been acknowledged more than once that there is a paucity of material about the Pentecostal perspective on human sexuality.[4] While Pentecostalism has been open to cultural changes, such as the use of media and its encouragement of a strong work ethic in a capitalist economy, William Kay and Stephen Hunt argue that:

> across its "various" streams Pentecostalism has largely remained counter-cultural in respect of preserving conventional moral positions, especially those related to sexuality and thus has taken a stand against adultery, sex before marriage, divorce (except on the grounds of adultery), and homosexuality.[5]

However, it is not Pentecostalism's conservative counter-cultural stance that draws our attention, but rather that historically these subjects related to human sexuality (for Kay and Hunt it was the subject of homosexuality, but it can also be extended to the other issues listed above) have "largely remained 'closed,' not needing discussion, and [have] usually only been dealt with as a matter of pastoral discipline."[6] This lack of engagement is once again reiterated by Michael Wilkinson and Peter Althouse, the editors of the eighth volume of the *Annual Review of the Sociology of Religion*, which was on the theme of "Pentecostals and the Body" (2017). They wrote in their initial call for papers in 2015 that "to date, there is no sustained examination of Pentecostalism and the themes associated with research on the body." Therefore, one of the main themes they have listed to be explored in their volume is "the politics of sexuality and gender roles—Pentecostalism as liberating and limiting for bodies, social control and gender roles, sexuality and notions of holiness/purity of body."[7] I believe the present discussion, as well as the aforementioned edited volume, seeks to remedy this lack of Pentecostal resources, albeit in a small manner. However, it must also be noted that within contemporary discourse, human sexuality has come to be taken as synonymous with discourses on homosexuality or LGBT rights. While these are legitimate contemporary concerns and issues that need addressing, the classical issues of identity and role of human beings on the basis of sexual differentiation equally need to be addressed from a Pentecostal perspective, which is precisely what this article attempts to do.

Narrative Identity

We argue that gender, sexuality, and marriage can be adequately treated under the thematic of narrative identity, following closely the model put forward by the French Protestant theologian/philosopher, Paul Ricoeur. Ricoeur argues that identity is always a response to "who," which is mostly in the form of "naming," although this "who" continually changes over the passage of time. Therefore, on what basis can we be justified in taking a single name of the subject throughout a life filled with changes from birth to death? Ricoeur's answer is because of its "narrative" structure. In other words, the answer to the question "who" is always "to tell the story of a life." Therefore the identity of this "who" must be a narrative identity.[8] Thus, identity, understood in narrative terms, can be called "by linguistic convention, the identity of the character"—in other words, a character in a narrative.[9] Ricoeur posits that this identity of a subject has two dimensions: identity as sameness (*idem*) and identity as selfhood (*ipse*) and it is the dialectic between *idem* and *ipse* that contains the identity of the subject.[10] Ricoeur argues that while *idem*-identity as sameness is what is permanent over time in the sense of a numerical identity, *ipse*-identity constitutes the changes over time. We argue that Ricoeur's narrative identity possesses a third aspect as well—the narrative role played by the character, which fulfills all the functions required by the constraints of the role. Thus, Ricoeur's narrative identity arguably implicitly possesses a three-part structure that responds to the following three questions respectively: a) *idem*, as what am I, or what about me does not change over time? b) *ipse*, as who am I even as I grow and change through time? and, c) character, as how am I supposed to live, or what role am I supposed to play in the larger narrative of life? The first question for us can be translated into the question of sex and sexuality—what am I? The second question refers to gender—who am I even as I change over time and am constructed by society? And the third question can point to marriage, the role played by the person in the larger family narrative. Ricoeur argues that "the identity of a person or a community is made up of these identifications with values, norms, ideals, models, and heroes, in which the person or the community recognizes itself."[11] Here it should be noted that the Shiksha Rath community belongs predominantly to various Hindu traditions and therefore their identity and roles are primarily informed by Hindu narratives. However, the work of Shiksha Rath introduces new narratives, new characters, values, and models, based on the Christian tradition, and this article also seeks to uncover how these new narratives have influenced the community.

With these preliminary points made, we now turn to the main section of the chapter, which raises questions about the sexuality, gender, and marriage of girl-children in India to which, following Tillich, we will posit an "answering" Pentecostal theology.

Sex, Gender, and Marriage of Shiksha Rath Women

Simon Brodbeck and Brian Black, in the introduction to their edited volume on *Gender and Narrative in the Mahabharata*, claim that "the *Mahabharata* is one of the definitive cultural narratives in the construction of masculine and feminine gender roles in ancient India, and its numerous tellings and retellings have helped shape Indian gender and social norms ever since."[12] They make a useful distinction between sex and gender that serves our purposes. They understand "sex" to be a biological identity, while employing "gender" to refer to a social identity. If "sex" makes someone male or female, then "gender," they argue, differentiates masculinity and femininity. Therefore, gender for them is culturally constructed even if sex is a biological universal.[13] Following this distinction, we want to begin with sex and sexuality. However, as said above, the discussion is not in the line of the common pursuit towards homosexuality and LGBT rights. The interesting question we want to pursue, albeit a classical question, is about the theological implications of the biological status of being female. In reverse, we want to begin by asking if there are implicit problems in being born female and possessing this sexual sameness throughout life. What are the implications and challenges of possessing a female biological identity in the Indian context?

On the other hand, gender seen as culturally constructed refers to the "who" question. Who is a feminine person in Indian society and how is her identity being shaped and constructed on the basis of her gender? While the term "gender," from the Old French *gendre*, now *genre*, derived from the Latin *genus*, originated as a grammatical term referring to "classes of noun designated as masculine, feminine, or neuter," since the fourteenth century it has also been used to refer to the "state of being male or female," which after the fall of Christendom has been dictated by medicine and the social sciences.[14] In other words, it is the discourse of medicine and social sciences that has shaped gender identity with its possibilities and constraints in the modern West. However, in the Indian context, it is the broader Hindu discourse that has shaped and constructed gender identity and set out who is a feminine person along with her identity. This goes back to the question of who am I, asked by feminine persons, which entails a deeper question—how do the Hindu traditions shape and construct the feminine gender and what are its implications for my life?

Finally, with regard to the role or function played by the feminine-character in the broader Indian social narrative, the primary role of women in the Indian social narrative is tied to her role in marriage. This connection is so strong that even when the girl is young, she is already seen through the lens of marriage and even betrothed at a very young age.

Of the thirty-one mothers from Shiksha Rath who were interviewed for this study, ninety percent of them (twenty-seven) who were married off below the legal age of eighteen say that being born female mattered a great deal to how life has turned out for them. Being a girl meant that they were to be married off and nothing else could be expected of them. Ramkali, who was married off at the age of thirteen, narrates about her marriage saying, "I was not ready for marriage, but after my mother had died while I was still very young, my older brother found a boy for me and asked me to get married." Sunita, who was married off at the age of fourteen, says, "I did not even understand what marriage was when I got married. My parents told me they would come and take me back after a month, but they never came back for me. I just listened to my parents and got married." None of the thirty-one reached university level in education. Over fifty percent of them (seventeen) did not receive any education at all, and another forty percent attended classes below fifth grade, with only three of the thirty-one women studying above sixth grade. Seventeen of them are working as maids, four as cooks, one gives beauty treatment from house to house, and three of them have small shops in the slum. Rekha exclaims, "I am working in eight houses now, and I am so tired of life." Most of them (twenty-six) said that they are not satisfied with the work they are presently doing. They believe that, if they had studied further, they could have gotten better-paying jobs and would have been treated with respect. Vimla best sums up the general feeling of the women: "I am not satisfied with the work that I am doing right now. I feel that had my parents allowed me to study further, today I could have done a better job and earned more."

Being born a girl-child, or having a feminine sexual identity, meant that they were to be married off at an early age, and so the families did not consider any value in educating them since they would be sent away to belong to another family. This also meant menial jobs for them along with much harassment. Their feminine sexuality disempowered them. What undergirds this treatment is not mere social pragmatism of getting the daughters married off, but a deep-rooted Hindu low view of the feminine sex.

Hindu View on Sexuality, Gender, and Marriage

Of course, affirming that there is no single Hindu view on anything is obvious, as there are multitudes of Hindu traditions, similar to any other world religion. This is more so the case in Hinduism, as each tradition with its gods, sacred texts, practices, and theology, also includes a theology of gender. However, given this diversity, is it possible to abstract from these traditions a Hindu theology of gender? Vasudha Narayanan, in her article on gender in *The Blackwell Companion to Hinduism*, affirms the diverse views within Hindu traditions. In her opening line, she contends, "gender is understood and acted out in different ways in the many Hindu *sampradayas* or traditions." She further argues, "The Hindu traditions have a wealth of materials which can inform us on how some human beings have understood gender in many ways over four millennia; narratives and arts which can contribute to the current academic discourses on gender."[15] In this work, she limits her discussion to a description of the gender of the devotee within the Tamil *Srivaisnava* tradition of the ninth century and bases her understanding of Hindu gender in light of the life and work of the poet Nammalvar. She particularly looks at his poems that are composed from the standpoint of a woman, which Nammalvar would recite in a woman's voice. Nammalvar becomes a young woman taking on the roles of different female characters of both the helpless devotee as well as that of a strong leader. From the classical Hindu texts characters such as Sita,

Radha or the gopis, and Lord Vishnu are portrayed by the young man. Narayanan asks, "In what ways does this role-playing inform us about gender?" To which she replies,

> some may argue that in the laments of the lovesick woman as well as in the ritual with Nammalvar, the portrayal projects a social, "patriarchal" relationship on to and replicates the male-female social power structure in the human-divine relationship. This indeed, is true in many instances, where the deity is seen as the supreme "Man" (*Purusottama*) and the woman's "lowliness" is exalted.[16]

But she quickly adds that this is only a partial view, as the voice of the helpless woman is only one of the voices the poet takes, and that he also takes the voice of dominant women such as a woman in love, a world-wise courtesan, as well as that of a mother. With this, Narayanan wants to prove that the voices of women are valued and privileged. However, what she fails to take into account is that it still took a male poet, Nammalva, to give voice to the feminine gender. Were the actual women of eighth- and ninth-century India not able to give voice to their own selves or did it necessarily require the masculine gender to give voice to them? Out of the twelve Alvar poets, Andal of the eighth century is the only woman poet. So, in spite of Narayanan's view of the positive portrayal of "women's voices," her perspective actually echoes the exclusion and helplessness faced by the Shiksha Rath mothers.

This is useful because then we can safely assume that the gender of the Shiksha Rath women is constructed in line with the social and cultural realities of their Hindu traditions. The above data on the women's experiences suggest that however idealistic textual Hinduism may be about feminine gender identity, Hindu women embodying these gender identities have been deprived of their dignity and have been disempowered.

The ideal woman is often portrayed in terms of the *pativrata*, the wife who is religiously devoted to her husband. One of the most well-known *Mahabharata* examples of the *pativrata* is Savitrı, who, by means of cunning, perseverance, and eloquence, outwits Death to save her husband. Another example is Gandharı, who makes loyalty to her husband her highest aim (*pativrataparayana*) by willfully blindfolding herself when she marries the blind Dhrtarastra, resolving that "she would not experience more than her husband could."[17] Another trope used for women is that of the courtesan. And in this role, although she does not play out the marriage ideal, it is still contingent on her sexuality and how she uses her sexual power over a man. "Srı, who in some ways resembles the courtesan (*ganika*) as depicted in the *Kamasutra*, chooses the man who pleases her most (this is the difference between victory and defeat), and features as a temporary and fickle consort, not as a childbearer."[18]

So we find that "the *pativrata* and *Sri* are two of the more prominent paradigms of femininity in the *Mahabharata*. Both paradigms present women as important complements to their husbands' success. Both are restrictive, only representing women in relation to their menfolk."[19]

Thus, we find that broadly within Hindu traditions the *idem*-identity of being female restricts the woman primarily to a complementary role as the *pativrata*, or wife, or its powerful counterpart as an aberration in the *Sri* as the courtesan. This restrictive view delimits all other possibilities. The woman is not viewed as a unique creation of God, who is an equal image-bearer, with creative possibilities.

Exploring a Pentecostal Theology of Human Sexuality

As mentioned above the contemporary discourse on sexuality, even within theology, has largely focused on responding to issues of homosexuality and LGBT rights. However, these are not the issues faced by the women of the Shiksha Rath community. With regard to the church's undivided focus on homosexuality, Elizabeth Stuart writes,

> while the church debates have become predictable...perhaps because the Holy Spirit has been moving elsewhere, theological reflection upon sexuality...produced a rich seam of theological discourse focused not only on homosexuality...but on human sexuality in all its diversity and complexity.[20]

So what is Shiksha Rath doing that can bring about a change in the lives of the girl-children so that they do not have to suffer the plight of their mothers? Thirty-two girls from the ages of five to fourteen were interviewed and surveyed for this article. Twenty-six of them said that they are happy to be girls and it was interesting to note that their social identity as being feminine was not seen negatively, yet many felt discriminated against for being a girl. One girl said she was unhappy because "she wants to be with her mother even after marriage but as a girl, she has to stay with her in-laws." Also, they can notice the gender differentiation. One of the girls complained, "Granny doesn't like girls, she says only my brother will continue the family line." All thirty-two of them want to work, and their dreams are diverse, either to be a doctor, teacher, dancer, artist, or engineer. Some said that if their parents do not support them, then they will fight for their career dreams and many of them want Shiksha Rath to be involved in negotiating with their families when it comes to these difficult decisions of marriage and career. One Shiksha Rath staff said, "We take groups of girls and spend time with them talking about different issues according to their age. For example, with the older ones, we talk about their careers, relationships, and dressings while with the younger girls we do activities and talk about different options for their career as well as about pursuing their hobbies."

So the question for us regarding these discussions on sexuality and gender is, what theology of gender is operative in Shiksha Rath that drives them to engage robustly with Hindu theology and the practice of gender differentiation faced by their girls?

First, the operative theology is one that affirms the creation of both the masculine and the feminine sex in the image of the triune God. While it does not pander to the call of equality of all genders, it deals with the precise uniqueness of the girl-child. Janet Soskice argues, "The as yet unsung glory of Gen. 1:26–27 is that the fullness of divine life and creativity is reflected by a human race which is male and female, which encompasses if not an ontological then a primal difference."[21] Beattie argues that "the account of the goodness of creation and of the human male and female made in the image of God requires a delicate balancing act between the affirmation of sexual difference as part of that original goodness."[22] The *idem*-identity of sexuality, of being a girl-child, explicitly differentiates the kind of life the Shiksha Rath children lead and the future they anticipate. This theology, sensitive to sexual differentiation, has enabled Shiksha Rath to encourage the girls to rethink what it means to be girls, different from boys, and yet wholly in the image of God, and thus full of feminine possibilities. As we saw above, two of the more prominent paradigms of femininity in the *Mahabharata* are *pativrata* and *Sri*, and yet both of these ideals are dependent on the menfolk, be it husband or male. This is precisely because the Hindu imagination does not have the notion of the woman being in the image of God, independent of the male folk. One way forward is to reimagine a Pentecostal Hindu theology of sexuality in which women can be directly connected to the divine, independent of the male.

Second, in Shiksha Rath, we take full advantage of the *ipse*-identity that opens up the girl-children to be reshaped by alternative empowering narratives. If the primary *ipse*-identity (the changing identity) of the girls is shaped broadly by the Hindu narratives and practices, then the teachers and leaders of Shiksha Rath wisely use their opportunity with the girls not only to address their problems but also to offer biblical material in the form of stories and narratives, including as expressed through art, drama, and theatre, as alternative visions of being of feminine gender. Stories of Ruth, Esther, and Hannah from the Old Testament, as well as the stories of Mary and Martha and Mary Magdalene from the New Testament, serve as powerful narratives of empowered women, which when shared with the girls enable them to be receptive to be reshaped by these narratives. Here the stress is not on imperatives and rules, as identities are seldom developed by such forceful constraints. Rather, it is a unique partnership with the Holy Spirit, in which while we share the narratives, we allow the Holy Spirit to do his work in enabling the girls to get embedded in these new narratives.

Here a question can be raised to Pentecostal theology. Would it be open to developing a theology of religion on different themes, including sexuality, which would take an interfaith approach? Such a theology would bring together narratives from both Christian as well as other religions' texts in order to seek an understanding of sexuality directed by the Holy Spirit. Would this provide a genuine platform for the development of a Pentecostal theology of religion on gender from the ground up? This is not a completely new idea within Pentecostal theology. In Amos Yong, we have a Pentecostal theologian who claims that emergent churches are already participating in these forms of interfaith engagement in that they "emphasize genuine dialogue, encourage visiting other sacred sites and even participating in their liturgies, and insist on learning about the lives and religious commitments of others."[23] On the basis of Eddie Gibbs' and Ryan Bolger's *Emerging Churches*, Yong argues that "these activities are informed by the conviction that there is much to be learned from other cultures, even to the point of being evangelized by those of other faiths in ways that transform Christian self-understandings."[24]

Finally, about the social role and character played by these girls in the larger social narrative, as shown above, the girls from childhood are steered to a single role and function, as a wife in a marital role. While this ideal does not go against the Pentecostal theological position of the primary role of a woman, we would like to broaden this understanding in light of the girl-child being in the image of God. If the Holy Spirit is actively involved in shaping and reshaping the unique roles of the girl-children so that they fulfill their unique destiny, then a "single standard fit" of "marriage" will not do for all. It is here that we at Shiksha Rath are sensitive to the Spirit's leading for each of these girls so that we can support them in the directions they are led regarding their futures, in which of course marriage is a central possibility. However, we want to be careful that we do not become the handmaiden of a Hindu theology that advocates women to be treated as Sunita and to suffer without consideration. Yet, this discovery is not made by the leaders of Shiksha Rath for the child. Rather it follows a Trinitarian model in which the girl, along with the Shiksha Rath leadership and the Holy Spirit, equally working together, are on a journey for the girls to find their dignity and roles in society. In our view, it is here in these moments of practical empowerment that the grounded Pentecostal theology of sexuality, gender, and marriage blossoms. While this is an initial attempt to abstract reflectively a theology from practice, much more must be done to work towards maturing such a theology.

Conclusion

This exploration of how the Spirit discloses the inherent image of God in female sexuality indeed reveals the godly destiny of the girl-child. The Spirit-given charismata operational in the service of the workers enables the growth and nurture of the godly destiny in the girl-child. We hope that the study of these themes has not only enabled us to begin an attempt at a Pentecostal theology of human sexuality, but also explicitly demonstrates the role of the Holy Spirit in restoring the dignity of the girl-child in Shiksha Rath.

To end this presentation, a recent story in a mainline Indian newspaper continues to reveal the plight of the girl-child in India. "A 12-year-old survivor of rape, who recently gave birth to a child making her possibly Bengal's youngest mother," has to transfer out of her school as she was being accused of bringing a "bad name" to the school. The reasons given for her expulsion are: a) she would discuss her "sexual exploitation" with her classmates, and they did not want such a "dirty girl" to study along with their children; b) they were questioning how a girl could even be raped in this manner; c) why was the family not more protective of the child? and, d) male faculty members feared that she might level false allegations of physical assault against them. However, her aunt said, "she was born on July 1, 2005, and isn't even 12 yet. She still plays with toys, and it's me who is taking care of her baby. Even now all she is concerned about is having chocolates and cold drinks."[25]

6.

Girls' Education and Sexuality in Burkina Faso: The Contribution from Pentecostal Churches and NGOs

Philippe Ouedraogo

Abstract

This chapter will locate the book's theme in the context of Sub-Saharan Africa with true stories told by women themselves about their own lives. Their stories took place in a study, through a rigorous narrative method carried out over six years in Burkina Faso. I will highlight the root causes of girls' low education and the implications of different actors such as individuals, churches, non-governmental organizations (NGOs) and governments. I will conclude by relating how many actors were led by the Holy Spirit to address this issue to save lives.

Introduction

Human sexuality is a global theme, with different interpretations and implications depending on one's continent. The universal reality based on the norms God revealed in the Bible, where it says, "What God created was good" tends to be misused. The biblical statement of truth regarding sexuality was diverted soon after creation through sin. The human departed from the purpose God created him for, and that led to the perversion of sexuality.

In our context of West Africa, gender discrimination is highly visible. One place it occurs is in education. The main obstacles that lead to girls' low enrollment in education are the socio-cultural factors that inhibit girls' access to education. Here is what I found.

Socio-cultural Factors that Inhibit Girls' Education

It has been argued by most scholars of Africa that gender issues affect the education of girls and women. The research from the Educational Research Network for West and Central Africa (ERNWACA) in 1998 suggested specific socio-cultural factors that cause gender imbalances in education in this region. Girls and women are highly valued for their reproductive capacities and for their domestic and farm labor. Families, cultural imperatives and socioeconomic constraints have a dramatic impact on girls' lives, often causing early school abandonment. Reasons put forward at the family level involve domestic poverty which makes them unable to pay for school fees, uniforms, and other expenses.

The family has to plan and select whom to send to school. It could be the eldest—a girl or a boy—and families who possess very few resources hope to receive a beneficial return for the whole family from this one child's education. The rates of early abandonment are higher among girls than boys because the culture favors boys' education rather than girls,' as the girl has a lot of household work to do before and after school which prevents her from studying in the best conditions. Some families prefer household work over schooling for their daughters: cooking, looking after younger children while the mother is working, and looking after the animals in the fields to increase family revenue. King and Hill agree that:

> In certain settings, religion, as well as socio-cultural factors (such as norms delineating the societal, economic, and familial roles of women), strongly influence parents' choices by imposing a heavy cost on nonconformist behavior. These may bear significantly on schooling decisions[1]

Their daughters' household labors and cultural norms represent an immediate return to the survivability of the family. Thus, sending girls to school and paying for their education is viewed as a waste of time and a loss of scarce family resources. While the girl is at school, the low-income family copes with the manual labor which she has left behind. Brock and Cammish state:

> Consequently, if a girl is to have education, there are often severe cultural costs to be met, notably, a price to pay for going against established social norms and, in particular, challenging the traditional authority of males. Such problems tend to be more severe in rural areas, but even in towns and cities where prospects of paid employment for educated girls may exist, many parents still fear the possibility of their daughters being alienated from a traditional lifestyle by contact with 'French colonial' education and its associated values[2]

However, low-income families who understand the value of equality among children in the research area do send their girls to school. This good attitude involves a great cost to these families because traditionally boys do not do as much household work as girls. Boys tend to imitate the father, who is not allowed by the culture to do much of the household work, such as cooking for the whole family. Yet in subsistence living, daily chores are labor intensive. Low-income families must overcome the dominant culture and its view of girls' role in daily survival if they are to send their daughters to school.

Early marriage is another social reason why girls abandon their education early. Within the traditional religious systems and among traditional Muslim Burkinabè parents, it is normal to pledge girls at an early age, sometimes from birth, to get married to a certain man whom the girl herself has neither chosen nor accepted. These arranged marriages then take place at ages as early as twelve to fourteen years old, limiting girls' primary and, more especially, secondary education, while boys are immune to such gender-bias in education. Meanwhile early, unwanted pregnancies and worries about sexual advances force teenage girls to get married. Here is a living story I collected from a focus group:

> I ran away from a forced marriage and sought refuge at the church for three years. This was before I got married to the man of my choice. Through the church literacy program, I can now read the Bible and Bible studies. After I ran away, the church pleaded my case with my family who accepted me back. Before that, I was disowned by my family because I refused to marry the man they had chosen for me. Traditionally this is an offense that needed restoring. (Focus Group, 22 February 2005)

I have chosen to examine these factors together because of the links that exist between culture and religion, tradition and history.

A human rights movement in Burkina Faso, the MBDHP, reported that the practice of early forced marriage is an on-going reality in the nation, despite legal protection for girls and much information provided by NGOs as well as awareness-raising campaigns[3] The evangelical and Catholic churches do not support the practice of early marriage because they advocate monogamy and mutual respect as the basis of mate selection for both girl and boy when they become adults. Furthermore, evangelical churches require couples to undergo the statutory marriage at the Town Hall before receiving a blessing in church. Marriage banns are posted in the church and at the town hall a month before the wedding ceremony to ensure that there are no impediments to the union.

The custom of early forced marriage is often rooted within traditional beliefs, such as an Islamic tradition where polygamy is a norm in family life, including the pledging of infant girls to be married at a very young age. In this context parents who are economically poor and have respect for these traditions pledge their daughters in marriage and then receive a dowry while the daughter grows up. To preserve the dignity of the family or their religious convictions, such girls are then forced to marry. This practice persists to the present day.

As late as 2007 Jean-Victor Ouédraogo reported on education in the Kain Department, located in the northwest region of the country in the province of Yatenga. Kain became a department in 1982, with 720 square kilometers and a population of about 11,000. The Kainan people are comprised 98 percent from the Dogon ethnic group and the remaining 2 percent from Fulani, Mossi, and Bela ethnic groups. In the official paper *Sidwaya,* Ouédraogo reported that education in general, but especially girls' education, had been relegated to a secondary position in that region. According to Bakiono Bamoa, the principal of Kain School, the Dogon have a sexist vision of girls: "Girls are enrolled in great numbers in the first year of primary school, to be taken out of the school a year before they complete the primary stage—that is, five years later—to be given away in marriage."[4]

In Dogon areas, girls are pledged in marriage from birth. School teachers watch this phenomenon with sadness. One primary teacher said, "Not long ago, a girl from my class was given in marriage to Mali when she went back for the Christmas period,"[5] indicating she did not return to complete even that school year. "The population does not appreciate the value of education. What is important for them is to go and work in gold mines and livestock farming. They do not invest in the long-term benefits of education."[6] The Prefect commented that another phenomenon they regularly face is the kidnapping of women. "For them, a 'courageous' young man is one who can take a girl and run away with her without anybody's notice, even if that is against the girl's and her family's wishes." This sort of behavior is part of the Dogon culture, said the Prefect (Ouédraogo). It should be noted that the evangelical church and Christian NGOs are not highly active among the Dogon in the education sector of the northern region.

I have included this finding to illustrate how cultural factors affecting education persist among communities, and also to point out that the church presence there remains weak. The Yatenga Province is predominantly traditional, with 90 percent of the population Islamic.

But moving on from the Dogon culture, there are other discriminations elsewhere.

In the Sahel region, the national radio reported that a teacher advocated for a girl to be able to carry on her education after she was given in marriage.[7] In Sénou Province girls of twelve, thirteen or fourteen years of age were being given in marriage, but the school system helps such girls, even if married, to carry on with their schooling. The teacher who was interviewed said that three years ago he met a brilliant girl in the last years of primary education and pleaded with her family and the in-laws to allow her to continue her education after marriage. Both families agreed that the young girl could carry on with her secondary schooling.

Keeping girls in school in such areas is still a big problem. Teachers are often presented with livestock as a bribe to allow the girl to leave school. Girls' early marriage is seen as a quick means of enhancing family income. When there is financial pressure, younger girls are the ones given away into early marriages because the in-laws will pay a large dowry for a young girl. Thus, early marriage of their daughters enhances the family's resources. There is also peer group pressure on the unmarried girls in any given cohort after one of them marries. Not getting married quickly then becomes a source of shame in the culture, as early marriage is tied to traditional customs in the Sahel region.

These findings confirmed the conclusions of Brock and Cammish about the socio-cultural impact of girls' education in the cases they studied:

> Early marriage is common in most of the cases studied, and this normally leads to early pregnancy. In some cases, there is a high incidence of early pregnancy outside the marriage. Either way, early pregnancy has a strong cultural dimension that would need to be contested through some form of education if the negative effects (including educational) are to be overcome. Early marriage inevitably shortens girls' schooling. Those who commence school late and repeat one or two classes may well reach the traditional age of marriage before they reach the end of the primary cycle[8]

In the Center region, a church leader echoed what the teacher said in Sénou province. This church leader believes that the obstacle is felt more in different parts of the country.

> Basically in the Central Plateau Region people understood that sending boys to school was a good investment. But in areas such as the northern region, north-east and west not all parents see the importance of sending their children to school. These obstacles may also be due to the geographical location of the school, as

there aren't enough schools around. Another problem is that many of these children leave school without being prepared to integrate into the productive labor force. We then need to think about secondary schools that will allow these girls and boys to increase their studies and be able to find jobs. The evangelical and Catholic churches have encouraged girls' education. For instance, local church leaders and missionaries have opened their homes to receive girls who had difficulties and needed help.[9]

There are many instances where a pastor or his wife reported welcoming girls who have asked for help into churches and their homes. When girls run away from their family who want to force them to get married, some run to the church for refuge. They decide to become Christians and ask the church to advocate on their behalf to the family and local authority for freedom of marriage and religion. A pastor's wife in the Center North of the country, during a face-to-face interview, reported:

> Those girls usually come to us from religions besides Christianity that will pledge them in marriage without their approval. First, when the girls come to us, we pray to God and ask for his protection over their lives. Even if we have to go to court, we go with them. My husband and I do not hide the girls when they come to us for help. We advise the girls to put their trust in God. We tell them to speak to their parents about their reasons for running away from home. The reason is that they need the freedom to choose the husband and the religion of their choice.

> Some girls run away because their parents want them to marry an older man without their consent. Those who do not want to be forced into an unwanted union run away from home and usually end up in the local pastor's family seeking freedom. The number of girls we assisted is between sixty and seventy. When they come, they have different needs. Some like freedom while others want to become Christians. Others who come for the sake of freedom end up becoming dedicated Christians before they find a husband.[10]

These moving testimonies emerged from listening to an open-ended conversation with a pastor's wife inside a local church. She related how culture affects the vulnerability of some girls of that region.

> The girl who recently got married stayed with us for four and a half years. They usually stay for two to three years. If they find a husband sooner, they stay with us for more than one year. With prayers and God's help, we can be of some help to them. When girls come to us and stay, we have to provide accommodation and food for them. Neither their parents nor public services provide them with material help. All the basic needs are met by the church and the pastor's family. Our support comes from the blessings in serving God. The first girl who came to us ran away from her newly married home where her parents had forced her to go. She disliked the way she was given into marriage and came from her village to stay with us. We were told that she is not interested in converting to Christianity. She used to sell goods in the

market, and through lots of advice, her character changed completely for the better. She was able to get married later and with her husband, went to a Bible school and today is serving God. But her background was difficult and different to what she is today in society. She had a good testimony by the grace of God.[11]

The above narration indicates the socio-cultural factors that limit girls' and women's education. I will now consider initiatives taken by individuals, families, churches, NGOs, and the government to address these obstacles to overcome them.

Actors for Girls' Education in Burkina Faso

Churches and NGOs have played a major part in contributing to the education of women and girls in Sub-Saharan Africa.[12] It could be accurately said that religious groups such as the Roman Catholic Church and evangelical churches started education programs well before the government. If the current debate about human sexuality sees elements of the Christian church as part of the problem, it is also true to say that the Pentecostal churches, NGOs and families made a significant contribution to women and girl's education in Burkina Faso. It was the Church who first set up facilities, and it was church members who began to open their homes to welcome women and girls in need. The public and the individual beneficiaries appreciated such safe and welcoming nets.

From the testimony of a church leader who was an eye-witness, the Assembly of God (AOG) involvement in education was led by God. God wanted the church to have good foundations even before the AOG talked about formal education in 1948.[13] It needs to be mentioned here that most missionaries at that time were American English-speakers, while the official language of the Upper Volta was French.

At that time Pastor Dupret from France had a conviction about starting schools.[14] He described how he received the vision from God for the schools, though not all his board members agreed with him in this project, especially concerning the inauguration of a secondary level of education. He even showed the eye-witnesses the place where he said that God had spoken to him, telling him to open the schools on that site. Pastor Dupret was convinced of this idea. Sixty years later that church influences 50% of the private evangelical schools. The 2006 results paper shows that 33 AOG schools represented 77.91% of the national primary schools.[15] The national records in 2006 had 99 private Protestant schools, of which 50% are related to the church, individuals or

NGOs who opened schools with the Christian ethos. This indicates the important role the church is playing in formal primary education. The remaining 50% of schools come from other denominations and church leaders, families and associations.

The AOG church has also opened several secondary schools. Two are specifically for girls; others are mixed for general and technical studies. NGOs such as l'Association Nationale pour la Traduction de la Bible et l'Alphabétisation (ANTBA) developed non-formal education nationwide, while l'Association Evangélique d'Appui au Développement (AEAD) integrated both non-formal and formal education with a potential for rapid growth from nursery to secondary levels following the introduction of innovation at the national level. As already mentioned, because of their specific relevance to the case studies these contributions helped to reveal the larger picture of the contribution of the evangelical churches and organizations in offering women access to education.

Ibrango,[16] a school principal in the northern region of the country, sees education as the basic tool for instructing while at the same time sharing the gospel. In his opinion, education is the most powerful tool that has proved itself for socio-economic and spiritual development. A closer look at the public sector reveals people that went through the evangelical schools, especially those founded by the AOG. All the office workers who came out of evangelical schools are instruments of light for the gospel across the nation. You will find Christians heading government departments who are in a position to be a witness for the gospel.

Further, there were no gender distinctions in Dupret's program. He was a man with the vision. Many of these girls are married to today's church leaders. The instructions they received helped them to establish harmonious families.[17]

The church leader Pastor Gouba found his wife in the church school and got married fifty years ago. He noticed that girls' education was very necessary for both a physical and a spiritual sense. Educated women can help other girls learn a skill and can also be of great help to their husbands.[18] Non-formal education predated formal education. Chronologically, girls' and women's education existed before the creation of formal schools in the late 1940s.

Former evangelists witnessed to the second generation Christians in Burkina Faso so that the very first reading and writing classes were taught in brief training sessions. Women were trained on the job at the mill, by the well, and in special classes. New believers were sent to the main towns of the Mossi Empire to share the Gospel of Christ. The churches emphasized the family from the beginning, so women were trained alongside their husbands by the wives of missionaries to learn how to read and write and assist their husbands. At the same time, they were trained with the purpose of reaching other women and girls with the gospel. This non-formal training which led to the creation of the first Bible school in Koubri came well before the formal education of 1948. Since then seven other Bible Schools have been opened across the country: Bethel Salbisgo, Ecole Pastorale et Agricole at Banakélédaga, Bon Berger Djibo, Tégawendé Kaya, and Betsaleel at Tenkodogo, Institut Biblique Supérieur (IBS), which then became the Faculty of Theology of the Assemblies of God of Burkina Faso and Oholiab for lay leadership training. These schools are opened to train men, women, and children for Christian ministries.

Pastor Sibiri Simporé, a church executive member, reported the following:

> American missionaries started with the education of girls and women in general. The first missionary ladies were learning the local language by spending time with their African mates. Pastor Harold Jones and his wife started that ministry within the church he was attending. The missionary lady taught things of which there was no prior knowledge in the village. Girls' homes in Tenkodogo were established, to which girls came from the East to be trained. Other centers were built in Ouagadougou and around. The church then opened the girls' education center in Loumbila. Girls' education started in the few existing churches even before the church-run schools began to operate. Girls' education was among the priorities of the church. The church always wanted the new believers in the faith to be literate. It has always been seen as helpful in fulfilling their vision of reaching the country with the gospel.[19]

We have the testimony of our church leader of the SIM/EPE church in the East of the country. Since the beginning, the village cursed new Christian believers, and no member of the village was willing to offer their daughter to marry a Christian young man. The first missionary set up a Bible school for girls, to give them the freedom from family-forced marriage. During the 1960s there were not enough Christian girls, and that Bible school offered a double benefit. One was to free them from forced marriage and teach them biblical values and practical skills; but also to provide them a haven, as the girls who became Christian were considered cursed, by their families. The mission opened the first Bible school for girls, and the church added others to help advocate freedom for the girls.[20]

Pastor Hamidou added:

> In our culture among the Gourmatché ethnic group, the young girls are pledged to marriage before their birth. The so-called expected family-in-law starts bringing gifts to the one who pledged, and when a girl is born, she is automatically pledged as expected. The family to whom a girl is pledged will start bringing support up until the girl is fifteen years of age. This situation contributes to a social problem that the churches choose to address. The church also fights against the practice of excision. Parents put their girls in concentration camps to force them to practice excision, and the church then becomes a place of refuge.[21]

The SIM/EPE churches have set up five units to care for the girls in the Eastern region. For these girls, Bible schools provide literacy training and skill learning. Two Bible schools are located in Piella, one in Fada Ngourma, and the remaining two are in the Tapoa province in Diapaga. We often invited resource people such as the head of the police to come and speak about women's rights because in those regions women are offered like objects. Therefore, the government works in collaboration with the church to help women avoid forced marriages. In Madaga the church is making an effort to assist girls who left school, or have not been at all, to a have an opportunity to learn how to read and write in their native language.

In the formal sector the church has five primary schools and the girls there are favored to carry on with their work with the helping goodwill of some, and there is little financial support. We do our best with very little, and God blesses the work.

All the girls who went through these centers become true mothers knowing how to read and write in their language. They can help the family economy with their skills in agriculture, sewing, weaving, livestock, soap-making and painting. Others become literacy teachers, becoming great support both to their family and society in general. The church contributes to eradicating barriers to girls' education and is working in partnership with the Association of Educator Mothers (AEM). The girls come voluntarily to these programs. They make a small contribution, but it is mainly the church and its friends and partners who run these girls' centers.

For Pastor Hamidou the vision is, "to allow [girls] to be better equipped after their training. Because of the shortage of resources the church is not able to equip them with tools after their training. We are often frustrated to see them leave. With skills in sewing, soap making, and others, we wish to help them establish their businesses and hope to teach in other languages such as French."[22]

Kientega[23] and Gouba[24] argued that mixed schools provide a better balance in gender issues while girls' schools expose girls to greater sexual temptation. This idea is supported by a former girl working in primary education with the government,[25] though some have argued that a single phase of girls-only education prepared them to concentrate on their studies. From the evidence gleaned from visiting and researching in both types of schools, the case is still debatable.

In addition to individuals, families, and church actors, I requested an appointment with the Ministry of Women Promotion to hear the official stand in terms of gender, sexuality and girls' education. The Minister, Céline Yoda, requested her Secretary-General, Mrs. Clémence Ilboudo, to meet me. Mrs. Ilboudo's comments on behalf of the Minister may be summarized, "The Ministry cares for all women and girls and children and collaborates with other ministerial departments." In addition to the policies of the Ministry of Education, Mrs. Ilboudo agreed that families and communities are the basis of the state. Asked about the obstacles to girls' education, she was concerned about the wide gap that exists between boys' and girls' enrollment in schools. "A girl, in general, is a child and parents have to decide for her. It is also a challenge if one goes to school to be employed in the public sector." She argued that being educated is first of all in one's best interest, helping to increase one's capacity. But she noted that it is more difficult for girls and women to do so because cultural factors hinder their freedom. In the traditional setting one believes that girls and women do not need academic knowledge apart from cooking and being a good wife. Girls' families expect them to become housewives rather than an agent in development.[26]

Within Burkinabè society the roles of men and women differ. The social system wishes the boys to keep their name and inheritance and stay in the community. The girl is a migrant. She will spend a little time in her family and later join another clan. Her family does not think that if she becomes educated, she can benefit her family. Apart from spontaneous gifts to her family, her most important contributions will go to her husband. When a family is facing a choice, especially in the case of a polygamous unit, the balance moves quickly in favor of the small boy rather than the girl. The United Nations Educational, Scientific and Cultural Organization's (UNESCO) Education for All (EFA) Report in 2009 noted:

> Poverty and other forms of social disadvantage magnify gender disparities. For example, in Mali girls from poor households are four times less likely to attend primary school than those from rich households, rising to eight times at the secondary level.

Referring to Universal Primary Education, the 2009 EFA Report put it differently:

> Children from poor areas, slums, and other disadvantaged groups face major obstacles in access to good quality education. While children from the wealthier 20% of households have already achieved universal primary school attendance in most countries, those from the poorest 20 % have a long way to go.

Household economic poverty is one challenge, among others, that affects a girl's success in school. Failures at school, bad physical health, not being able to access the right information, and the risks faced on the way to school are factors named by the Ministry of Women's Promotion as hindrances to girls' education.[27]

Girls, furthermore, are not prepared to cope with sexual harassment. Once a girl becomes a victim [of rape] she will bear the visible mark [of pregnancy] and bring dishonor to her family. Such situations lead to social conflict among different families in society: because she is the daughter, she can disgrace the family through early pregnancy, while boys can pretend to get away with it. Keeping the girl in the family and not sending her to school can help avoid bringing shame to the family. Assie argued that "...the wish to protect daughters from undesirable influences appears strongest in areas that are still very traditional."[28] Girls are at risk of sexual harassment and abuse by male teachers who do not have good moral standards. The teacher may commit adultery with the girls and still get away with it. To protect their daughters and their family from this shame, parents in traditional cultures may keep their daughters home rather than send them to school

The UNESCO (2009:5) EFA Report noted:

> Once girls are in school, their progress is often hampered by teachers' attitudes and gender biased textbooks that reinforce negative gender stereotypes. These school-based factors interact with social and economic factors that influence school performance along gender lines.

The same applies to women in the sense that they are not free to enroll themselves in adult education without their husband's permission. When he does not permit her to enroll, the wife has no choice. Besides, she has a lot of household work that limits her concentration on learning. Bearing children can also constitute an obstacle to women's education. Very often, to study properly, she needs to bring a babysitter into an adult literacy class, for example. In the beginning, like the girls, women are highly motivated; but completing the program becomes very difficult, especially when there is no additional food to feed the children who accompany their mothers to the adult training programs. The Ministry supports the view that to overcome these obstacles, a woman needs to enroll, attend for the whole program, and also succeed in acquiring the desired skill. If all three steps are not fulfilled, the process remains incomplete.

The Secretary-General of The Ministry of Women's Promotion also raised the problem of Female Genital Cutting (FGC). There is hardly any scriptural evidence in Islam and none in the Christian faith to support this practice. The Imams and traditional chiefs cannot back up this practice from the basis of their religions. But what arguments will a woman put forward when her husband sends their daughter to be excised? Without knowledge and education, she has little argument to counter the order from her husband. If she were able to read the Family Code regulating these issues, or the Holy Scriptures, she could argue from what these books say. But without knowing what the books say, nor how to read them for herself, she is left without arguments and is obliged to acquiesce, though such practices are illegal in the country.[29] It should be noted that the practice of excision is not tolerated among Christian families, who accepted the national decision to combat such practices even before they became law.

For Mrs. Ilboudo, the churches are the best places to promote and invest in gender and women's education. Christian congregations have increased the number of girls' schools, colleges, and training centers in the nation, making even the government aware of their impact. There is also the spiritual dimension, and these schools have the reputation of producing high-quality results. In church services and programs, men and women come under one roof and sit together during meetings many times a week. This setting provides socialization for women. In other religions, no such opportunities exist for women and men to mix regularly during the week in worship places. The church does hold different models of gender behavior which points to its disparities in interpreting the Scriptures. This naturally influences women's conduct. Few women today are without faith, but accepting the faith of the husband without critically reflecting why she does so could also lead to spiritual illiteracy.

The Role of the Holy Spirit in Girls' Education

After identifying several factors that inhibit girls' education and actors that made a significant contribution to resolve them, we will now consider impact stories of lives that have been transformed by the power of the Holy Spirit through Christian education.

Jokébed Damoaliga works in the government health department as a teacher in the national teacher training school for nurses. She revealed that being the person she is today is the result of her going to the Young Girls' College at Loumbila from 1972–76 and spending two years at the Protestant College from 1977–79. She asserted that she had received a great deal from these schools. I wanted her to clarify her view, but she insisted simply that the spiritual environment itself influenced her life greatly. She said, "I went there as a teenager, years that witnessed many changes in my life in physical, psychological, moral, and spiritual senses. In these different schools, I had a favorable climate that allows keeping a spiritual fellowship with the Lord."[30]

Priscille Zongo, now working in diplomatic service, went to the same church-run-school as Jokebed, as well as to other private and public and private schools, and she agrees with Jokebed that the Biblical aspect of her education greatly impacted her life.

> The spiritual impact of education greatly influenced my life. It is true that my father was a pastor and he taught us the Bible. But it was only in Loumbila that I had my personal experience as a believer in Christ. Teachers encouraged us to pray and I experienced the baptism in the Holy Spirit. I could say that I was spiritually built in Loumbila. Who I am today spiritually is the result of the impact I had in my life in Loumbila. It was there I learned how to live a life of prayer.[31]

These personal testimonies and stories are selected from among others recorded in my book, *Female Education and Mission*,[32] illustrating the nature of girls' education and sexuality in the context of West Africa. There have been large influences in Burkina Faso by Pentecostal churches and NGOs, such as the evangelical relief organization AEAD, which have proven track records in addressing many obstacles.

I hope to have prepared the ground for further research by presenting a reflection on the education of girls and women provided by the evangelical churches of Burkina Faso and other NGOs. I trust that others will build upon this study and use the framework of qualitative research into education, or some of the information given in this overview, in other disciplines for the benefit of girls and women, not only in Burkina Faso but also in other parts of the developing world.

7.

Sexual Exploitation of Children in the Philippines and the Role of Pentecostal Churches

Lulu Suico and Joseph Suico

Abstract

This chapter examines the case of sexual exploitation in the Philippines and analyzes Pentecostalism through its basic theological views and its attitudes towards social issues.[1] The Global Slavery Index reports there are nearly 36 million victims of human trafficking worldwide. Most of that 36 million are from Asia. One of the major problems in Philippine society today has been the growing number of child prostitutes and sexually abused children. Yet, the government does not seem to be keen on finding a proper solution to this crisis. At present, the focus is on the war on drugs while the problem of sexual exploitation of children has not been adequately addressed.

A basic assumption of this chapter is the definite role of the Church in addressing the problem under consideration. As God's agent of change, the Church has the responsibility to defend the cause of the exploited children. The Church being "salt and light" should make its presence felt more strongly. Its influence should affect society until injustices are rectified and oppression is dealt with.

This study also probes why Pentecostals are perceived to be indifferent towards the issue of sexual exploitation of children. Does the basic doctrine of Pentecostals direct them to socio-economic and political action or inaction? The Pentecostal church in the Philippines will need to seriously reflect and evaluate its role in order to effectively alleviate the situation.

Introduction

The sexual exploitation of children has become a tragic and global phenomenon. In 1996 at the Conference of World Congress against Sexual Exploitation of Children held in Sweden, UNICEF reported that "an estimated one million children (mainly girls but also a significant number of boys) enter the multi-billion-dollar commercial sex trade every year."[2] Twenty years later, global statistics on the sexual abuse of children have both exploded, heightened by increased travel and internet use, and blurred, by the same means. However, what we know is that by 2016 the International Labor Organization (ILO) counted nearly 36 million victims of human trafficking worldwide. Of that 36 million, a high percentage are children, and nearly two-thirds are from Asia.[3]

Several factors contribute to the rapid growth of children becoming sexually exploited. Studies show that poor economic condition is one of the leading causes of children being forced into prostitution in the two-thirds world.[4] Without intervention from both government and non-government organizations, millions of adults and children will continue to be forced into bonded labor, sex trafficking, slave-like conditions, and child soldiering in Asia.[5]

This chapter examines the case of sexual exploitation in the Philippines and will analyze Pentecostalism through its basic theological views and its attitudes towards social issues.

Overview of Sexual Exploitation in the Philippines

The Philippines, a country in Southeast Asia, is composed of 7,107 islands and has a population of nearly 107 million, of which a high percentage suffer from debilitating poverty. Although the World Bank puts the figure of those who live below poverty at about 20%, the Secretary of the National Economic and Development Authority (NEDA) named Php42,000 as "a decent income at least to live above the poverty line," and 88% of Filipinos live below that level.[6] There is a high percentage of unemployment and underemployment.

The capital city and its suburbs, Metro Manila, are overpopulated, with approximately 34.6 million people. There is a growing number of very poor people living in garbage dump areas. The World Bank Report indicated that in the mid-1990s, there was a "significant increase in income inequality with the Gini coefficient[7] increasing from 0.45 to 0.5 in three years" and the rural economy weakened more.[8] Inevitably, the high incidence of poverty in rural areas led to urban migration.

Almost half (44.98%) of the country's total population are children below eighteen years of age.[9] The nation's poor economic condition has left many of these children in a difficult situation. The city of Manila is home for 50,000–75,000 street children,[10] but it is not known how many of these street children are sexually exploited. There were concerns even in 1996 that the number had tripled in the previous five years, up to 60,000 from 20,000 in 1991.[11] UNICEF reports estimate 60,000–100,000 sexually abused and exploited children all over the country. The End Child Prostitution in Asian Tourism (ECPAT) and the Department of Social Welfare and Development (DSWD) give the lower figure, about 60,000.[12] The lack of available data to substantiate accurate figures is part of the difficulty of working in this field. For example, current figures for sex trafficking worldwide range from 21 million to 45 million.[13] This is a very wide margin of error; yet, both numbers are intolerable.

The nature of sexual abuse and exploitation in the Philippines takes the form of prostitution, pornography, pedophilia, trafficking, bonded sex labor (or white slavery), incest, rape, and cybersex trafficking. Well-documented reports show that children were sexually exploited and coerced to engage in prostitution in the cities of Angeles and Olongapo where the former United States military bases were located.[14] Writers and civic organizations have argued that the presence of US military personnel led to the establishment of sex trades in these two cities.

In Olongapo City, it was the People's Recovery, Empowerment and Development Assistance (PREDA) Foundation who exposed the sexual exploitation of children by both the local authorities and US military personnel. PREDA's report revealed that the majority of prostitutes and dancers working in clubs were children.[15] In 1983, a particular case of sexual abuse committed by a US Navy chief officer on a local nine-year-old girl was disclosed by Father Shay Cullen who is the founder of PREDA. Since then, several cases of sexual abuse committed against children, ages 4–16, were documented and brought to the attention of local authorities and even in some international forums.[16]

Another place noted for sex trade tourism is Pagsanjan, a town in the province of Laguna, 62 miles south of Manila. The province is famous for its hot springs and its main tourist attraction, the Pagsanjan Water Falls. The place was visited by foreign pedophiles as early as the 1950s, but foreign pedophilia took a huge toll in the seventies and eighties.[17] Kevin Ireland described Pagsanjan as the "pedophile capital of the world"[18] and gave the following account:

> At the height of the tourist boom in the late 1970s and early 1980s, Pagsanjan was estimated to have 3,000 young boys ("pom poms") involved in providing sex to visiting tourists. At that time, some 500 to 600 foreign visitors would be present on ordinary days and up to 2,000 on weekdays and holidays. It was estimated that half of these tourists were pedophiles; two-thirds of them were Australian and the rest Americans and Europeans, with some Japanese and Chinese from Hong Kong and Taiwan. The demand for young, male sex partners was so strong that it attracted boys from neighboring towns and provinces.[19]

Although it is not clear where Ireland got the idea that Pagsanjan was the pedophile capital of the world, his account of Pagsanjan's case was corroborated by documented reports from the local government and by journalists, as well as NGOs such the Council to Protect the Children of Pagsanjan (CPCP). The alarming increase in the number of young boys who joined the pedophilic activity moved the concerned citizens of that town into action.[20] As a result, the CPCP was formed in 1981. However, CPCP faced much opposition from the parents of the children, pimps and those who were in the sex trade business.[21] This resistance eventually slowed the campaign of CPCP. Most of the parents opposed CPCP because they did not want to lose the benefits which foreign pedophiles heaped upon them. CPCP's Ronnie Velasco pointed out that these pedophiles "treated the families very well, giving them gifts such as television sets, cars, money, even buying houses for them, in exchange for sexual favors from the children." This practice has aptly been called double exploitation because the children are exploited sexually by the pedophiles and monetarily by their families. Velasco further states that parents were not aware of the extent of the sexual involvement of their children until a police raid in 1988 which discovered appalling evidence from the foreign pedophiles' safe house:

> The occupant of the apartment was an expatriate. Since coming to Pagsanjan in 1981, he kept meticulous records of local children. Some children had up to ten 3 x 5 index cards, each one neatly typed backgrounds on each child, with ages, address, body shape, and what type of sex was obtained from the child. On the back of each card was the amount of money paid to each child, and other information concerning genital size, circumcised or not.[22]

Beginning in the early 1990s, there was again a considerable rise of foreign pedophiles and sex tourists visiting the country. To date, the city of Manila, which has the largest number of street children, remains a haven for foreign pedophiles. The exploitation of young boys and girls continues to take its toll. The Department of Social Welfare and Development (DSWD) reported the number of child prostitutes in the Philippines was 20,000 in 1987.[23] The number is now between 60,000 and 100,000 *new* child prostitutes each year.[24] DSWD shows the profile of sexually exploited and abused children in Manila and Pagsanjan:

- 74% of the total population are male victims
- 36% of the children victims come from a family with four to six members; 28% come from a family with seven to nine members.
- 34% are between the ages of 13 to 15; 28% are from 10-12 years; 5% are

between 0–3 years old.
- 36% have parents who are separated.
- 76% of the cases are not filed in court.[25]

This profile shows there are more male than female victims in these two areas. It also reflects that victims are mostly teenage boys from either dysfunctional homes or poor families. The lack of advocacy for the victims could explain why most of the cases are not filed in court.

Being one of the 'sex tour destination' countries in Asia,[26] the Philippines was regarded as the fourth country with the most number of prostituted children. Whether or not this comment is verifiable, it has generated a negative image of the country and has spurred several non-governmental organizations (NGOs), government organizations (GOs) and civil society organizations (CSOs) to coordinate among themselves in facing the issue of child prostitution. The general feeling among these groups and concerned citizens was to rally the Filipinos to strategize and deal with the root cause of the problem. The root cause has to do mainly with the economics of survival.

The country's long socio-economic crisis has had an excruciating effect on the basic unit of society – the family. The sad state of Filipino children and their families is overwhelming. Many children throughout the country are engaged in exploitative labor and more continue to join. The Child Protection in the Philippines (CPP) reports that:

> The statistics are growing each day. These clearly depict the immense hardship to which Filipino children are subjected. Unfortunately, the family that is supposedly the primary source of the children's sense of trust and security is itself beleaguered. In most instances, it can no longer adequately provide even the children's most basic needs like food, education, housing, and an atmosphere of love, affection, and nurturance. Its capacity to protect the children and enhance their development and participation rights is likewise affected.[27]

The fact is that the majority of Filipino families are living in abject poverty and are not capable of giving proper nurture and protection for their children anymore. The lack of material resources incapacitates them for providing a future for their children. Also tragically unfortunate is that even the national government cannot provide a safety net for the Filipino family. To service the country's huge foreign debt, the government has had to cut the budget for basic services.[28] The present situation of the country is that its political and socio-economic crises create an exploitative environment for the most vulnerable member of the society—the children.

Factors that Led to the Increase of Sexually Exploited Children

Most researchers agree that the combination of socio-economic, political, religious, and cultural factors have triggered the increase of sexual exploitation of children.[29] As described above, research shows that despite several institutions and organizations working to address the problem, the number of exploited children is still increasing. We will now analyze the current theories and diagnose why, in spite of many efforts, the problem still exists.

Socio-economic and Political Factors

The economic crisis of the country that brought high levels of poverty and unemployment affects every Filipino family. There is a widening gap between the poor majority and the rich few.[30] The landed and rich few control and manipulate the country's businesses and industries. Thus, less opportunity is given to the poor. In rural areas, landless farmers continue to suffer from underdevelopment. As the country's economy continues to deteriorate, slums, shantytowns, and numbers of street children keep growing. There is a close link between unemployment, urban migration, poverty, less access to education and population growth.[31] All these factors put a child in a vulnerable situation. The migration of family from rural to urban to seek for a better life removes the support system and security given by the extended family.[32] Unfortunately, the children are the first to be affected. Urban migration is the prime cause of the mushrooming of slums in Metro Manila areas. In this scenario the rapid growth of street children is inevitable. The majority of these children work as scavengers, hawkers and prostitutes. The ILO's report on Child Labor Issues explained:

Poverty is the greatest single force which creates the flow of children into the workplace. Acute need makes it nearly impossible for households to invest in their children's education, as the price of education can be very high and most 'free' public education is, in fact, expensive for a poor family. Poor households also tend to have more children....[33] The high cost of education and the need to work to survive take many children away from school. Impoverished children who lack education and skill may find prostitution an easy way to earn more money than selling newspapers and cigarettes on the street. While it is already hard for adults to find a job, it is more difficult for young children. For a hungry child, a day's meal is more important than preserving his or her body against sexual abuse. Parents too, allow and sometimes coerce their children to engage in this kind of work in exchange for material benefits.[34] In most cases, older children, especially from poor and large families, are the ones who are engaged in this kind of trade. Chris and Phileena Heuertz write, "The desperate poor may even go so far as selling their children into this brutal and abusive profession just to find money to make it through one more day."[35] According to Robert Linthicum, most of the child prostitutes in Manila are "purchased from their parents to be sex slaves."[36]

There are also cases when children are sold for reasons other than impoverishment. Some fathers sell their children because of material greed or to sustain their own vices. An example of this is the case of a young girl sold by her father to former congressman Romeo Jalosjos, who was arrested in 1998 and eventually jailed and sentenced to two life terms for sexually abusing her.[37] This particular circumstance and the release and presidential pardon of Jalosjos 13 years later[38] shows that what is best for children is not given priority and has become a sacrificed value.

Poverty is implicated in incest against children, too. Caroline Moser found in poor Filipino neighborhoods, "Adverse economic conditions put additional pressure on human relationships, increase conflict, and even violence between household members sometimes results."[39] Likewise, Josefina Gutierrez of the Philippine Children's Ministries Network (PCMN) states, "There are indications that socio-economic status has a relation to incest: unemployment of fathers, the physical structure of the home where privacy is difficult to attain, the absence of mothers."[40] The DSWD Statistics show a high figure of cases of incest in the Philippines. Violence in homes also pushes children to run away and live on the streets, where they are at high risk of exploitation. Based on the studies done by Moser and Gutierrez, socio-economic crisis and/or poverty produce dysfunctional homes that become an unsafe place for children and may even push them to prostitution. A case in point is a victim of incest who now works as a prostitute in Manila. She does not like the job but says, "It is better to get paid for it than to have to go on doing it with my stepfather for free."[41]

International migration is another factor that contributes to family disintegration. Every year, hundreds of thousands of contract workers leave the country to seek employment abroad; in 2016 the number was estimated at 2.2 million.[42] Most of these contract workers leave their family behind for a long period. The children are usually left to the care of the spouse or, if both parents work, to the nearest relatives. This kind of arrangement leaves the children vulnerable to unsafe conditions. Unfortunately, it is the absentee parent who puts their own children at risk. This could be one reason for the increasing incidence of incest. There is a great number of women and/or mothers who work as domestic helpers and nurses in other countries.

While it is true that poverty is a big factor in pushing children to prostitution, it is necessary to recognize there are additional reasons for the rapid growth of sexual exploitation of children. Muntarbhorn has argued, "It is not poverty *per se* that drives children into exploitative situations; it is poverty plus other factors that are at work."[43] Sex tourism, criminality, government corruption and even a racially discriminatory attitude on the part of the tourists are some of the reasons. Similar to Muntarbhorn's argument, Ireland attributed the increase of sexual exploitation of children in the Philippines to the "burgeoning demand for prostitution and for children for sex and that this was stimulated and developed into an industry as a result of the military bases and tourism promotion."[44] He further stated that,

> Without these two factors, prostitution and the sexual exploitation of children in the Philippines would undoubtedly have still occurred. It is extremely doubtful, however, that it would have developed to be so organized, so profitable or so pervasive.[45]

In addition, there is evidence that commercialization is "a more important catalyst than poverty."[46] Some countries capitalize on child prostitution to attract more tourists. It can also be said that money and power play prominent roles behind the growth of sex tourism in the two-thirds world. According to Ron O'Grady,

> It is the economic imbalance between the relatively wealthy tourist and the shocking poverty of the poor people in the farms and slums which makes prostitution flourish in the third world countries.[47]

As poor countries draw on sex tourism to earn more dollars, the wealthy pedophiles take advantage of the situation to satisfy their perverted lust and sexual fantasies,[48] which they could not do with freedom in their own country.[49] In addition, sex tourism provides an opportunity for brothel owners, pimps, prostitution gangs, and syndicates to make big business. Power and the discriminatory attitude of individuals contribute to the commercial sexual exploitation of children. Judith Ennew, who conducted a study on this issue, remarked, "Sexual exploitation is part of the wider spectrum of domination, in which rich exploit the poor, males females, whites other ethnic groups, and adults children."[50] Rich tourists, materialistic pimps and syndicates, and corrupt government authorities use their power to exploit these children. Likewise, the parents, friends, and relatives exert their power over these children to comply with adults' dark wishes. It is worth noting the attitude of some pimps who look down upon the uneducated and docile rural folks. They deceive and persuade these parents to allow their children to work in the cities as waitresses or domestic helpers, only to be locked up in brothels. Ennew also noted that the increase in the trafficking of young girls to marry men from developed countries could be attributed to the notion that Filipino women are "compliant, faithful and passive."[51] Clients who were interviewed by other researchers in the Philippines support this notion.[52] This racist attitude towards Asian women is discussed by O'Connell Davidson in her research:

> White Western sex tourists consider that their whiteness, in and of itself, is enough to make them irresistibly sexually desirable to 'Third World' women and girls. They comment on the 'fact' that all women in the countries they visit want to marry a Western man. Since they want to be wanted for more than a 'green card' or its equivalent, they tell themselves that their white skin is 'valued' for other reasons, and that to be white skinned is to be socially constructed as sexually desirable in countries they visit.[53]

These tourists justify their coming to Asian countries for sex tours since they narcissistically believe that women and young girls in Asia are truly attracted to them.

A Case Study: Philippine Tourism and Criminality

The Tourism industry in the country was greatly developed in the 1970s and early 1980s by the former President Ferdinand Marcos, primarily not to boost the economy but to improve his poor image in the outside world.[54] Marcos established the Department of Tourism and spent millions of dollars on building five-star hotels and cultural and art centers and on beautifying tourist spots all over the country. However, hotels were not earning much because "occupancy has been so slow."[55]

Until 1986 when he was exiled, Marcos' government allowed sex tourism to flourish. This brought a heavy influx of sex tourists and foreign pedophiles into the country. Incorporating the sex business into the tourism industry created a demand for children in the sex trade.[56] Many children were recruited from the provinces and were brought to Manila. They were promised nice jobs with a good salary. Instead, young girls were visible in hotel lobbies, brothels, and private houses.[57] A shopping mall known as Harrison Plaza Manila was a regular hangout for hundreds of boys who serviced mostly Japanese tourists.[58] These Yen-rich tourists often come to the Philippines not only for business purposes but also for sexual pleasure. The growth of sexual exploitation of children in Pagsanjan was also a result of this tourism development. Even after the Marcos regime fell, the next leaders of the country maintained the tourism industry, including sex tourism, as a source of foreign exchange.

The growth of sex tourism brought with it the escalation of crime, violence, and corruption inside and outside the country. Globalization contributes to the problem of commercial sexual exploitation of children because it facilitates the expansion of international organized crime; sex trade and child trafficking across national borders have increased.[59] The pervasiveness of prostitution cannot take place without the involvement of powerful figures in the country, from the military and law enforcement to local and national government.[60] Ireland pointed out that the former head of the Department of Tourism owned several motels and massage parlors and was given illicit special privileges.[61] Indeed, "corruption of police and political leaders is one of the most aggravating factors in the spread of child prostitution" in the country.[62] PREDA asserts that police authorities and politicians give protection to the perpetrators in exchange for huge amounts of money, as part of a larger system of corruption.[63]

Weak Enforcement of *Child Protection Law*

Weak enforcement of the *Child Protection Law* and non-cooperation of the police to crack down on sex syndicates worsens the problem of sexual exploitation of children. Even if the new *Child Protection Law* imposes harsh penalties on the perpetrators, no foreign pedophiles and gangs have been convicted as of yet. Usually, foreign offenders are deported and nothing more. On the contrary, it is the powerless children involved in prostitution who face arrest and sometimes harassment by local authorities.

The difficulty of stopping the sexual exploitation of children is mainly ascribed to lack of political will to implement the law against child prostitution and the apathetic attitude of the government against the plight of these children. The children remain in a disadvantaged position. This kind of structure is very oppressive and favorable to the rich and powerful who continue to dominate and exploit the poor and the weak. Julia O'Connell Davidson's view affirmed this analysis by saying that "the multiple oppressions involved in [child] prostitution...arise from unjust laws and...deeper systemic forms of social and economic marginalization."[64]

The increasing incidence of sexual abuse and exploitation of children in the Philippines since the middle of the 1970s to the present is quite significant. Though a number of non-governmental organizations (NGOs), governmental organizations (GOs), civil society organizations (CSOs) and Christian development organizations are now working to rescue and help these children, more and more children, especially the street children and those who come from poor areas, are forced to join the sex industry.

Given this background in which a large number of children are at risk, the Pentecostal churches in the Philippines are perceived to be ineffective in addressing the issue of childhood sexual exploitation. To be true to its mission and calling, the Christian church might be expected to play the role of an advocate and defender of vulnerable and powerless groups, like the children, in society. It is important to test and assess the perception that the Pentecostal Churches are ineffective in dealing with the problem of sexual exploitation of children.

Theological Assumptions

God's Intent

Children can easily be neglected and ignored simply because they are children. However, God never intended for children to be exploited and abused. God has a special concern for children, especially those who are at risk. He constantly reminds his people to care for them—defend the weak and the fatherless (Psalm 82:2–3; James 1:27). God intended children to be cared for and nurtured in the family. Scripture supports this in the foundational Old Testament passages of Genesis 2:24 and Deuteronomy 6:4–9, and again in the New Testament in Ephesians 6:1–4. In situations where this basic unit fails, or for some reason the capability to nurture and protect the children is absent, the Church as the community of faith has to take the "responsibility to provide protection and nurture"(Deut 6:4). This is God's intention from the very beginning. Chris Wright explains, "the major reason for the special care commanded for widows, orphans and strangers [is for] those who lacked the natural inclusion and protection of a household.[65] The Christian Church, Wright believes, corresponds to "the nation of Israel" as God's people who were given the task of "providing social care and inclusion" to the displaced member of a family.[66]

The Judeo-Christian view regards sexual abuse and exploitation of children as a sin against God and a crime against humanity.[67] Patrick Parkinson argues that "child sexual abuse is a violation of the scriptures' general commands about the misuse of the gift of sexuality" and that it has "devastating effects on children."[68] Children created in God's image are being reduced to commodities and objects. Their rights are violated and their dignity not respected. The Lausanne Covenant on Christian social responsibility states, "Because humankind is made in the image of God, every person, regardless of race, religion, color, culture, class, gender or age, has an intrinsic dignity because of which he should be respected and served, not exploited."[69]

Jesus expressed his concern for children by saying that for anyone who causes them to stumble, "it would be better for him to have a large millstone hung around his neck and to be drowned in the depths of the sea" (Matthew 18:6). These words sound a warning to anyone who sexually exploits children, including those who allow such grave sin to happen. The Old Testament also records that God opposed this practice, and he warned his people: "Do not degrade your daughter by making her a prostitute, or the land will turn to prostitution and be filled with wickedness" (Leviticus 19:29). Likewise, God's judgment will come to those who "traded boys for prostitutes" and "sold girls for wine" (Joel 3:3), and for "father and son [who] use the same girl" (Amos 2:7). He strongly expressed his anger whenever children are taken advantage of (Exodus 22:22–24).

A Model for God's Kingdom

In the Gospel narratives of the New Testament, Jesus treated children with great importance and affirmed their value (Matthew 18:1–9; 19:13–16; Mark 9:33–37, 42; 10:13–16; Luke 9:46–48; 18:15–17). In one instance, he allowed them to come to him. He embraced and blessed them even though his own disciples hindered them. In Mark 10:14, it says that Jesus was 'indignant' at his disciples' treatment towards these children. Jesus accorded dignity to these children whom his society treated with discrimination.

It is significant that Jesus presented the children as a model for everyone who wishes to enter the kingdom of God. In Matthew 18:3, he said, "I tell you the truth, unless you change and become like little children, you will never enter the kingdom of heaven." Michael Eastman, of Frontier Youth Trust, is insightful:

> Our Lord presents a small child, as a way of understanding the kingdom (to understand the kingdom you have to understand it this way); as a way of encountering the kingdom; as a way of relationship with the king (Whoever accepts a child accepts me and whoever accepts me accepts the one that sent me) and as a way of receiving the kingdom.[70]

Children are "more trusting, more ready to come to a loving Savior, and more open to the inbreaking of God's rule in Christ" than adults.[71] Children possess nothing that will keep them from entering the kingdom. This contrasts with the rich young ruler, seen in the same Gospel narratives, who was not willing to sell his possessions and follow Christ (Matthew 19:16–29; Mark 10:17–29; Luke 18:18–29). Children have no status and they are not concerned about it at all. Jesus made it plain to his disciples that "where God reigns, the unimportant and the powerless are the recipients of the eschatological blessing of the kingdom."[72]

Holistic Mission

Holistic mission is well described by Jesus' proclamation in Luke 4:18 and 19. "The Spirit of the Lord is upon me, because he has anointed me to preach the good news to the poor. He has sent me to proclaim freedom for the prisoners and recovery of the sight to the blind, to release the oppressed, to proclaim the year of the Lord's favor." Jesus' ministry is directed towards proclaiming the good news and addressing the social, physical, and emotional needs of individuals. The Brussels statement on evangelization and social concern declared, "Because God bestows human dignity on all people, everyone, regardless of their status in life, deserves the church's full attention. Jesus' own growth as a child (Luke

2:52) and his earthly ministry demonstrated a deep concern for every aspect of human life (Mk. 1:25–26, 29–31, 40–42 and 6:30–40). To follow Jesus' example, the community of faith must, therefore, address spiritual, personal, social, economic and physical situations."[73]

If indeed the Church follows Jesus' example, a ministry cannot be confined only to preaching and teaching the good news. The Church, reflecting Jesus, addresses not only the spiritual but also the social dimensions of the gospel. The mission of the Church includes both evangelism and social action, which are "inseparably interrelated."[74] Its task is to dispense spiritual and social care to people.[75] Bryant Myers describes spiritual or "soul care" as the "development of personal faith… and commitment to truth and teaching of the biblical command to love God and your neighbor as yourself;" while he defines "social care" as "community service, the importance of social action, helping the poor, and correcting injustices in society."[76] Spiritual care also includes prayer and reading and living out God's Word.

The Church, to be true to holistic mission and genuinely caring for the community, cannot separate itself from active involvement in social, economic, political, and other issues in society. The prophetic role of the Church is to confront the evil structures in society. Structures that allow and even provide for the oppression, exploitation and sexual abuse of children are evil beyond measure. To fulfill its mission, the Church needs to play its prophetic role and speak out against these structures. The Church "is in a unique position to articulate what is wrong, and why it is wrong."[77] The Church's prophetic role seeks to bring transformation that promotes truth, justice, and righteousness in and for the community.

As God's agent of change, the Church has the responsibility to defend the cause of exploited children.[78] To bring change in the community, the Church must deal with injustices and stand up against them.[79] God demands justice, particularly for the powerless, like children.[80] This is clearly stated in the scriptures: "Do not deprive the alien or the fatherless of justice or take the cloak of the widow as a pledge" (Deuteronomy. 24:17; cf. 27:19). This mandate implies that justice must also be accorded to victims of child trafficking and bonded sexual labor to pay the debt of the family. Advocacy, lobbying, and creating awareness are important to bring change in the community. "The church must understand the biblical commands to engage in advocacy for the children who have no voice."[81]

The Church is also called to be "salt of the earth" and "light of the world" (Matthew 5: 13–16). The escalation of child sexual exploitation reflects the moral decay of society. To be "salt" means to preserve society from social, moral, and spiritual corruption. To be "light" means to lead people who are blinded by sin to see the difference between right and wrong. The role of the Church being "salt and light" is "to challenge and change corruption, misrule, and evil in the world affairs in general, by example and influence."[82] While the Church is itself a community, it can make its presence felt in a larger community by upholding justice and the righteousness of God.

Attitudes of Pentecostals toward Socio-Economic and Political Issues

The Pentecostal Movement in the Philippines

Pentecostalism in the Philippines, like Protestantism in general, has always been associated with the U.S.A. All major Pentecostal denominations in the U.S. and some minor ones have sent missionaries to the Philippines, beginning in the 1920s. Almost a century later, there are many Pentecostal churches, mostly located outside the city or town centers. The Pentecostals' strong emphasis on the miraculous and divine healing is a major factor why people are attracted to its faith and practice.[83] Another draw is Pentecostals' tendency to be "member-oriented," which results in effective mobilization of lay leaders in recruitment activities (evangelism). In contrast, classical and more established churches allow elite clergy to monopolize power. The Pentecostal churches are known to provide opportunities for the empowerment of their members through the gifts of the Spirit. This means that any member in the congregation has an equal opportunity to "move in the Spirit," through gifts such as prophesying, giving the interpretation of tongues, healing, or discerning of spirits.

Among the autochthonous Philippine Pentecostal churches, the most prominent is the Jesus is Lord Church (JIL) headed by Bishop Eddie Villanueva, a former radical activist, communist, and atheist.[84] The church started as a Bible study group for college students at the Polytechnic University of the Philippines (PUP), where Villanueva used to teach. His experience in leading people to protest against the evils of capitalism when he was an activist helped him found a vibrant group of young people willing to sacrifice their time and efforts to advance the Kingdom of God. Today JIL has grown into a worldwide multi-ministry network, establishing churches in Asia, Australia, Europe, Africa, the Middle East, Canada, and the United States of America mainly amongst Filipino immigrants.

In socio-political involvement, JIL has been very visible. For instance, Villanueva and his group publicly endorse a certain candidate during presidential campaigns, up through the 2016 election. Moreover, he runs and hosts a weekly television show which discusses current socio-political issues from a religious perspective. He also writes a weekly column for one of the major national newspapers. With these vehicles, he communicates the position of JIL on issues confronting both the Christian church and society. So far, JIL has been involved in presidential elections, campaigns against smut in the film industry, and various government policies. Villanueva was the only church leader among the Evangelical churches who openly called for the resignation of President Joseph Estrada in 2000. A few months after the JIL leader spoke out, Estrada was ousted amid public protests ("EDSA 2") and later found guilty of corruption. In addition to speaking out, Villanueva started an organization called the Philippines for Jesus Movement composed of several Pentecostal and Evangelical churches. This multi-church group continues to be vocal regarding social and political events and candidates. Because JIL is autochthonous, it is not dependent on any kind of missionary leadership or even partnership[85] and can authentically engage in Filipino issues as Filipinos.

Pentecostal Doctrine[86]

Karl Marx was a materialist. As a materialist, he believed that the economic system acted upon individuals' thinking and determined their beliefs. Max Weber held the opposite view, that religious beliefs can be a major influence on economic behavior.[87] Does the religious belief of Pentecostals direct their socio-economic and political action? What shapes their day-to-day political thinking? What are the factors that contribute to the development of a Pentecostal attitude toward socio-economic and political issues and in particular the issue of sexually exploited children?

There has been a perceived indifference of Pentecostals toward socio-economic and political issues, at least in some regions and time periods, including the Philippines in this century. This indifference has been attributed to various reasons. Following are five common views:

End-Time Views

One of the most common criticisms against Pentecostalism is its emphasis on "premillennial eschatology," which is a specific view of how the world ends. One outcome of this view is the sense that it is futile to try to transform social structures into a just environment. Kyle McDonnell, a Roman Catholic theologian, believes that "the popularity of an apocalyptic eschatology among Pentecostals is a major source of their withdrawal from social action."[88] McDonnell concludes that this theological emphasis has impaired the social vision of Pentecostals resulting in a reactionary social stance or a "general non-involvement in programs of social improvement."

The strong emphasis of the Pentecostals to live personal moral lives has also made them turn away from the social gospel. As McDonnell described it, "They take pride in looking upon their church as their hospital, social center, educational center, and sanctuary."[89] The result is that the Pentecostals in a given society take little interest in politics and often do not participate in the voluntary associations of the community.

These analyses, however, are not without opposition. Doug Petersen, for example, bewailed how the movement is misunderstood. While it is true that Pentecostals traditionally taught a premillennial eschatology, their practice did not necessarily reflect indifference to present realities. Petersen argued, "Stereotypes of Pentecostals as 'otherworldly,' pathological, or fanatical obscure one of the movements' strengths, which is divine healing."[90] Juan Sepulveda agrees and says that, to understand Pentecostals better, it is important to recognize that while Pentecostal eschatology is a rationale for their experience, it is not intrinsically connected with the experience itself.[91] Dayton also, quoting Faupel, says, "[Pentecostalism] has on occasion supported a vision of social reconstruction."[92]

In the early years of the movement, it is a fact that Pentecostals had an affinity with some forms of social concern. Although evaluating them is not easy, Dayton brings to our attention the various forms of the movement's revolutionary impulse of social responsibility.[93] The following is a tabulation of Dayton's findings:

> (1) The early statement of faith that came out of Azusa Street Revival regularly published in *The Apostolic Faith* alludes to its commitment to "missions, and street and prison work." (2) The radical social vision expressed by the chronicler of the Azusa Street Revival Frank Bartleman included articulations of his conviction against capitalism, the abolition of any form of slavery, and other oppressive social

structures of his time; (3) Songs that contain a message of social protest were used in some Pentecostal groups, with the theme usually centering on the "special role of Christ with the poor."(4) The role of women was viewed as "one of the striking features of Pentecostalism." This is readily evident in the ascent of women to positions of leadership in the movement. And (5) many interpreters of the movement have observed the frequent appearance of pacifism in early Pentecostalism.[94]

In the same way, Petersen has maintained strongly that Pentecostal theology is not solely other-worldly. The Pentecostal experience prepares the adherents not only for the future but also for the present.[95] How far this view is echoed and reflected in various Pentecostal churches around the world requires an extensive set of empirical studies. Regarding the Philippines, this question is addressed by the analysis in this research.

Dualistic Vision of the World

Historically, from the Middle Ages to the seventeenth century, the churches in Europe were holistic in their approach to ministry. During the Enlightenment, this holism fell to a divorce between religion and social ethics.[96]

Juan Sepulveda (1988:299), speaking from the Latin American context, sees Pentecostal theology leaning toward a dualistic vision of reality. This creates uneasiness and confusion in the face of social oppression and injustice. Priority is given to personal conversions and church growth, while oppression and injustice are spiritualized. The perceived indifference of Pentecostals toward social, economic, and political issues has been attributed to this dualistic otherworldliness. A configuration of this dualism is explained by Sepulveda:

> All reality is marked by the opposition between the spiritual dimension, the place of the divine presence and the source of all good; and the material, marked by the sign of sin and therefore the source of all evil. The opposition between spirit and matter is represented cosmologically in the opposition between the church and the world.[97]

This kind of cosmological and anthropological dualism runs through all Pentecostal theology, claims Sepulveda.[98] Sepulveda's view is to some extent supported by Howard Kenyon of U.S. Assemblies of God who said, "The Assemblies of God (USA) has long defined Pentecostal experience and doctrine, but it has continuously sidestepped the task of delineating [sic] a suitable ethic of right action for its constituency."[99]

This neglect has mirrored similar limitations within the Assemblies of God churches in the Philippines.[100] For many Pentecostals in the Philippines separation from "this world" is often equated with true spirituality based on Paul's exhortation to the Romans "not [to] conform any longer to the pattern of this world...." (Rom 12:2).

Fundamentalism and the Great Reversal

Evangelicals reacted against the so-called 'social gospel' at the end of the 19th century and certainly by the 1920s. Any progressive social concern, whether political or private, "became suspect among revivalist evangelicals."[101] Pentecostals moved with the Evangelicals in this major shift, as Pentecostalism and Methodism shared doctrinal roots in the Holiness Movement.[102] As Sider says, "One can only evangelize persons, not social structures."[103] Pentecostals generally believe social change is only possible through personal conversion and incorporation into the community of faith. Structural change—economic norms, social welfare, political systems, etc.—is not usually part of their agenda. "Effective social change often takes place at the communal and micro-structural level, not at the macro-structural level,"[104] according to many Pentecostals. Once personal salvation is achieved, a change in the person's life is readily noticeable—healing effects on family life and on his or her physical health and well-being, for example. While Pentecostal churches do not usually prohibit their adherents from participating in the "affairs of the world," they offer no concrete guidelines.

Aversion to the Roman Catholic Church

Having been "born again" and delivered from extra-biblical teachings, there is a tendency among Pentecostals to take the opposite political position from the Roman Catholic Church. This is widespread. In Latin America, Protestants tend to be automatically opposed to Catholic policies, practices, and political identifications or alliances. This opposition "arises partly for classical theological reasons and partly because Catholicism symbolizes integration into a complete socio-religious system"[105] in these regions.

Mutual Rejection

Historian Vinson Synan insightfully observed a mutual rejection between the early Pentecostals and their culture. "The Pentecostals rejected society because they believed it to be corrupt, wicked, hostile, and hopelessly lost, while society rejected the Pentecostals because it believed them to be insanely fanatical, self-righteous, doctrinally in error, and emotionally unstable."[106]

In the Philippines, disillusionment with politics during the dictatorial regime of Marcos fueled Pentecostals' alleged indifference towards society. During the 1986 EDSA[107] Revolution, while hundreds of thousands of Filipinos filled the streets, most Pentecostals felt all they could do was pray within the confines of their churches. Even the Philippine Council of Evangelical Churches (PCEC), which includes most Pentecostal denominations, did not take a clear stand during the revolution.

Pentecostals also feel that key areas in society are sources of threat and anxiety. Participating in a 'Jesus March,' which is basically a worship parade for Christians, is viewed as more beneficial than joining a protest march against tax increases or school fees.

Elements in the surrounding culture that are shared by activism-averse Filipino and South American Pentecostals include, "Spanish colonial heritage, overwhelming Catholic majority, poverty, American influence in the twentieth century and the experience of dictatorship governments."[108] David Stoll, in studying Central American Pentecostals, believes the marginalization and extreme poverty they have experienced make them passive in responding to socio-political issues.[109] Pentecostals themselves affirmed this observation:

> Most Pentecostals do not give priority to systematic reflection on problems related to social structures. They place more attention on the ways people experience those problems in their own lives and communities. Pentecostalism, for the most part, has not existed until recently among "well educated" people who are able to reflect more systematically on structural dimensions of social justice. Pentecostals do not read the New Testament as placing a high priority on structural change; rather they read it as emphasizing personal conversion and commitment to the communities of faith, and through that process affect social change.[110]

Maldonado also observes, "Political withdrawal or passivity seems more characteristic of Pentecostals converted by missionaries than of those who have an autochthonous or indigenous origin."[111] Balancing this,

Martin notes that, "In spite of the Pentecostals' apolitical stance, they are not necessarily committed to quietism or to conservatism."[112]

Conclusion and Recommendations

Conclusion

The growing number of child prostitutes and sexually abused children has been one of the major problems in the Philippines. Yet, the government does not seem to be keen on finding solutions to this crisis; and neither, for reasons described above, does most of the Pentecostal church. The enormity of the task in solving the problem requires the collaborative efforts from various cause-oriented groups and sectors in the community. The statistics described in this paper show that interventions made by individual organizations and agencies alone are not sufficient to tackle the problem. Support from all sectors of society is needed.

Pentecostals' lagging participation slows the process of solving the problem. Some Pentecostal leaders claim that addressing the issue is not the task of the Church but of the para-churches and NGOs, revealing a non-holistic mission, as well as the belief that social concern does not have equal status with evangelism. Pentecostal theology, however, incorporates both.

The Church being "salt and light" should make its presence felt more strongly. Its influence should affect society until injustices are rectified and oppression is dealt with. The potential of the Church to address the problem of sexual exploitation of children, however huge the problem may be, cannot be underestimated.

The Church's spiritual mandate includes authority and power to spread the good news—"to proclaim freedom for the prisoners...to release the oppressed" (Luke 4:18). People look up to the Church as an institution responsible for spiritual care. The Church in many ways is expected to take the initiative of making sure justice and righteousness rule the country. Because of this high respect, the Church has a voice and can speak on behalf of the voiceless and be listened to.[113]

Recommendations

The study shows the seriousness of the problem of sexual exploitation of children in the country and therefore reveals much more effort will have to be exerted to alleviate the situation. There is a dire need to gather resources and consolidate the efforts of different groups and agencies for more effective results. It is necessary for the church to become aware of what is happening to the plight of the children in the country. Community civic groups like the Council to Protect the Children of Pagsanjan (CPCP) will greatly benefit if they get the support of the Church. The Church can help by explaining to the parents who oppose the project that what the civic groups are doing is for the welfare of their children.

The Church should endorse the actions of NGOs, CSOs, Crime Watch groups, and other agencies that labor for the cause of these children. The possibility to work with other faiths in tackling socio-political issues like sex tourism, corruption, and weak enforcement of Child Protection Laws is crucial. Advocacy and lobbying are equally important to put government policies into place that will fit the basic needs of the families and improve the quality of life of the children.

The Church must plan for feasible alternatives to get the children off the street and away from prostitution. The evangelical churches that already have a ministry to children at risk must include the sexually exploited children in their program. Because of the gravity of the problem, ministry to the sexually exploited children must be given priority in the churches' development work. Long-term and sustainable programs should also be considered instead of just limiting the work to feeding and relief distribution. Since the Church has a great potential to rehabilitate, heal and restore the psychologically damaged and traumatized children through the power of the gospel and the ministry of the Holy Spirit, it should also open its door to these children.

A good starting point in prioritizing ministry to the sexually exploited children is to create awareness on the plight of children at risk through workshops and seminars. Churches lacking resources should collaborate and network with agencies and organizations that are already established in this area.

Theologically, the challenge for Pentecostal churches is how to integrate evangelism and social concern. Social responsibility, in general, need not be viewed as being inherently disconnected from the proclamation that Jesus Christ provides a saving way of life. As Orlando Costas wrote, a biblically-based understanding of mission "is not so much concerned whether we proclaim, make disciples or engage in social, economic and political liberation, but whether we are capable of *integrating* all three in a comprehensive, dynamic and consistent witness."[114]

To effectively address the problem of sexual exploitation of children in the Philippines, the Church will need to evaluate its role, strategize, and put into immediate action the plan written in their statement of concern. The Pentecostal church in the Philippines should extend its reach—establishing a theology appropriate to the context in which people are being abused and exploited.

8.

Resilience and Spirit-Empowered Communities: Stories of Overseas Filipino Women Workers in Pentecostal-Charismatic Churches

Doreen Alcoran-Benavidez and Edwardneil Benavidez

Abstract

Studies have identified that vulnerabilities of women overseas workers are greater than those of men. In the case of the Philippines, the number of female overseas Filipino workers (OFWs) was higher than that of males in 2015, and the number of women OFWs who have experienced abuse is also greater than of men. The experience of abuse among women OFWs adds to their already heavy load and the stress of being away from their families. However, whether they continue being overseas contract workers (OCWs) or decide to return home, women OFWs needed to cope with their situations and become resilient so that they could continue to carry their responsibilities to their families. This article presents stories of resilience among women OFWs who suffered abuse, how they coped with the situation, and how they were able to stand up again to their feet. Also, as the Filipino identity is influenced by religion or faith, this study explains how the involvement of these OFW women with a Pentecostal or Charismatic church contributed to their resilience and how the church can further help them.

Introduction

Many domestic workers are beset by problems that affect their mental health. Currently, literature, media, and interventions emphasize the vulnerability and problems of migrant workers, often in the context of abuse and violence. But there is little insight into the factors that positively affect their well-being and eventually resilience.

In this paper, we present some factors that potentially contribute to the resilience of Filipino female domestic workers who are connected to Charismatic or Pentecostal churches. Using a qualitative research design, results show that respondents perceive their experience abroad as relatively good, while they also experienced high levels of stress, abuse, and violence. The workers used a variety of coping mechanisms to deal with stress. Socially-oriented coping strategies and spirituality play an important role in developing resilience for these women, as personal coping strategies. These terms will be defined below.

Domestic workers represent a significant share of the labor force worldwide, and domestic work is an important source of wage employment. Domestic work is a so-called 3D job (dirty, dangerous, and degrading), and workers often have short-term contracts or no contract at all.[1] In recent years, the number of workers exposed to abuse and violence has increased. The major reason for this is globalization and bad migrant labor policies in receiving countries.[2] Although efforts have been made to draw attention to the situation of migrant workers, the protection of their well-being remains very challenging.[3]

In this study, we focus on the resilience of female overseas domestic workers from the Philippines. We explore a range of factors that enable their resilience and play a role in dealing with migration-related stress.

The Migrant Domestic Workers

A domestic worker is a "wage-earner working in a (private) household, under whatever method and period of remuneration, who may be employed by one or by several employers who receive no pecuniary gain from their work."[4] Domestic workers are mostly adult women who voluntarily migrate from one country to another to find work in the domestic service sector. Women may be especially drawn to overseas domestic work because of gender stereotypes associated with this type of low-skilled labor.[5] They are often recruited from the most vulnerable populations in poor countries, where labor migration has increasingly become a structural survival strategy for migrants and their families.

The Philippines is one of the main countries of origin of migrant domestic workers.[6] Migration in the Philippines is primarily driven by poverty and the need to explore other sources of livelihood. Most Filipino migrants describe their reason for migration as a personal decision based on familial needs. Migration is further facilitated by the Philippine government's [labor] export-oriented policies.[7]

In many destination countries, domestic work is not considered part of formal work, which means it is performed outside the realm of labor regulations and social protections.[8] The living-in and irregular nature of their work isolates domestic workers and makes them especially vulnerable to abusive working conditions and associated adverse effects on their well-being, as reported in a range of studies.[9] Issues frequently cited in these studies include marital problems, worrying about children at home, loneliness, homesickness, and poor working conditions. Psychological and physical abuse by employers are commonly identified as stressors by migrant domestic workers. As a result of all these factors, migrant domestic workers constitute a vulnerable group in terms of psychiatric morbidity.[10]

However, little is known about factors that help to prevent, reduce, or cope with stress and mental health problems among migrant domestic workers.

The Resilience of Filipina Domestic Workers

Theories of strengths and resilience provide insights that are useful in generating knowledge on how migrant domestic workers deal with the many stressors they face. According to Saleebey, the strengths perspective and resilience literature "obligate us to understand that however downtrodden, beaten up, sick, or disheartened and demoralized, individuals have survived, and in some cases even flourished."[11] This observation appears highly relevant in the context of migrant workers – despite the hardships they face, many are able to adequately deal with stressors. Moreover, a significant number of workers continue to look for opportunities abroad.

Resilience is believed to protect well-being by minimizing the negative effects of stress and promoting successful adaptation to changes.[12] Two types of protective factors can be distinguished: (a) personal resources, which are characteristics of an individual such as personal coping strategies, and (b) social resources, which are characteristics of relationships and support networks within or outside the family.[13] These two factors are the variables considered in this chapter.

Several studies which focused specifically on the well-being of migrant populations found high resilience to be related to improved well-being and lower depression scores.[14] Some researches shed light on factors that might support resilience among the migrants. A study by Wong and Song suggests that workers whose appraisal of being abroad was positive, particularly those who perceived migration as providing more financial and material gains, had better mental health.[15] Keezhangatte identified factors that contribute to the resilience of Indian domestic workers in Hong Kong, including meaningful reasons for migration, membership in small groups, the nature of their work, and income.[16] Other studies reveal social support and religion as important factors in the well-being of migrant women.[17]

We aim to provide further insight into the resilience of female domestic workers. Particularly we will explore how being part of a religious community—specifically a Charismatic or Pentecostal church—helped them overcome stress and traumatic experiences.

Method

The study made use of a qualitative research design. Qualitative research approaches allow the researcher to identify variables by interpreting the meaning of the phenomena under study from the perspective of those who are involved in and are experiencing the phenomena.[18] Data were collected using open-ended questionnaires aimed to identify the perspectives of female OFWs, first, about their work abroad; second, about their experience of difficulties or abuse(s); and third, about their personal and social-resources coping strategies, including how the community of faith helped fortify their resilience.

The questions were presented in both English and Filipino, and respondents answered in either or both languages. Respondents are former and current female migrant workers who had finished at least one contract as a domestic worker abroad and who are also members of Charismatic or Pentecostal churches. A total of 10 female migrant workers completed the questionnaire. After reading the responses from the questionnaires, follow-up questions were asked to clarify and further elaborate the respondents' answers. For respondents who are not in the Philippines, online communication was used. Respondents who are in the Philippines were interviewed. Key participants were also interviewed using a semi-structured interview questionnaire. With the data collected, we have identified personal resources and social resources for coping strategies of female OFWs in the study and explain how these factors contribute to their resilience.

Findings

Perspectives on Overseas Work

In the Philippines, migrating for the sake of the family runs through the script of migrants, men and women alike. The ten respondents in our study took it upon themselves to work abroad in the hope of improving the economic well-being of their families. These women came from poor families, and they saw working abroad as a domestic worker as the only avenue through which to help their families have a better life. The reasons given by the respondents are economic in nature or related to providing support to family members. Angelyn shares, "My problem was really about how I would support my two children since I am a solo parent."[19] Also, Gina narrates, "My father was sick and he needed to undergo medication. Going abroad was the only way I knew that could help us be able to help him."[20]

Awareness of the Risk Involved

When asked about their apprehensions regarding going abroad, all respondents identified their being away from their family, particularly their children, as their main concern. They were worried about how their children would survive without their mother. This anxiety was overcome by three factors. First, extended family members, like the grandparents of the children or their aunties, gave their assurances that they would provide additional care for the children left behind. Respondents also identified the church community as a family that may also look after the welfare of their children. The second coping mechanism that respondents employed was to rationalize that their being abroad was primarily for the future of their children. And third, respondents believed that God was allowing them to go abroad. They all shared that they prayed earnestly and asked God for guidance when they were deciding whether to go abroad.

Initially, only one of the ten respondents mentioned that she was anxious about the possible risk of being abused. After probing further, all shared awareness of the possibility of abuse. They had all heard stories of abuse. Also, all participated in the Pre-Departure Orientation Seminar (PDOS), a required seminar provided by the government for OFWs in which educating about risk and how to cope with it is one of the objectives. In spite of this awareness, all the respondents still pursued going abroad. They explained that the success stories of people they know who went abroad prevailed over the stories of abuse that they seldom hear. They saw the economic progress of OFWs they know, and for them, that was more real than the risk of being abused. Respondents who had previously experienced abuse were the only ones who addressed their vulnerabilities and the difficulty of the situation. In the area of the possible risks of women working abroad, neither extended family members nor the church was able to help them become more informed about their vulnerabilities, the risks they might encounter, nor how they might face those risks.

Personal Resources Coping Strategies

Respondents were asked to share how they cope with stress during their time abroad. The most frequently reported coping strategies are praying and reading the Bible. Crying and resting or sleeping were the most frequently cited ways of dealing with stress. Other strategies involved talking to others, including friends, children, and partners. The participants further emphasized family as an important source of strength that enabled them to deal with problems. They explained that thinking of and communicating with their families helped them through hard times and gave them joy and happiness. Rowena shares, "Talking with your children makes you strong; you keep in mind that all your sacrifices are for them.[21]

In addition, the respondents stated that spirituality and religiosity formed a major source of strength for them. Prayer was described as an important way of coping with problems. Faye states, "My employer is always hurling many hurtful words at me. I cannot do anything; I just cried and prayed for strength.[22] Grace also narrates, "I called my family as a way of coping. They told me, 'Be tough and always pray,' and sometimes we pray on the phone."[23]

We also find that endurance and acceptance were important elements of workers' coping strategies. They tried not to think about their problems and to 'just bear it.' Teresita explains, "While we were abroad, we worked very hard, but we would always think of the time that we can go home and be happy again. I prayed to God to help me persevere."[24] Aileen also shared, "When my employer gets mad, I really wanted to talk back, but I didn't because I was afraid to get fired. I just endured it. I prayed for the Holy Spirit to give me self-control."[25]

Another recurrent theme in the interviews was the need to be flexible and to maintain the ability to adapt. Teresita shares, "To go to [an]other country is a privilege but you will experience culture shock. But we Filipinos are tough, creative and resourceful. We could easily adjust to any situation that we are into. We could easily adapt to situations abroad."[26]

Several respondents indicated that they used practical coping strategies, such as learning the language of their employers. Grace explains, "Before, I always got scolded by my employer because often I did not understand what he was talking about. What I did is to list down the most frequent words he is using and learn them. My relationship with my employer improved because I learned how to speak Chinese."[27]

Social Resources Coping Strategies

Employer-Worker Relationship

Receiving material and financial gifts and the feeling of being part of the family showed a strong connection with resilience. According to Faye, "The job is very demanding, but as long as my relationship with my employer is good, it's okay for me."[28] The payment that workers receive plays a fundamental role in the employer-worker relationship. This is especially relevant considering that many workers experienced problems with nonpayment and delayed payment and the fact that regular payment was crucial to the workers' ability to send remittances to their families in the Philippines. Rowena explains how receiving payment meant to her, "You feel good thinking that your family can eat whatever they like at least once a week."[29]

Social Support

Our study shows that workers mostly received social support from Filipino friends in the country of destination, but family members were an important source of support as well. Workers who received support from their mother or father reported higher resilience. The following statements from participants provide insight into the importance of social support. Angelyn shares, "I have no one to help me; I'm alone. Every payday, I spend all my money on overseas calls. I called my mom; I always cry my heart out to her."[30] In the absence of social support, the respondents feel helpless. Ginalyn shares, "If you are abused and not allowed to go out, you cannot connect with people and you feel helpless because you cannot ask for help."[31]

One respondent described how contact with other migrant workers helped her through hard times in Hong Kong. Grace narrates, "The good thing that my employer, together with her whole family, as well as her siblings and their family, visit their mother every Sunday. They have Filipino domestic helpers too, and we talk about our employers. It also helped. It helped me to release my anger; it helped me to release stress, reduce it."[32]

Church Membership

The respondents indicate that they are or were members of a Charismatic or Pentecostal church while being overseas or were active members of a church before going abroad. The participants explained why migrant workers mostly join churches. According to them, the church provides emotional and social support and nurturing, especially to newcomers in the country. Also, friendships are easily established through the church's discipleship programs.

Coping with Experiences of Abuse

When asked about their experience of abuse, only two respondents (Angelyn and Ginalyn) say that they experienced abuse. One experienced physical abuse, and one verbal abuse. While all of them talked about experiencing long hours of work, lack of sleep, not getting days off or rest, deprivation of food, and verbal abuse, most of them do not consider these as abuse and view abuse as limited to physical abuse. They felt helpless when forced to work extended hours while very hungry and very tired while at the same time being verbally and physically abused. They cry every night, they could not tell their family in the Philippines, and all they could do was to pray to God for help. For all the respondents, praying gave them strength to endure the hardships that they experienced. Praying strengthened them because it helped them to feel they were not alone in their suffering, believing that God was with them. God was their *kadamay*, a person who suffers with the other. God became like a social support to them, a shoulder to lean on in their times of need. Another way prayer strengthened them is that, while they may be helpless due to circumstances, they earnestly believe that God is not at all helpless, but rather he is able and active in doing something to help them. This belief gives them hope that their situation will eventually change, and praying strengthens that belief and hope. Knowing that God is working, they became sensitive to possible solutions to their situations and were willing to act, with God's help. In retrospect, as the respondents prayed to God in their experience of crisis, they view their experience of abuse and hardship as an instrument that made their relationship with God stronger.

The respondents' church membership also helped them cope with their situation. One respondent received a daily ration of food from a Filipino church in Hong Kong. That church regularly gives sandwiches, particularly to Filipino domestic workers. They even rescue domestic helpers who need help to get away from their abusive employers. The church as a social support is also where women who experienced abuse could find other women who had the same experience. There, they console one another and may talk about practical ways they can cope or get out of their situation.

Discussion

Personal Resources

Findings show that connectedness to others, especially family, plays an important role in migrant workers' ability to cope. This indicates that the family bonds that have driven women to migration, simultaneously serve as a means of coping during migration. Findings of this study also reveal the importance of feeling connected to God through prayers, suggesting that a considerable number of workers see God as a part of their social network in the sense that they maintain a relationship with God through praying and reading the Bible. The close connection we found between spirituality and coping among Filipino migrants has been previously described by Cruz[33] and Nakonz and Shik.[34] This is a reflection of the strong religiosity among Filipinos. Religiosity continues to affect workers' behavior and attitudes abroad and possibly become even more influential in the context of migration.

With regard to patterns in coping behavior, Nakonz and Shik indicate that religious coping strategies used by female migrant workers from the Philippines generally aim at emotional adjustment to the situation or transference of responsibility to a higher entity.[35] They argue that religious coping strategies reflect preferences for self-discipline and passivity.[36] Many studies show that passive, emotion-focused coping styles are more likely to be employed when a situation seems uncontrollable and that lack of control is related to adverse effects on well-being.[37] In the case of our respondents, entrusting to God their hopeless situation through prayers may be viewed as passivity. However, while in a situation where their control is minimal, believing that God is in control may also be viewed as an active coping strategy. This belief, in the case of our respondents, gives them strength to act, knowing that the one truly in control is on their side. As mentioned above, every opportunity to have a reprieve from the situation was also seen as a provision from God.

Social Resources

Several studies show that social support is beneficial to well-being and provides a buffer against stress and mental health problems.[38] Our study suggests that support from family is beneficial to our respondents' well-being and contributes to resiliency. All ten respondents said that connection to their children, spouses, and parents helps them fight homesickness and persevere in their work away from home.

Being part of an organization, such as the church, also appeared to be strongly related to the resilience of the respondents. This finding reflects the social support that workers received through such organizations. The positive impact of group membership is consistent with Sanchez and Gaw's observations regarding the collectivistic character of Filipino culture, wherein family, peer groups, and regional affiliations are highly valued.[39]

Pentecostal/Charismatic View of the Spirit and Resilience

The view from Pentecostal and Charismatic theology that the Holy Spirit is a comforter, an advocate, and a source of empowerment in times of suffering may contribute to OFWs' resilience toolkit. Further, Pentecostal theology views the Holy Spirit as empowering believers to be witnesses of Christ to the world. Becoming a witness entails suffering, but the presence and the empowerment of the Holy Spirit enable the witness to face and overcome suffering. With this perspective, when a domestic worker decides to impose discipline upon herself, it may be a passive response to a situation wherein she has no control. But it may also be the active response of a believer empowered by the Holy Spirit to witness to her employer (i.e., the opportunity to show self-control and kindness to people undeserving of such). The experience of Grace may illustrate this:

> While my employer was scolding and cursing me, I was praying in tongues. Then I suddenly went into tears because I was seeing a big cross instead of my employer, and I was not hearing the cursing of my employer. I felt the presence of God and that he was working in my life. I decided to become more devoted in reading the Bible. I read even very late at night after my work. I bring my Bible anywhere I go, even when I accompany my employer to the mall. My employer saw my devotion and she began to change.... I finished my two years contract and my employer talked to me and asked forgiveness for all she has done. She wants me to renew my contract with them.... With much thinking and praying, I agreed to renew my contract.[40]

From a Pentecostal-Charismatic perspective, the Holy Spirit helped Grace to feel the presence and work of God in her life. This may also be viewed as the work of the Holy Spirit in her life as a witness of Christ, allowing her employer to see the work of God in her life.

The perspective on the Holy Spirit mentioned above may also be used as a framework for church communities to continue to respond to the needs of OFWs in need. Church communities empowered by the Holy Spirit may be a source of comfort for OFWs in need. The empowered church is enabled by God to demonstrate his love and power as it becomes active in helping OFWs, particularly women domestic workers who are in need.

Conclusion

This study provides insight into the resilience of Filipino female migrant workers from Charismatic and Pentecostal Churches. Our study indicates that although migration is a stressful experience for migrant workers, many are willing to accept and deal with the stressors and problems they face in order to pursue financial security and earn a livelihood for themselves and their families. Escaping poverty and improving quality of life appear to be the main drivers for seeking migrant work. The support they experience from the church helped them develop their faith in God, which is a helpful coping mechanism they can access in times of need and stress. The Pentecostal and Charismatic communities also became their social resource to cope with the challenges of their life as migrant workers.

9.
African Sexuality in the Context of HIV/AIDS
Joshua Banda

Abstract

In what has become a dual struggle, Africa is fighting for its life against HIV/AIDS and against what some see as a new wave of European colonialism. Rights agendas conflict at the international level. African nations possess empirical evidence for effective AIDS prevention, and the proven-effective protocol includes behavioral interventions that are also culturally appropriate in most African states. However, wealthy outside nations oppose the behavioral strategies and prefer a sexual rights agenda that is foreign to most of Africa. Tying donor money in the fight against AIDS to a cultural imposition of progressive sexual values, the battle has gone to the United Nations, where it often takes the form of coercive language tucked almost invisibly into UN policies. This chapter outlines some of the layers of that dual struggle and asserts the validity of both the empirical evidence against the spread of AIDS and the sovereignty of the African state.

Introduction

If John Mbiti's description of Africans as being "notoriously religious"[1] is anything to go by, there exists an inevitable, albeit at times disconcerting, interplay between the efforts of implementers of global health programs and those of the massive faith community from the majority of African States.

In this chapter, international polity is discussed, taking into account the active global promulgation of a conventional public health message that includes the promotion of reproductive sexual health values (termed as "rights") and initiatives targeted at adolescents.

Spiritually based sexual behavior change is discussed in the specific context of sampled congregation-based programmatic interventions in a medium- to high-density population area, located on the south-side of Zambia's capital city, Lusaka. Cursory references and reflections on anecdotal insights gleaned from selected global fora serve to illustrate the complex matrix at play in the global arena, as the rights agenda is, in the author's view, churned out systematically in multiple nations.

The candid narrations herein show how some entities promoting conventional public health approaches have tended to raise sustained apprehensions towards spiritually-based sexual behavior programs. However, the sheer complexity and pervasive pandemic nature of HIV requires sober engagement and recognition of the comparative advantage brought to the table by various multi-sectoral actors, and presumably all, in genuine endeavors to save lives. This chapter is premised on the latter, as a hopeful assumption. It attempts to chart a course towards bridging the widening gap of the distinctive approaches cited. The global terrain is highly sophisticated. The following encounters assist in shedding light in this respect.

Global Sophistication

In June 2008, I was privileged to travel, for the very first time, to the United Nations General Assembly (UNGASS) High-Level Meeting for Heads of States and Other Representatives of Member States. Aside from the main General Assembly sessions, I participated in a Civil Society hearing that featured a presentation from a Civil Society activist who called for the global recognition of prostitution as "legitimate labor." From where I sat, I followed the discourse rather uncomfortably, knowing this was not an isolated voice at such fora. One had to see it in light of the systematic campaign by a myriad of interest groups, select non-governmental organizations (NGOs), and various well-resourced Western funders including United Nations (UN)-associated entities that have been known in some instances to sponsor lobby groups that advocate specifically for a human rights approach in the context of HIV prevention. On face value, there may not appear to be any cause for concern, until one hears the specific set of so-called "human rights." One activist in particular took a swipe at religious organizations and labeled them guilty of "moralizing" generally and stigmatizing, in particular, "sex work," which activity she vehemently defended as legitimate.

My comment in response to the said postulation was partially captured by Dr. Allison Herling-Ruark,[2] who, I later learned, was an observer in the terraces at the time of the session and was kind enough to send me the following email later that evening:

Bishop Banda,

I am at UNGASS, and just heard your very powerful comments. I just wanted to applaud you for saying those things. I have been waiting for someone to make *any* mention of sexual behavior—it is amazing how everyone gives the same comments over and over, and yet so much is not discussed at all. (I am here as a civil society observer, so don't have the opportunity to make comments anywhere.) FYI, I am sitting in the overflow room, not the main room, but there was enthusiastic applause from a number of people, mostly Africans.

For those of you who I am copying and don't know what Bishop Banda (of Zambia) said, here are my rough notes (and he is the ONLY one I have heard say most of these things): "What can be done to translate info into knowledge, and knowledge into behavior change? There are certain approaches that must change. There is lots of new evidence that must guide our programs. A one-size-fits-all approach doesn't work—some things that I hear promoted as a one-size-fits-all solution here [at the UN] will not work for Zambia. In Zambia, we have evidence that moral and religious teachings have played a very important role. We would like to put it on record that there is a role for FBOs and moral and religious teaching. We need sexual behavior change, and moral and religious organizations can promote sexual behavior change. Northern organizations need to listen to local organizations, to those of us working on the ground." I know that is very rough—if you have a copy of your comments that you could share, I'd love to have it. As a note to all of us, I was pleasantly surprised by this language in the 2001 UNGASS Declaration: "By 2005, ensure that a wide range of prevention programs which take account of local circumstances, ethics, and cultural values, is available in all countries, particularly the most affected countries, including... [those programs] aimed at reducing risk-taking behavior and encouraging responsible sexual behavior, including abstinence and fidelity...." Had I had a chance to make a comment, I would have loved to ask the Assembly why there has been NO discussion of those kinds of programs or that goal at this meeting.

Depressed at UNGASS. (Allison)

A bit later Dr. Edward Green (Dr. Ruark's co-author) sent me his own commendation regarding the recorded comment. Ruark and Green's impassioned quest for different voices to be heard in the response to AIDS is laudable, especially given that we live at a time that the then-Deputy Chairperson of the African Union, Mr. Erastus Mwencha, in one instance described as a period when "many nations in the North appear to be turning towards Sodom and Gomorrah.["][3]

Rights Agenda—The Neo-political Path

In a study titled "Interrogating a Rights-Based Approach to HIV Prevention," Ruark and Green were apt in pointing out that "the field of HIV/AIDS, like other health and development fields, is dominated by a so-called human rights-based approach" which while possessing "many valuable aspects...has also taken on other meanings."

The afore-going is especially evident in the observable global interest the subject has generated. Building on this observation, I will highlight illustrative anecdotes that exemplify some of the key concerns raised by Ruark and Green. I will show in which respects the rights-based approach has taken on "other meanings." In so doing, I will affirm their assertion that these maneuvers have essentially been redefined as "rights." Notably, Green and Ruark stated:

> It may or may not be news to you that behaviors such as prostitution, risky sex, and drug use are now deemed "rights" by many of those working in HIV prevention, including by such organizations as the World Health Organization and UNAIDS, which is the United Nation's AIDS organization.[4]

At the United Nations Special Session held on June 8–10, 2011, which was focused on universal access to treatment for HIV, nearly every Western nation that made their statement to the General Assembly included some sort of call for member States to recognize the rights of Lesbians, Gays, Bisexuals, Trans-genders and Inter-sexual (LGBTI), injection drug users, and sex workers, along with open demands that member States where such practices are legally prohibited should decriminalize them. Inevitably, negotiating a consensus document as a corporate outcome of the session was extremely challenging. In the final analysis, out of 104 points in the political declaration from this sixty-fifth session of the UN General Assembly, number 29 read as follows:

> Note that many national HIV prevention strategies inadequately focus on populations that epidemiological evidence shows are at higher risk, specifically men who have sex with men, people who inject drugs and sex workers, and further note, *however, that each country should define the specific populations that are key to its epidemic and response, based on the epidemiological and national context.*[5]

When the formal reading was finally presented to the floor of the United Nations, Brazil and Mexico were the movers for support of the resolution, while Iran and Syria were allowed to voice objections. Therefore, the variation in the last half of the above provision stated fittingly, "that each country should define the specific populations that are key to its epidemic and response, based on the epidemiological and national context." The two States argued for this variation on the basis of epidemiological, sociological, cultural and religious factors. It ought to be plain to most readers that this exception balances the scenario appropriately and makes sound common sense.

In respect to the contestation surrounding the above resolution, Ruark and Green are correct in noting that "it is unusual (and possibly unique) for the political agenda of human rights to be elevated to a major theme for disease prevention, as it has been for HIV/AIDS.[6]

Beyond the sector of disease prevention, it is of great concern to observe the further elevation of sexual preferences, for instance, to the same level as the inalienable rights of children, women, and persons with disabilities. A case in point is a visit in February 2012 of the United Nations most senior representative, then Secretary-General Ban Ki-Moon who, while paying glowing tribute to Zambia on various positive economic developments recorded in recent years, also went on to say shockingly the following, in his first ever address to the people's representatives in the Zambian parliament:

> Now you have embarked on a transformation agenda – a process for a new people-driven Constitution that will be a foundation for Zambia's progress, a Constitution that will stand the test of time. This offers Zambia an opportunity to lead once more by enshrining the highest standards of human rights and protections for all people – regardless of race, religion, gender, *sexual orientation* or disability.[7]

So politically correct and inclusive! Observably, the specific reference to "sexual orientation" is telling.

Prior to the Zambia visit, Mr. Ban Ki-Moon made a similar call before African Heads of States and their Foreign Ministers at the African Union Summit in Addis Ababa in January 2012. Then before departure for his next State visit which was scheduled for the Democratic Republic of Congo, a "closed door" meeting was held with human rights groups in the Zambian town of Livingstone on Sunday, February 26, 2012, which, it must be indicated, attracted widespread disdain from the Zambian public.

So, what are these human rights in reality? Why are they being re-defined in this fashion? What should the church do about this global campaign? Will it be possible for the church to stay focused on the holistic transformation of society while the rights drama plays out? What are the eventual implications for the church's basic understanding or interpretation of human sexuality in general and state polity as well as international politics in particular?

Human Rights: A Cursory Overview

In a paper presented in Stellenbosch (2010), I mention human rights as generally understood to refer to the rights and freedoms to which all human beings are entitled.[8] The most comprehensive compilation of fundamental human rights is the United Nations' Universal Declaration of Human Rights (UDHR) having developed in the aftermath of the Second World War, in part as a response to the Holocaust, and culminating in its adoption by the United Nations General Assembly in 1948.[9] In modern society, it is widely held that basic human rights include civil and political rights as well as economic, social and cultural rights.

Owing to the limited scope of this presentation, we will not delve further into the various theoretical distinctions that exist regarding these rights. Suffice it to say that the division of human rights into three generations[10] was initially proposed in 1979 by the Czech Jurist Karel Vasak at the International Institute of Human Rights in Strasbourg. It is said that he used the term at least as early as November 1977. Vasak's theories have essentially taken root in European law, as they primarily reflect European values.[11]

In the context of Africa, one needs to familiarize with the African Charter on Human and Peoples' Rights (also known as the Banjul Charter) which is an international human rights instrument that is intended to promote and protect human rights and basic freedoms in the African continent.[12] The African Commission on Human and Peoples' Rights (ACHPR) is a quasi-judicial body given the task to promote and protect human rights and collective (peoples') rights throughout the African continent as well as to interpret the African Charter on Human and Peoples' Rights and consider individual complaints of violations of the Charter.

Some Lessons from One of Zambia's Constitutional Processes

From December 2007 until August 2010, I served as Chairperson of the General Constitutional Principles Committee of a 500-member statutory National Constitutional Conference (NCC), mandated by the then

Zambian Parliament to examine, debate and adopt public proposals to alter the Zambian constitution which had been earlier drafted by a Presidential appointed Commission. As Chairman of the General Constitutional Principles Committee of the NCC of Zambia, I presided over committee sittings convened to cover specific terms of reference as mandated by the NCC, to exhaustively examine and recommend the adoption of underlying constitutional principles (inclusive of directive principles of State policy) to be enshrined in the normative section of the new Zambian constitution and upon which the rest of the substantive constitution was to be based. The committee consisted of 44 members including eight Honorable Members of Parliament (MPs), among whom was the then Vice President of the Republic of Zambia, who was also Minister of Justice.

One of the most engaging sections of the draft constitution focused on whether to place the economic, social and cultural rights in a substantive part of the constitution (in this case, the bill of rights, making them justiciable) or to have them under directive principles of state policy where they would be non-justiciable. The final decision was for the latter.

In the public arena, general debate calling for the inclusion of the said rights in the bill of rights raged on, but notably led by donor aided civil society organizations, some of whom it was feared in certain quarters, may have been projecting their funders' agenda. This was more so in response to the fact that the NCC draft attempted to strengthen the marriage clause by specifying that marriage in Zambia should be between two adults (minimum age:18^{13}) of the OPPOSITE SEX. The draft specified further that SAME SEX marriages would stand prohibited. Although there were no specific public statements locally opposing this direction, the ensuing policies from many donor countries represented in Zambia indicated undercurrents that are likely to gain intensity in terms of pressure surrounding human rights issues.

This kind of pressure is likely to go on for a long time in Africa for as long as the budgets of African States are hugely reliant on donor aid. For instance, in the wake of global resources that are channeled into Africa to fight HIV/AIDS, there has been a growing call from donor countries for African states to adopt fully (as highlighted earlier) a rights-based approach in all HIV interventions.

A case in point happened in September 2010. In my role as Chairperson of National AIDS Council of Zambia, I hosted His Excellency Festus Mogae, former President of Botswana, who was then

Chairperson of a high-profile organization known as Champions for an HIV-Free Africa, made up of a group of former Presidents of several African countries. In a scheduled meeting with civil society representatives, the following submission was top on a list of 5 items the civil society presented:

> Legal and policy environment for Most at Risk Populations (MARPS)...there is a disconnect between the legal and policy environment: the penal code criminalizes most behavior the MARPS are engaged in, i.e., sexual contact between members of the same sex, injection drug use, commercial sex work, etc.[14]

What is becoming abundantly clear is that it's the highly emotive issues associated with sexual lifestyles that are more likely to continue topping the advocacy and policy agenda in many African States. Other topical matters likely to gain momentum include abortion easy-access and a values modification program now termed, "comprehensive sexuality education for young people."

In this chapter, I limit the consideration of the sexuality debate only so far as it relates to international state polity in the context of what I have termed the *new human rights crusade*, which in practical terms boils down to *"sexual orientation"* and related 'rights' issues, now inextricably tied to donor aid. In this regard, the environment in many African countries has become fairly charged as nations are subtly pressured into reassessing their laws and intent on having them to indicate expressly where they stand on LGBTI issues.

For instance, in Zambia, homosexuality is the *de facto* axis hotly at the center of the said political debate for some time now and does not appear to be waning yet. Here may be the possible reason why.

The law in its current form criminalizes homosexuality and related unnatural acts as per the following stipulation in the Penal Code Chapter 87 of the laws of Zambia where section 155 provides:

> Any person who has carnal knowledge of any person against the order of nature or (c) permits a male person to have carnal knowledge of him or her against the order of nature; commits a felony and is liable, upon conviction, to imprisonment for a term of not less than 15 years and may be liable to imprisonment for life.

Various players in the global community are pressurizing for a wholesale decriminalization of this and similar laws, yet such attempts are opposed strongly by a predominant majority of citizens. Admittedly, the matter is "thorny" and "has not been absent from various considerations and treatment in academic journals and theses."[15]

Conditional Donor Funding and a Narrowed Human Rights Approach

One of the most defining public pronouncements made in recent times that further illustrates how high on the global priority list the LGBTI agenda has ascended, is the high-level statement made by then Great Britain's Prime Minister Cameron at the 2011 Commonwealth gathering in Australia, where he threatened that "...countries that ban homosexuality [risk] losing aid payments unless they reform.[16]

The Guardian News Paper reported, however, that Mr. Cameron was quick to concede that "deep prejudices[17] in some countries meant the problem would persist for years. Mr. Cameron stated plainly that Britain was "putting the pressure on,[18] though "it was not a problem that would be solved by the time Commonwealth leaders are next due to meet, in Sri Lanka in 2013.[19] He made this statement while warning Sri Lanka "to improve its human rights record or face boycotts of the 2013 Summit."[20]

Further, the *Guardian* carried the following continuation of Cameron's remarks at the 2011 Australia Commonwealth meeting of Heads of government:

> Ending bans on homosexuality was one of the recommendations of a highly critical internal report on the future relevance of the Commonwealth, written by experts from across the member nations. "We are not just talking about it. We are also saying that British aid should have more strings attached," Cameron said on BBC1's Andrew Marr Show in an interview recorded at the Summit in Perth. "This is an issue where we are pushing for movement, we are prepared to put some money behind what we believe. But I'm afraid that you can't expect countries to change overnight.[21]

A similar call was made by then-USA Secretary of State, Hillary Clinton, and which story was anchored as follows on the BBC:

> The US has publicly declared it will fight discrimination against gays and lesbians abroad by using foreign aid and diplomacy to encourage reform. Secretary of State Hillary Clinton told an audience of diplomats in Geneva: "Gay rights are human rights." A memo from the Obama administration directs US government agencies to consider gay rights when making aid and asylum decisions.[22]

Battling with Sexual Liberalism

On July 25, 2012, the *Washington Post* carried a lead story headlined, "Conservative Christians Working on HIV/AIDS See Burden of Sexual

Liberalism." Part of the article written by Jabin Botsford had the following caption:

> A room full of prominent development, health and faith leaders listened and then clapped politely as a leading Zambian evangelical pastor told the Georgetown University-hosted conference that African nations work with Western non-governmental organizations (NGOs) has "had a downside." That downside, said Bishop Joshua Banda of the Assemblies of God, is the pro-choice "slanted manner" of health outreach.[23]

I was on a panel discussion at the Georgetown University-hosted faith-based AIDS summit (on the sidelines of an International AIDS Conference) with three high-profile individuals namely, Rajiv Shah, Administrator of the United States Agency for International Development (USAID), Lois Quam of the United States Department of State, and Rick Warren (top American Evangelist) of Saddleback Church. Children's AIDS Fund, Catholic Relief Services, and World Vision jointly convened the meeting. We were each allocated a topic to deliver in 5 minutes. My topic was "The Role of the Faith Community in Leveraging HIV/AIDS Work for the Health of the Whole Person—A Zambian Perspective."

The first of four slides in my presentation introduced the following three areas and ways which, I explained, the Zambian faith community was utilizing to leverage HIV/AIDS for the health of the whole person: 1) provision of treatment and care services in health institutional settings, owned and run by the faith community (The church in Zambia has had a well-acknowledged legacy and backdrop of home-based care initiatives since the early stages of the AIDS epidemic); 2) advocacy activities for holistic health care provision targeting the whole person; and 3) increased community links through massive volunteerism within the churches. These volunteers personally and consistently reach families in various communities where churches are located. As a result, robust and sustainable rapport is developed with needy families. It becomes like an "open door" into people's hearts. The breadth and depth of this outreach by the Zambian faith community and the length of time it has been sustained is beyond the ability of human energy alone. It is a sign of the Holy Spirit at work within and through the faith community that people connect person to person, and physical, emotional, spiritual and relational healing occurs.

On the second slide, I highlighted a challenge, namely, a clash between the faith approach and the conventional public health sexual reproductive health rights approach. The clash is inevitable because of the variance that exists between the two approaches. I then proceeded to the third slide to illustrate the point by narrating an incident in Zambia where a named large international NGO (headquartered in the West) had been compelled by the Ministry of Health to withdraw from a rural province of Zambia where it had been operating for some time. This was because the said INGO allegedly conducted 490 illegal abortions on young girls, on the pretext that the girls in question had had 'unwanted' pregnancies. The organization in question was reported to have conducted the abortions as part of a routine campaign on adolescent sexual reproductive rights. They claimed it was the girls' social right to access the said abortion services.

On the third slide, I argued that this 'rights' or 'purely medical/public health' the only approach was a category error on the part of the INGO because in Africa generally, and Zambia in particular, the first point of call for a young girl who happens to get pregnant unexpectedly, is her family. Granted, she may be 'chided' initially by the family for breaking chaste tradition or simply failing to uphold values, including abstinence from premarital sexual involvement. However, in the final analysis, the family will rally around her and encourage her to keep the pregnancy until she is able to safely deliver the baby.

Much like what the conservative Christian view holds, the acceptable norm in the majority of cultural settings in Zambia is *pro-life* rather than *pro-abortion*. This is enshrined so deeply in Zambian society that the Ministry of Education has enacted a policy provision for young girls to still return to school if ever they got interrupted due to an unexpected pregnancy. Thus, an unexpected pregnancy does not necessarily become 'unwanted!'

In that vein, one can understand the gravity of the matter in attempting to run a *pro-abortion* campaign in such a cultural setting. My point on the panel, therefore, was to indicate that it was culturally insensitive for INGOs to promote reproductive sexual health values in total disregard of the norms of the local people. I argued that the impunity with which these approaches are promoted in both rural and urban settings is morally disrespectful and inappropriate. I concluded that if mutual respect were not the basis for the sharing of global resources in the health fraternity, it would be best for donors to keep their funds. The applause that followed took me somewhat by surprise. However, therein commences our discourse on the battle with sexual liberalism in the wake of the global efforts to curb the spread of HIV/AIDS. This battle is stiff. Yet,

I am convinced of the rightness of our course; and guided and aided by the Holy Spirit, we are far from weary or faint in our love for the people of the continent of Africa and in our conviction to fight for their lives against the spread of HIV/AIDS and of international agendas that are not a good fit for the African context.

Launched in 1999, Love-Life is a campaign said to have been South Africa's largest national HIV prevention initiative for young people, which combined a "sustained high-powered campaign with nationwide community-level outreach and support programs to promote healthy, HIV-free living among South African teens."[24]

However, in a critical review of the program, Kylie Thomas (2004) noted that Love-Life's highly visible campaign may not have achieved its intended AIDS prevention goals "as it obscure[d] rather than address[ed] the issues that shape[d] gendered identities and determined the course of the epidemic in South Africa..."[25] AIDS Practitioners from Port Elizabeth interviewed said the campaign, despite having been heavily funded, directed its energies towards promoting its sexual values and the sexual independence of young people rather than positively combating the AIDS Pandemic.[26] Rena Singer of the Mail and Guardian wrote:

> The same is being asked of many of LoveLife's other AIDS-prevention programs: a television show that flew seven young South Africans to destinations around the world; a journey to Antarctica for another half-dozen youths; and an advertising campaign that has left many South Africans confused. LoveLife maintains that its controversial and unorthodox campaign is designed to make teens more positive and future-focused under the assumption that these qualities will lead them to act more responsibly and avoid exposure to HIV. But after more than five years and R780-million [equal to $56.5M in U.S. dollars]—more than half of it from the Kaiser Family Foundation and other non-profit organizations in the United States—the HIV infection rate among young South African teens remains disturbingly high. About one in ten teenagers is HIV-positive and about six million people are infected.[27]

Love-Life Switzerland[28] is even more illustrative of the sexual liberalism approach as its official website, along with a prominent 2014 Love-Life campaign banner, features the following *"love manifesto"*:

> I love my body. That's why I protect it. To enjoy life, I need my body. I protect it from sexually transmitted infections like HIV: if I'm single, cheat on my partner, or if a relationship has just ended, I use condoms and play by the *safer sex rules*. In a faithful relationship, after getting ourselves tested, we can stop using condoms.
>
> I have no regrets. And I'll keep it that way.

Mostly you don't regret what you do, but what you don't do. Whether it's an adventure, talking to someone – or safe sex. But I make sure I can always say: I have no regrets.

Another opening message read:

I love my life. I live it to the full. I live as I please and love whoever I want. After all, I only have one life. It's up to me whether I enjoy it or not. I make my own choices and take responsibility for them.

Here is how the full site opens:

The new love life campaign, "no regrets," does just what it says on the tin: *it's all about joie de vivre and worry-free sex*. The campaign shows that enjoying life and your body needn't cause you [to] worry – because if you keep yourself safe, you won't have any regrets." The love life manifesto sums up the message of the campaign. Anyone who says yes to the love life manifesto also says yes to themselves – and can enjoy their life and their body without any regrets.

After the above the message, a number of pictorials follow. Let me attempt to describe them: first an explicit picture of a man and woman in a bath-tub, in each other's arms (with foam all over), leaving the imagination to guess what else. Next to the picture, right below, is a video, ready to run – (play/ pause option in place). The scenery has a half-dressed young lady, sitting on the edge of the bed with both hands near the mouth—somewhat tightly clasped against her cheeks (sort of surprised at something she has just sighted!) Her eyes are in the direction of a partially undressed gentleman, whose trousers and underwear are lowered down to somewhere below the knees, as he appears to be advancing towards her.

So, could this be the new face of AIDS prevention? The point is clear: Sexual liberalism has taken over a good segment of the initially well-meant public health message.

In a riveting chapter titled "How the global AIDS response went wrong,"[29] Green and Ruark (2011) rightly diagnose the heart of the problem with some aspects of the global AIDS response as that of "mistaken priorities." Here is an example they register:

Thus, the first experts in AIDS prevention, mostly gay men and members of the family planning community, agreed about the priorities and guiding values of AIDS prevention. Relying on the triumvirate of condoms, HIV testing, and drugs (for treatment of STIs and later HIV) avoided awkward, thorny issues of changing (or restricting) sexual behavior. If the harmful consequences of sexual behavior could be mitigated or prevented through medical and technological solutions, there was no reason to address sexual behavior itself. A risk-reduction approach had seemed to work among Western MSM, although how well it worked is now in question (Stoneburner and Low-Beer 2003), and indeed HIV infections among U.S. MSM are today on the increase. But a risk-reduction approach already had the allegiance of the U.S. MSM.

The assessment above illustrates in one sense the key challenge of Western social policy that is essentially based on a form of radical moral relativism, whose negative impact is apparent globally. It is a moral, ethical failure with adverse implications that permeate beyond the health sector into the socio-economics. It is a dilemma for which, in this discourse, an alternative namely, spiritually-based ethical change is proposed.

It must be noted, though, that the sexual liberalism battle is not just waged by non-religious or secular entities *per se*. There is a society called Liberated Christians ("Cyber swing and Polyamory Resource Center and Other-centered sexuality") with an address in Phoenix Arizona, USA, which has a blog where a posting read: "Abstinence and the purity propaganda can harm Youth.[30] A front banner on the official website indicated that the said 'Liberated Christians' group "promote[s] positive intimacy and sexuality including non-monogamy or polyamory.[31]

Another front banner on the site indicated that this society is involved in "exposing false traditions of sexual repressions that have no biblical basis" and so forth. Unlike *Love-Life*, there appears to be no direct mention or reference to HIV/AIDS. However, it is a typical illustration of the complex social matrix Western funders and programmers have to contend with in the quest to deliver life-saving interventions globally.

The church needs to partner credibly with key stakeholders and service providers in the global AIDS fight so that its strengths can be leveraged, and the global community can benefit from its values. The United Nations' Human Development Report (2011) stated: "Sustainability is inextricably linked to basic questions of equity — that is, fairness, social justice and greater access to a better quality of life."

I argue that these questions of equity, fairness and social justice are not executable unless the basic values of the populations receiving aid are appropriately considered. Many faith-based organizations in donor-aided countries have enormous advantage and knowledge to combat religious extremism that could impede legitimate efforts to combat AIDS. However, FBOs generally, and churches, in particular, have to be engaged more resourcefully by funding agencies to enable the positive deployment of demonstrable comparative strengths, even though some may not suit conventional or traditional public health approaches.

Moving Forward

A Matter of Dignity and Justice

It will be noted that the named conditional funding approaches described thus far are reminiscent of a prejudicial construct that essentially minimizes the worth of the African peoples. Stereotyping chiefly by Western media continues to portray wrongly the African continent as being outdated in their attitudes to same-sex behavior and lifestyle. It amounts to a redefinition of 'human rights' that, as stated earlier, are now re-prescribed conditionally for donor-aided nations.

This amounts to a violation of the dignity of the African people and a total disregard of their human worth. The normal course of justice demands fair play in which people are respected for who they are and therefore allowed to determine their own position on pertinent matters.

A Clash of Viewpoints on Human Autonomy

It may well be contended here that what is at play is essentially a 'clash' of viewpoints regarding human autonomy. For instance, the Western concepts of *human rights* and *tolerance* are deeply located in an *individualistic* understanding of human autonomy that is at variance with the African value of common good that is deeply rooted in African culture. In this respect, some pertinent questions raised in a similar context by Chris Sugden,[32] Doctor of Canon Law, can be asked, including, "whether human rights are universal and are to be imposed *sui generis* in different cultures." Another line of inquiry for further reflection is: How is the question of cultural defense of human rights to be addressed in the face of such unguarded universal claims by donor countries? Is "inclusion" to be understood in Africa as it is in the West as the inclusion of limitless individual preferences; or is it to be related, more Africanly in Africa, to "the common good?" Where is the balance to be found between individual agency and common good?[33]

A New Scramble for Africa?

Earlier, I preempted the question of why human rights are being "redefined" in this fashion. I dare say that it is a power play towards setting the global agenda consonant to donor interests. If not cautioned, these acts will amount to a new scramble for Africa that could render the infamous earlier scramble child's play by comparison.

In a masterful narration, Martin Meredith reported the following about the "Scramble:"

> During the Scramble for Africa at the end of the nineteenth century, European powers staked claims to virtually the entire continent. At meetings in Berlin, Paris, London and other capitals, European statesmen and diplomats bargained over the separate spheres of interest they intended to establish there. Hitherto Europeans had known Africa more as a coastline than a continent…[34]

If the little-known Africa attracted that much foreign interest then, how much more interest will the current Africa that has been extensively explored, draw? It is clear that the human rights agenda appears to be merely adding impetus to a much bigger global agenda. Ruark and Green caution rightly, that "we should not need the impetus of AIDS to make protecting human rights a matter of prime importance and urgency. The danger is that the cause of human rights may be used to justify investing significant resources in programs that have little or no prevention impact on HIV infections.[35]

It is desirable then that Africa prioritizes what is most important to her, without outside interference. This will give her the chance to construct her own relevant approaches towards matters of sexuality, informed by her own felt needs and priorities.

10.

Good News from Africa: Is a Person's Sexual Behavior Influenced by Their Attitude and Behavior towards God? A Voice of Evidence

Joshua Banda

Abstract

This study investigated (1) the impact of congregation-based interventions as HIV/AIDS programs, and 2) how abstinence and marital fidelity function within the larger picture of overall strategies to combat AIDS. It examined the community work of the Circle of Hope Family Care Centre, a congregation-based HIV/AIDS support group initiative undertaken by the Northmeade Assembly of God Church in Lusaka, Zambia. The main research question was: Is a person's sexual behavior influenced by his or her attitude and behavior towards God? Two subsidiary questions were: 1) what are the factors that affect a person's sexual lifestyle? 2) Does attendance at church-based HIV/AIDS programs cause a change of behavior in a person's sexual relationships?

A triangulated methodology was used, which required the collection of both quantitative and qualitative data. The experimental design included a purposively selected intervention group and a control group. Both groups were studied by employing baseline first, and follow-up measures after three months. Quantitative data analysis was carried out in two stages. The first is cross-tabulations to examine the relationship between safer sexual behavior and socio-economic variables. For the statistical analysis, chi-square tests of independence were conducted at the bivariate level, and the differences were determined at $P < 0.01$ and $P < 0.05$ significant level. Next, major predictors were carried out with the help of logistic regression analysis.

The results of the logistic regression analysis showed that those who participated in the interventions were 4.1 times more likely to report having adopted new behavior or modified old behavior, specifically to live positively, than those who did not attend the interventions. Similarly, participants in the faith-based interventions were 2.3 times more likely than those who did not take part to report having adopted safer sexual practices. Further analysis revealed that those participants were 1.8 times more likely to report abstinence from non-marital sex than those who did not attend.

The conclusion is that church congregations have an immense comparative advantage to influence sexual behavior through increasing captive audiences constituting the churches' presence in the community. Additionally, their morally based interventions such as abstinence and marital fidelity show significant impact on sexual behavior change and have potential to turn the tide of HIV/AIDS, as the tested models are replicable, scalable and sustainable. In this vein, a description of how the study intervention was set up is necessary.

The Main Intervention: Life Transformation Seminars (LTS)

The main intervention for the study was conducted through the convening of twenty-four Life Transformation sessions using tailor-made Life Transformation Seminar (LTS) curriculum, compiled specifically for this purpose. Each session ran for approximately one hour. Invariably participants stayed longer than one hour, as the sessions took root and as people became more acquainted with each other.

The material content for the LTS was compiled from the Bible and incorporated key tenets of the Christian faith from a spiritual formation perspective, as is common in practical teachings of many Zambian Pentecostal Churches. Although the participants varied in terms of religious affiliation, the Pentecostal norm was chosen as a distinctive norm and pattern of delivery, as it was the environment in which the HIV initiatives under exploration, grew. The biblical content was supplemented by motivational anecdotes from publications of five Christian motivational teachers.

Using predominantly biblical content was a purposive step to test the hypothesis central to the study, that attendance to such a congregation-based program alters the sexual behavior of the participants. In particular, no specific mention of HIV was included so that LTS participants would be exposed to content that generally is, as much as possible, close to the norm in church services in Pentecostal congregations. Surprisingly, HIV-related matters would still emerge from time to time during discussions.

The LTS was designed to run over a period of 12 weeks (approximately three months), starting shortly after the initial survey was administered. Completion of the LTS training coincided with the follow-up survey measure at the conclusion of the applicable modules.

A summarized outline of the material is available, to demonstrate a possible replicable model for congregations. There were nine topics divided into three modules sets (I, II and III), each containing three topics and each topic delivered in two-part tiers, as the sessions were conducted twice weekly for the applicable period. After each module set, the intervening week was structured as an 'open' session, meeting once only, in a double-session format of up to two hours maximum (on a Friday) where the participants gave feedback on the previous module's lessons and shared personal stories (testimonies). Thus, there were a total of 3 open sessions, delivered in weeks 4, 8 and 12.

The format adopted for all the sessions was a basic interactive approach normally utilized in church Life groups: First, there are the opening formalities of salutations, prayer, and brief worship/song time. Then a leader introduces the topic of the day and gives the teaching. This is followed by a semi-structured and robust question and answer time. However, this order remains flexible enough for participants to interject at any point and ask a question or seek clarification. The song and worship time also comes again at the end of the session. It has been said, "The engine of Pentecostalism is its worship...the heart of Pentecostalism is its music."[1]

The baseline survey performed at the commencement of the LTS (N [number enrolled] = 122) was administered by research assistants and conducted simultaneously with and separate from the baseline survey for the control group (N=135). Participants in both the study and the control group were from the Makeni community. Three months later the follow-up measure was administered to the participants who completed the study (N=102) and the control group (N=114), through the same method of data collection as the initial survey.

Focus Group Discussions (FGD)

Since the targeted group for the FGDs were the existing support group of the Circle of Hope (COH) which usually meets monthly, a variation was made for them to meet bi-weekly during the period of data collection for the study. A total of 6 sessions were held, with an average attendance of 85 out of the nearly 100 registered members. The spectrum of discussions as per FGD guidelines was directly and topically related to HIV and covered subjects of health, congregation-based program perspectives, and sexual behavior. The next section is based on the results of the study. It discusses the results of the logistic regression analysis.

Overview of Results

Sexual Behavior and Practices in the Functionality of Abstinence and Marital Fidelity

Summary—Key Findings:

The results of the logistic regression analysis show that those that participated in the faith-based Life Transformation Seminars (LTS) were *4.1 times more likely* to report having adopted new behavior or modified old behavior, specifically to live positively, than those who did not attend the faith-based seminar. Similarly, those that participated in the Life Transformation faith-based Seminars were *2.3 times more likely* than those who did not participate in the seminars to report having adopted safer sexual practices. The results further reveal that those that participated in the Life Transformation seminars were *1.8 times more likely* to report abstinence from sex than those who did not attend the seminars.

In this section, *abstinence* and *marital fidelity* are considered. A look at the determinants of sexual behavior revealed by logistic regression testing shows significance that is instructive. For instance, at the baseline stage, there were no significant differences between the intervention and control groups. However, at the follow-up phase, several significant differences emerged between the two groups. Participants in the intervention group evidenced a significant change in behavior, as some reported having abstained from [non-marital] sex while others reported having significantly modified their behavior towards safer sex practices. Specifically, 26% and 51% of respondents reported having abstained from non-marital sex at baseline and follow-up, respectively. In the control group, by contrast, 74% and 49% of the respondents reported not having abstained from sex at baseline and follow-up, respectively. There was an increase in the percentage of respondents who abstained from sex in the Intervention group and a reduction in the percentage of respondents who had not abstained from sex (non-maritally) in the control group. This shows that the intervention was effective.

Findings are consistent with earlier evidence gathered through a study led by David Atkins and Deborah Kessel of Fuller Theological Seminary, who established that attendance at religious services predicts marital fidelity. The study appropriately explores how various dimensions of religious life, including prayer, closeness to God, faith, and religious activities relate to alteration of infidelity practices. Their finding is that church attendance is the particular religious factor that most protects marriages from infidelity.[2]

In the early years of efforts to combat HIV, there was a general skepticism regarding the efficacy of faith-based prevention approaches, particularly abstinence. This was largely due to a lack of documented interventions and verifiable evidence to demonstrate such efficacy. Between 2003 and 2008, financial resources from the United States of America Government through the Presidential Emergency Plan for AIDS Relief (PEPFAR) assisted in boosting FBO efforts, which resulted in the expansion of programmatic interventions with the capacity to document best practices.

The current study is among the first to seek to specifically assess the impact of specifically Pentecostal congregation-based interventions while elucidating the practical functionality of abstinence and marital fidelity. The preliminary findings suggest that scaling up these interventions holds potential for significant gains towards stemming new HIV/AIDS infections.

Further, these findings are in consonance with evidence from at least three consecutive rounds of the Zambia Demographic and Health Survey (ZDHS). A comparison of the ZDHS of 1996, 2001 and 2007 showed signs that more young people (both males and females, aged 15–19 years) delay sexual debut and remain sexually abstinent for longer than before intervention programs.[3] It is yet necessary minimally, to place this finding against the well-known historical backdrop of early apprehensions that met the promotion of abstinence (and in some cases marital fidelity), both of which approaches gradually came under intense public scrutiny and criticism, as they were repeatedly dismissed for being allegedly "non-evidence based and unrealistic." However, data demonstrate that only 12.3% of females and 16.2% of males had made a sexual debut by age 15 in 2007, compared to 22% of females and 39% of males in 1996. This reduction of 10–20% is significant and coincides with the intervention period.

This finding lends further credence to the growing body of literature published in some peer-reviewed journals showing that Abstinence and Being Faithful (A&B) behaviors, especially the latter (i.e., mutual marital fidelity, partner reduction), are among leading factors that impact HIV prevalence and incidence rates at the population level. Evidence from Uganda[4] and Kenya still ranks the strongest at present. Policy and practice must be duly informed by such evidence.[5] The significant optimism towards the ideal of sexual abstinence as a key measure for AIDS prevention in this regard is well founded.

In an in-depth analysis of data from the 2001–2002 and 2007 Demographic and Health Surveys, Kembo (2013) concluded that there had been significant changes in "selected sexual behavior and practice and HIV indicators among young people aged 15–24 years."[6] Particularizing the first indicator which dealt with *abstinence* among "never-married young men and women aged 15–24 years,"[7] Kembo explained:

> This indicator refers to the percentage of never-married young women and men aged 15–24 who have never had sex. The results presented...indicate that overall in Zambia the percentage of abstinence among never-married young men and women aged 15–24 years increased significantly by +15.2% ($p = .000$) and +5.9% ($p = .001$), respectively, between 2001–2002 and 2007. A comparison by area of residence reveals that this increase was only significant among young persons aged 15–24 years residing in urban areas as compared to their counterparts who lived in rural areas. The percentage of abstinence among never-married young men and women aged 15–24 years who resided in urban areas increased significantly by +27.1% ($p = .000$) and +9.3% ($p = .000$), respectively, from 2001–2002 to 2007.[8]

Linking his conclusions, in this respect, to programmatic implications drawn, Kembo posited that the "...delay of sexual debut among young people has been well embraced in Zambia and should continually be promoted and sustained."[9] Further, he observed that "research has shown that the delay in sexual initiation is an indispensable aspect in HIV prevention programs,"[10] adding that "promoting abstinence has been an important strategy that has led to the delay in sexual activity among young people in Zambia."[11] In the same breath, Kembo counseled aptly that "programs aimed at combating HIV and AIDS in Zambia should deliberately seek to address the higher risk of HIV infection among young women aged 15–24 years relative to their male counterparts."[12]

In the study on Uganda, Green and others compared neighboring countries such as Kenya, Ethiopia, Zambia, and Zimbabwe. They suggested that a comprehensive, behavior change-based strategy, ideally involving high-level political commitment and a diverse spectrum of community-based participation, may be the most effective prevention approach.[13]

This comparative evidence opens a window of opportunity for the global community to reprioritize sexual behavior-change interventions. This study has capitalized on that window of possibility with hope and espouses further as per Green and others summation that "According to modeling by Stoneburner and Low-Beer (2004), behavior change, particularly partner reduction, since the late 1980s in Uganda appears to have had a similar impact as a potential medical vaccine of 80% efficacy."[14]

We turn now to consider marital fidelity. In the literature review section of the study, the UK-based NGO Advert and the U.S.-based Center for Disease Control (CDC) are identified as global entities that, among many, have advocated the ABC approach towards AIDS prevention. The "B" focuses on Being Faithful to one sexual partner. In the church congregation circles, this is understood as being faithful within the context of marriage. Respondents in the intervention group evidenced a significant change of sexual behavior, directly addressing the main research question as well as the subsidiary questions.

In this study, marital fidelity is identified as a functional outcome that can contribute significantly towards curbing new HIV infections, particularly given multiple and concurrent partnerships being ranked among the six key drivers of the AIDS Epidemic in Zambia's National AIDS Strategic Framework (NASF, 2011–2015). However, what is the extent of multiple concurrencies and its related complexities?

The ZDHS (2007) found that only 12% females and 24% males surveyed believed that "most married men they know only have sex with their wives." Only 32% Females and 35% Males believed that "most married women they know only have sex with their husbands." It has been noted that multiple and concurrent sexual partnership (MCP) behaviors and extramarital affairs are "under-reported in surveys, especially by women." Reporting concurrency is also understood to be negatively affected by social desirability or self-reporting bias as per the following comment: "If I must have another girlfriend, I mustn't make it public" (Zambian male, 20–25 years).[15]

It is worth observing though that the ZDHS (2007) results showed decreases in reported multiple partner frequencies in adults with decreases in the mean number of reported partners in the past year and also decreases in frequencies of extramarital sex in Males and Females.

And in youth 15–24, there was evidence of partner reduction. Noting once again that MCP is among the six key drivers of the Zambian HIV epidemic, it remains necessary to see MCP interventions as ranking very high on the prioritization list for ethnocultural and social factors upon which to anchor long-term positive responses to reverse the current HIV trend.

As stated in the Pan African Christian AIDS Network's (PACANet) April 2010 publication on Multiple and Concurrent Sexual Partnerships:

> Epidemiological modeling suggests that even a relatively small reduction in MCPs would break up extensive sexual networks and could significantly slow the spread of HIV in the sexually active population. Various research findings have shown that having concurrent partners greatly increases HIV transmission compared to sequential or serial partnerships because new infections can spread much more rapidly through the sexual network when its members are simultaneously connected. Therefore, the ultimate goal of all HIV prevention initiatives must be to reduce HIV incidence. And to maximize prevention outcomes around MCPs, the following two outcomes need to be prioritized: A reduction in multiple and concurrent partnerships—through social and behavioral change. A reduction in the transmission of HIV within multiple and concurrent partnerships as well as within known discordant relationships [where one partner is HIV-positive and the other is HIV-negative]—including through consistent, correct use of male or female condom use.[16]

A study bearing evidence from various National Population-Based Surveys on concurrent sexual partnerships and HIV Infection established that "men are more likely than women to have multiple and concurrent sexual partnerships."[17] The study, which represents a significant attempt to call attention to the "prevalence and correlates of sexual concurrency, as well as on the association between concurrency and HIV infection at different levels of aggregation"[18] also revealed the following:

> Many multiple partnerships in the past 12 months were not concurrent and...for men, the majority of concurrent partnerships (excluding polygamous marriages) overlapped for less than one year. In the pooled samples for sub-Saharan Africa, urban, more educated, and wealthier women and men are more likely to have had concurrent partnerships than their rural, less educated, and poorer counterparts. Circumcised men are also more likely than uncircumcised men to have had concurrent partners. Women and men who had concurrent partners were more likely to use condoms than those who did not have concurrent partners;

Whatever the permutations may end up being, a key practical consideration at programmatic and intervention level is to propel initiatives towards partner reduction, as that will, in turn, minimize the risk of spiraling new infections. "Partner reduction remains the predominant explanation in Uganda's early success story of the then drastically decreased incidences."[19] In an earlier publication, titled "Partner reduction is crucial for balanced 'ABC' approach to HIV prevention," Shelton contended that "behavior change programs to prevent HIV have mainly promoted condom use or abstinence, while partner reduction remains the neglected component of ABC."[20] The study is well abstracted as follows:

> The key to preventing the spread of HIV, especially in epidemics driven mainly by heterosexual transmission, is through changing sexual behavior. Interest has been growing in an "ABC" approach in which A stands for abstinence or delay of sexual activity, B for being faithful, and C for condom use.... Although "be faithful" literally implies monogamy, it also includes reductions in casual sex and multiple sexual partnerships (and related issues of partner selection) that would reduce higher risk sex. While most of the often-polarized discussion surrounding AIDS prevention has focused on promoting abstinence or use of condoms...partner reduction has been the neglected middle child of the ABC approach.

Green *et al.* cited "lower levels of multiple partnerships and reduced sexual networks in Uganda compared to many other African countries."[21] The comparative picture is painted skillfully as follows:

> By the mid-1990s, in general, Ugandans had considerably fewer non-regular sexual partners across all age groups. Population-level sexual behavior, including the proportion of people reporting more than one partner, were comparable in Kenya (1998), Zambia (1996) and Malawi (1996), for example, to levels reported in Uganda back in 1988–1989 (Stoneburner and Low-Beer, 2004). In comparison with men in these countries, Ugandan males in 1995 were less likely to have ever had sex (in the 15–19-year-old range), more likely to be married and to keep sex within the marriage and much less likely to have multiple partners, particularly if never married. Strikingly, the proportion of men reporting three or more non-regular partners in the previous year fell from 15 to 3% between the 1989 and 1995 GPA surveys. The latter figure was identical in both that GPA survey and the 1995 Uganda DHS (Bessinger *et al*.2003)

Green rightly observed that the "reported behavioral changes [were] consistent with the dominant AIDS prevention messages of Uganda's early response (i.e., 1986–1991), specifically: "stick to one partner," and the ubiquitous "love faithfully" and "zero-grazing."[22]

Spiritually Based Ethical Change—A Pentecostal Perspective

This study has generated evidence regarding significant sexual behavior change that occurred in a wide range of key variables following attendance at the Life Transformation Seminars. The content of the material to which various respondents and participants were exposed at baseline as well as at follow-up intervention levels was deliberately designed to be consistent with the basic foundational Pentecostal biblical doctrines and social teachings. The COH model, around which the interventions were woven, evolved over time in a Pentecostal congregation, the Northmead Assembly of God Church.

It is now established increasingly in Pentecostal studies that the adoption of the Protestant moral ethic, which involves the promulgation of principles of hard work, frugality and diligence as a "constant display of a person's salvation in the Christian faith,"[23] forms a practical base for a person's morality. At the heart of any spiritual experience is an evident ethical change. Personal morality, which must be distinguished from mere social change, lies at the foundation of this prospective change.

In a review of David Martin's *Pentecostalism: The World their Parish*, Peter F. Althouse suggested, "In conversion, a personal transformation occurs in which moral relativism and self-indulgence are rejected in favor of marital faithfulness, moderation, and responsibility."[24] Martin argued:

> Pentecostal conversion contrasts helplessness with empowerment, in which people without material wealth gain equality and worth. Like Latin America, women are encouraged to participate in leadership and are encouraged to take pride in their achievements. Church offers a place to find stable husbands who are peaceable and respectful. Pentecostals are encouraged to become individuals, thereby loosening traditional family ties.[25]

The dynamic particularity herein is deeply rooted in the biblical origins of Pentecostalism which show that the very essence of the promise of the Holy Spirit by Jesus Christ, the founder of the Christian Faith, was that his disciples (then and now) as per New Testament narrative in Acts 1:8 would be spiritually empowered to effect global ethical impact.

Luke wrote: "But you will receive power when the Holy Spirit comes on you, and you will be my witnesses in Jerusalem, and in all Judea and Samaria, and to the ends of the earth." A good while before the promise in Acts, Jesus, through what has come to be known as the great commission in the gospel narrative, gave the following abiding command:

> All authority in heaven and on earth has been given to me. Therefore go and make disciples of all nations, baptizing them in the name of the Father and of the Son and

of the Holy Spirit, and teaching them to obey everything I have commanded you. And surely I am with you always, to the very end of the age (Matt 28:18–20).

The very nature of Pentecostal Mission today motivates its followers to see themselves inherently as seeking personal ethical transformation as part and parcel of daily life. This is not an additive, but rather it is an integral part of the heart of the gospel message. It derives directly from the 'manifesto' in Jesus Christ's announcement at the commencement of his earthly ministry. The ideals of this teaching are now well developed as a central part of Lucan pneumatology[26] (Luke 4:18, earlier referenced) in which Jesus announced, "the good news…and… the year of the Lord's favor."

In calling attention directly to the "good news to the poor," "freedom for the prisoners…recovery of sight to the blind and letting the oppressed go free…." Jesus made clear a new day had dawned on his hearers. Jamieson *et al.* explained that "Jesus select[ed] a passage announcing the sublime object of his whole mission, its divine character, and his special endowments for it." They noted that Jesus' message was:

> Expressed in the first person, and so singularly adapted to the first opening of the mouth in His prophetic capacity, that it seems as if made expressly for this occasion. It is from the well-known section of Isaiah's prophecies whose burden is that mysterious "SERVANT OF THE LORD," despised of man, abhorred of the nation, but before whom kings on seeing Him are to arise, and princes to worship.[27]

The nature of dynamic, personal moral change proposed here and which to this day is expressed through millions of Jesus' followers, invariably results in social and moral order. That is, at the very heart of the gospel message is the ethical agency that produces transformation.

Robert Woodberry's extensive research on *"The Missionary Roots of Liberal Democracy"* proves the significant social impact of the gospel message propagated faithfully through the efforts of early Protestant missionaries. Applying what took place then to the current norm, Woodberry's rigorous work concludes that:

> Conversionary Protestants (CPs) heavily influenced the rise and spread of stable democracy around the world. CPs were a crucial catalyst initiating the development and spread of religious liberty, mass education, mass printing, newspapers, voluntary organizations, and colonial reforms, thereby creating the conditions that made stable representative democracy more likely, regardless of whether people converted to Protestantism. Moreover, religious beliefs motivated most of these transformations. Statistically, the historical prevalence of Protestant missionaries explains about half the variation in democracy in Africa, Asia, Latin America,

and Oceania and removes the impact of most variables that dominate current statistical research about democracy. The association between Protestant missions and democracy is consistent in different continents and subsamples, and it is robust to more than 50 controls and to instrumental variable analyses.[28]

This global research empirically demonstrated the transformative power of the gospel message over a wide range of social contexts. The findings of the current Lusaka–based study reveal similar impact and therefore confirm Woodberry's conclusions, given that the interventions employed and investigated centered on the gospel message and noting particularly the significant positive changes represented by the key variables and social indicators observed from both the quantitative and qualitative results herein.

It is reasonable to conclude also that the fertile environment of congregation-based interventions nurtures potential for long-lasting transformative behavior change that positively impacts the well-being of society.

Redefining Key Populations: A Further Voice of Evidence

Implications for Global, National, and Church Policy

Nomenclatures (Key Populations: A Case of Zambia)

Learning from the Uganda case, where the rapid decline of HIV was suddenly met with charged debates regarding what really caused the decline, some attributed the trend reportedly to condom use (C) and deaths, while others pointed to abstinence (A) and particularly faithfulness (B), yet not excluding condoms.[29] Unfortunately, while the debate raged on, incidence and prevalence began to rise again. So the matter is self-evident: focus must be maintained on high impact interventions which are evidence-informed.

Policy makers have the task to do in reality what is claimed on a myriad of well-written policy documents, which may at times remain unexecuted and thereby allow the epidemic to resurge. The issue in Uganda's case was not that the debate should not have gone on. It is that precious time and focus for a given period wavered and gave way to polemics.

In Zambia's case, the lesson from Uganda would be, proverbially, to 'keep our eyes on the ball.' A policy-level discussion that nearly shifted

Zambia's attention was regarding the classification of key populations. Key populations are defined in UNAIDS terminology guidelines as:

> 'Populations at higher risk of HIV exposure' refers to those most likely to be exposed to HIV or to transmit it – their engagement is critical to a successful HIV response, i.e., they are key to the epidemic and key to the response. In all countries, key populations include people living with HIV. In most settings, men who have sex with men, transgender persons, people who inject drugs, sex workers and their clients, and sero-negative partners in sero-discordant couples are at higher risk of HIV exposure to HIV than other people.[30]

The definition of "key populations" is very important.[31] However, in reality, some funders often appear to narrow it down to men having sex with men, sex workers and their clients, transgender persons and people who inject drugs. In most parts of Africa, this approach stirs up much controversy when it comes to funding proposals for the national response and what the programmatic priorities should look like.

It ought to be stated clearly that the HIV response simply cannot be reduced to nomenclatures and terminologies. Defined terms like *key populations* ought to be understood directly in the context of what is detailed and dictated by the nature and progression of the epidemic. The question to be asked in the case of key populations is, *who* or *what* is the particular population that is key to a given epidemic? Nationals of many affected countries would prefer more holistic attention given in reality by donor governments and other international entities to nationally prioritized aspects of the response. As these international actors work to reverse the devastating impact of the HIV pandemic, it is the contextual peculiarities that require prioritization rather than controverted and sometimes merely polemical matters.

In 2013–14, Zambia was engaged in a national exercise led by the National AIDS Council (NAC) to revise its National AIDS Strategic Framework. NAC seized the opportunity also to draw up a funding proposal to the Global Fund under a new funding model dubbed the 'Investment case.' Zambia rightly elected to optimize the opportunity in order to re-identify interventions with potential for highest impact in the HIV response.

A review of any document requires consultations at various levels, including sub-national structures in the urban and rural areas. For a process of this nature, the consultations involve engagement with international cooperating partners and donor representatives, civil society and churches.

It emerged in due course that the matter of "key populations" was regularly featuring in many of the stakeholder discussions related to the said NASF review process. In the majority of cases, representatives of international funding agencies would raise the matter. In one instance, a named representative stormed out of a meeting in protest, as Zambia was now seeking to redefine its own understanding of key populations, which appeared to be in slight variance with the conventional definition.

With the protest walk-out came verbal cautioning that Zambia risked losing the bid to have additional funding from the Global Fund, particularly if (in the view of the said official) it did not 'address key populations.' However, that is precisely what often begs the question. How does an attempt by a national task team to seek re-alignment of its HIV response based on its known local epidemiology, receive such a charged reaction from an international policy maker?

Being that it was an important policy matter, the author, then chairperson of the National AIDS Council, undertook a frank discussion with the NAC Board that eventually resulted in a redefinition of 'key populations,' tailored to Zambia's context of the epidemic. The relevant section of the R-NASF (2014–16) reads as follows:

> Zambia has prioritized implementation of High Impact Interventions focusing on reaching key populations as part of its strategy to reduce new infections and improve the life expectancy of PLHIV. The country, through NAC Council in 2014, has defined key populations as: People living with HIV; Women and children; Adolescents (10–14); Young people (15–24); People with disabilities; Prisoners; Sex workers and their clients; and Migrant and mobile populations. The expanded list is a deliberate attempt by Zambia to ensure that populations with historical and disproportionate lack of service access are identified and considered for programming.[32]

In the context of this research, the counsel to policymakers is to stay true to policies that are evidence informed. The full range of high-impact interventions yielding notable results must continue to be prioritized. A multi-sectoral response must, in reality, take into account all players on the ground, and Zambia has a wealth of well-organized and energized civil-society players as well as churches.

How Zambia's prioritization of key populations is addressed in the R-NASF (2011–2016):

Option B+:

1. These individuals are identified at all antenatal clinics where HTC is conducted during the booking visit (first visit). In facilities where ART is provided, these identified individuals will receive ART; otherwise, they will be referred to the nearest ART-providing facility (pre-existing ART facility or PMTCT facility that have been mandated to provide ART).

2. The individuals will receive support from networks of people living with HIV and AIDS, community health workers and Safe Motherhood Action Groups (SMAGs);

Discordance:

Couples counseling and testing is the mainstay strategy of Zambia's HTC guidelines and through this approach discordancy is identified at all HIV testing facilities and the HIV-positive partner is linked to care and the provision of ART under the 2013 guidelines;

Children (0–14):

The 2013 guidelines provide for all HIV-positive children to receive ART regardless of CD4 count; and,

All members of key populations who qualify for ART provision receive access to ART irrespective of their status or inclination.

Conclusion – Policy Implication

Global policymakers and national and religious leaders must heed the HIV crisis' call for action. In doing so, the epidemiology of the disease must instruct all concerned. Evidence must inform all policy efforts sustainably. And what do we know? We know that incidence is dropping quite rapidly in some parts of the nations affected. We know that essentially, if for argument's sake, HIV prevalence as well is averaging 7% in the Sub-Saharan region,[33] then we must agree that it means approximately 93% of the persons in these regions are HIV negative. A large priority in the fight against HIV, then, must be the prevention of its spread into 93%. Towards that goal, there is a growing body of literature published in peer-reviewed journals and some cases even just anecdotal evidence, showing that "abstinence and being faithful (A&B) behaviors, especially the latter (i.e., mutual marital fidelity, partner reduction)" are precisely among leading factors that impact HIV prevalence and the rate of new occurrences, at the population level.[34]

It is apparent that the biases against faith-based behavioral options still abide, despite the growing body of evidence that behavior change is central to winning the fight against HIV. The danger with labels and stereotypes is that they tend to belittle, howbeit indirectly, some of the available epidemiological evidence favoring behavior change approaches to AIDS prevention. Instead, the evident biases perpetuate a subtle, institutionalized stigma against prevention efforts and general programmatic strategies that may appear to be unconventional.

Necessarily, several questions arise: Could it be that time has possibly come for Western governments, in particular, to look afresh at the evidence being generated from Africa? Could it be that there is indeed a moral norm that might be rightly acceptable to societies in the global South, where, in Africa, "roughly nine out of ten people say religion is very important in their lives?"[35] Indeed, in Sub-Sahara Africa, where AIDS is highest, face-to-face interviews with 25,000 Africans confirmed, "Africans [are] devout and morally conservative."[36] Epidemiology and evidence-based preventions and interventions match with each other, then, and also with the culture of Africa.

Thus, there is need for a paradigm shift[37] in order for actions to refocus on "prevention and behavioral AB efforts,"[38] and there is need to note evidence of studies showing that "the trend in Africa is towards higher levels of monogamy and fidelity, and it is [likely] that HIV [infections] trend will eventually be downward."[39] This is good news!

And this is a call for all to hold hands and raise one banner: an HIV free global village at all costs!

11.

A Transformational Work of the Holy Spirit For Freedom from Gender Inequality In Nepal

Bal Krishna Sharma and Karuna Sharma

Abstract

Known for its natural beauty and religious plurality, Nepal is influenced by several socioeconomic and religious structures, including strong sexual discrimination. This creates disparity among the Nepalese that impacts them both individually and collectively in every aspect of their lives.

Discrimination against women causes religious suppression, economic imbalance, social inequality, and gender violence and injustice. Women are considered deeply inferior to men and, based on this, women are deprived of education, religious activities, and the freedom to make choices. From childhood till they become old, women are under the supervision of father, husband, and son. Even before she is born, a girl is branded as inferior. This is because according to Hindu philosophy, the birth of a son is regarded as opening the door to heaven or getting salvation; there is no corollary blessing associated with the birth of a daughter. This creates havoc in women's lives, physically, psychologically, and socially. Not having the privilege to freely participate in society as men do, women experience isolation and rejection. They experience low self-esteem, fear, shame, and inferiority, and this affects them both individually and as a group.

A transformational encounter with the Holy Spirit brings freedom and peace. Women facing gender discrimination and violence experience transformed lives as they respond to him. The Holy Spirit's empowering love brings inner healing to suppressed emotional pain. The Holy Spirit gives women freedom and a place in the community, which is a testimony of victory. Thus, the work of the Holy Spirit in transforming the individual and community is absolutely vital in the mission of God.

Nepal: Setting the Context

Nepal is an independent state in South Asia. A country of nearly thirty million people, it is bordered by two great neighbors: China in the north and India in the south, east, and west. The population of Nepal shows both Indo-Aryan and Mongoloid strains. Their blending, long history, culture, and civilization have shaped the character of the population.

A multi-ethnic nation, Nepal has more than 125 different languages and cultures, and several major religions. The religions include Hinduism, Buddhism, Animism, and Islam. Christianity is growing, but it is still not fully recognized by the government. Indeed, Christianity in Nepal is a persecuted religion.

Nepal was ruled by a monarchy or dynasty for centuries. In the middle of the twentieth century, that began to slowly and unevenly change. From 1960 to 1990 the king, an absolute monarch banned the fledgling multiparty democratic system that had been introduced a dozen years earlier. During the 1990s there was a revolution, and the ban on the multiparty system was relaxed. People then had a very high expectation of democracy; everyone believing their situation would magically change.

So far people have not had many of their expectations fulfilled. Citizens affiliate with various parties and some of the extreme parties have taken the way of violence. The political situation in Nepal is very unstable, and the government is not able to provide security to its citizens. Many live in fear and anxiety. The present political situation also highlights the gross neglect of political courtesy between the various parties. It seems the parties are there to pull down and fight one another. The political situation in Nepal is a threat to the norms of democracy. People feel that the principle of democracy is good, but those who are given the responsibility to implement the democratic principles are not mature people.

The earliest Christian contact with the land of Nepal took place in 1662 AD when Italian priests passed through Nepal en route to Tibet. The priests returned home and encouraged evangelization in the areas they had just been. In response, in 1703 the Roman Catholic Church assigned the Capuchin fathers to evangelize in North India, Nepal, and Tibet. These priests made their base at Patna in India, and several came to work in the Kathmandu Valley of Nepal, where they made converts for nearly 70 years. During a monarchy change in 1768, the priests and Christians were expelled, accused of being agents of European colonial power. For the next 200 years, a firm Nepalese policy excluded all foreigners and Christians.

As political changes began to occur around 1950, small congregations started to emerge in various parts of Nepal. Some of the earliest congregations were established in Nepalganj, Pokhara, and Kathmandu.

In the 1950s and '60s, only a handful of Christians were found in Nepal. During the 1970s churches began to grow in various regions. Christians were not allowed to preach, and conversion to Christianity was prohibited. The Nepalese law stated that conversion to Christianity meant one-year imprisonment for the convert, three-year imprisonment for the preacher, and six-year imprisonment for the one who baptizes. From 1960 until 1990 such laws were in effect and many Christians were imprisoned because of their faith, including severe persecution during the '80s. In 1990, after pressure by pro-democracy groups, the king lifted the 30-year ban on the multiparty system and soon afterward proclaimed a new constitution, with himself as a constitutional monarch and democracy as the new form of government. At that time, the church officially began to experience some freedom. However, the unofficial attitude of the government toward Christians remains the same. In some places, there are still arrests. Christians have been imprisoned. The government does not acknowledge a Christian presence, and it does not register Christian churches and organizations.

In spite of all these pressures, the church in Nepal is growing. There are small and large congregations all over the country. The church faces a significant challenge to witness to its neighbors and also to disciple its converts and develop quality leadership. Developing ministerial courtesy among the new churches and denominations is another challenge the Nepali church faces. There is a genuine concern among some of the leadership that in order to establish God's kingdom in Nepal we need to work together. Our united effort will convey a better message than our many single efforts. This does not mean we need to be uniform in everything we do. We need to have the unity of the Spirit. Our primary motive should be to establish the kingdom of God.

Human Sexuality in Nepal

About 85% of the population is rural. The literacy rate is 75% percent for males, but only about 45% for females. This—the availability of information/knowledge, and the discrepancy between males' and females' access to it—impacts the sense of personal power and power dynamics within couples, which impacts expressions and experiences of human sexuality. In addition, the social order in Nepal, both public and private, is organized along patriarchal lines: the dominant person in the relationship holds the decision-making power and respect. Samira Luitel says, "The Nepalese social system is based on patriarchal Hindu philosophy that empowers men and subordinates women. Women are weak and dependent on men and derive from men their social status."[1] This patriarchal system has evolved under Hindu customs and traditions over centuries. As a result, even though Nepal has modernized in some ways, it has failed to remove many of the barriers caused by sex discrimination and gender-based inequalities. Women play multiple roles that benefit the family, yet most do not receive the freedom to make any family decisions. Women are also socially and religiously deprived, which affects their entire personality, self-confidence, self-efficacy, and self-determination.

This chapter is not denying the contributions of the few Nepalese women who have gained positions of leadership in various fields. For example, women have recently achieved representation in constitution-making, especially in the first Constituent Assembly (CA). The second CA finalized the new Constitution in 2015, and soon after, Nepal's first female President and Speaker of the House of Representatives were elected.[2] Further, the nation declared 2016 as the Year of Women Empowerment. Yes, some women are playing crucial roles in building the nation. However, the number of women thus involved is still minimal. Most of Nepal still operates as if women are inferior. This gender bias creates intra- and interpersonal chaos, impacting the individual, family, and society, and bringing disputes and dissatisfaction in family relationships across much of Nepal.

Gender Difference in Nepal

In Nepal, a woman's sexuality is considered inferior to that of a man. Women are viewed as subservient and their bodies impure. Religiously, the *Tij* Festival and *Rishi Panchami* are widely practiced by the women of Nepal. Traditionally, these festivals require fasting, without drinking even water, for the forgiveness of women's "sins and bodily impurity." Women are truly seen as property, and men the rightful property owners.

Sexuality has become a powerful tool of patriarchy for controlling and subjugating women. It is said, "In a patriarchal society like Nepal, sexual behavior affects the entire life of a person. The dignity of a person in a society is based on his or her ability or disability to maintain the sexual behavior or norms of sexuality as expected by his or her community."[3] Thus, women are considered as an object sexually, as in other ways. They are not respected in society and have become a target of control and subjugation by men.

On the other hand, society seeks to control the sexual behavior of both men and women, as social construction plays a crucial role in maintaining the power dynamics of masculinity and femininity. Sexual behavior affects the entire life of a person because the dignity of a person is based in part on his or her ability to maintain the sexual norms of the community.[4] Sexuality is influenced by the interaction of biological, psychological, social, economic, political, cultural, ethical, legal, historical, religious and spiritual factors.[5] Women are still, to this day, considered impure. They are not even given proper education, including on subjects regarding reproduction or women's health. In a few cases when women have received an education of any kind, the traditional culture has not been noticeably impacted. Educated women face much the same oppression as women who have not received any schooling.[6]

The practice of rejoicing at the birth of a son and lamenting at the birth of a daughter is common in many communities. Women who have many sons enjoy some status in the family, whereas women having more daughters are placed in a lower status. According to Hindu philosophy, the birth of a son is regarded as opening the door to heaven or getting salvation. The son is called *putra* meaning one who brings out the ancestor from the ditch. Therefore, in order to acquire salvation, a son is necessary. Such religious beliefs compel people to value having sons rather than daughters. Nepal being a patriarchal society also means that a son inherits his parents' property, whereas a daughter goes to her husband's house. This practice discriminates against girls and women. When women do not share equal rights in property and other privileges, gender discrimination is intact. The value system of society thus strengthens discrimination against women.

Women face discrimination, familial bullying, and domestic violence. They can be subjected to restrictions and abuses that they don't believe they can combat.[7] Violence against women is defined broadly as "any act of gender-based violence that results in, or is likely to result in, physical, sexual or psychological harm or suffering to women, including threats of such acts, coercion or deprivation of liberty."[8] It encompasses physical and sexual abuse perpetrated against a woman or female child by persons known or unknown to her, such as spouses, partners, boyfriends, fathers, brothers or strangers.[9]

Deprivation of Women in Various Sectors in Nepal

Religious

From the early centuries, religious beliefs and practices assigned a low status to women, bringing discrimination. Caste and inequalities are still prevalent in Nepal, which leads to social exclusion for individuals in lower castes and ethnic groups, making them high-risk groups.[10] The view of women being impure dates back to the ancient period. Women are deprived of taking part in various religious ceremonies. On certain days (during the menstrual period), women are considered impure and are not allowed to get involved in daily chores. They are not even allowed to enter into their *puja ghar* (worship center), because it is assumed that their impurities will defile the holy place. Thus, women are kept aside from religious activities such as entering *puja ghar* temples and taking part in important religious functions.

In some places in Nepal during the time of menstruation and child delivery, women are considered impure, so they are kept outside of the house in a secluded place known as *chhaupadi*. Though there are attempts to eradicate such practices, these attempts have not yet been entirely successful. This practice of *chhaupadi*, found mainly in mid and far western Nepal, isolates and separates women from others in many spheres of their daily life. In this tradition, women are not allowed to enter their houses, touch other persons, cattle, vegetables, or plants during menstruation, nor are they allowed to drink milk products. They generally stay in separate hut or cattle shed for five days and are allowed to use only *chhaupadi dhara* (a separate well or stream). It is believed that if anyone violates the practice of *chhaupadi*, the god and goddess will be angered and give them shorter life, the death of livestock and destruction of crops.[11] Women feel discriminated by practices such as *chhaupadi*, restriction from entering the temple or speaking aloud, and being completely dependent on male power.

Social

Socially, male members of the family enjoy first right in all religious and cultural functions.[12] There is a saying that a woman is always under the control of a man: during childhood, she is under her father; after marriage, she is under her husband; and after having children she is under her son. She is dependent on males and does not have any power to choose. Low economic and social status make women more vulnerable to domestic abuse. The constant pressure to produce a male child, shame for having a girl, and exhaustion from multiple childbirths have a negative impact on women's psychological health.[13] Child marriage is another social custom which affects the system of society. In Nepal, early marriage remains a persistent problem that affects children, particularly girls, highly.[14] In rural Nepal, whether in hills or plains, child marriage is still very much practiced. Once the girl child is married, there is no opportunity for her education, and early childbearing brings many physical, financial and emotional difficulties.

Education

The first education system in Nepal was only available to elite families. Women are deprived of education. The belief that "women who get education become witches" made many think twice before getting an education. This, as a result, affected the lifestyle of women. According to the Nepal Living Standards Survey (NLSS-III 2010-2011), the female literacy rate in Nepal is 44.5%.[15] Many Nepalese still consider women as backward, despite the government introducing several rules, regulations, plans, and policies to increase women's empowerment and literacy rate. Daughters are considered to be someone else's property because they will get married and eventually go to their husband's house. For this reason, women are not encouraged to get an education; rather, they are made to do the housework in addition to taking care of their younger siblings. UNESCO has identified two main challenges for the educational sector, namely access to (secondary) education in general and for girls in particular, as well as the quality of the education.[16]

Health

The health status of women remains lower. The book, *Contemporary Nepal*, citing the report of Nepal Fertility Family Planning and Health Survey (NFPH), states that 78% of girls in Nepal get married when they are 10 to 19 years old, and early pregnancy is prevalent. They are prone to pregnancy complications which hinder fertility, mortality, morbidity, and undesirable health status.[17] The legal age of marriage is 20, for both men and women.

Economic

Women in Nepal share a much lower economic status than men. Women are major labor contributors in agriculture, mostly without pay. In addition, they have the primary responsibility in household chores, also without pay.[18] Even though Nepal is now giving importance to women's empowerment, yet many people are still deprived of opportunities. Women have less access to property, income, inheritance, and credit and often have little control over their own or the household's earnings.[19] Women are less educated and more likely to be engaged in non-skilled work, rather than be employed in better paid professional, technical and management related jobs. Poverty is one of the major causes of indifference about gender. Because of poverty, many women struggle due to hunger. Taking care of the whole family and meeting their needs leads many to live in poverty. Secondly, due to poverty, women are not receiving the right education and opportunities to improve. Even the parents of a girl child think that spending money on a girl child is a waste, as she will get married and go to another's house. Therefore, education is not given importance. A girl child is taught household chores from childhood. Girls are kept in charge of taking care of their younger brothers and sisters.

The above discussion reflects the situation of Nepalese women in particular, though women in other nations experience gender disparity also. Gender issues are real, and they need to be addressed. How the Holy Spirit can bring freedom to women in Nepali society is something we need to discuss.

As stated earlier, Nepali society did not have the opportunity to hear the gospel of Christ until 1950. The gospel of Christ has restored the dignity of humanity in general and women in particular. Caste-ridden society in Nepal has been experiencing discrimination and humiliation in their lower caste status. Even ethnic groups from the upper castes have faced such discrimination. But discriminated groups have found dignity and acceptance in the Christian community. Let me describe a short case study that portrays what I am trying to communicate.

Case Study of Transformation

Rama Tharu comes from a downtrodden society. She and her family members live in a village, and they have a small plot of land and some cattle. They toil day and night for their survival. People in their community have alcohol-drinking habits, and they spend their limited grains to make alcohol. They drink alcohol almost daily. They have developed the perception that if they do not drink, they cannot work in their field. Therefore, Rama's husband also became a habitual drinker, and eventually an alcoholic. This drinking habit ruined the lives of the family. Her husband started abusing her verbally and physically. There were misunderstandings and arguments almost every day, which affected their relationship as husband and wife. Rama started feeling sick because of malnutrition. Moreover, she always felt humiliated and left behind. Her voice was silent; she was unable to protect herself against her husband and his cruel behavior.

One day, Rama heard the good news from one Christian believer. She accepted Christ and was healed from her sickness. She was relieved from her burden and felt the touch of God in a miraculous way. She was completely transformed and renewed, and she experienced peace and joy for the first time. Despite struggle and pain in life, she never gave up in her life, and she received inner healing. Both her soul and her body were healed. Seeing her changed life, the husband and household accepted Christ as their Savior. The life of Rama has become an inspiration to many, as people have seen the light of God reflected through her life.

Rama's husband received short-term Bible training after coming to believe in Christ, and he was then called to the ministry. He began to pioneer a church. Since their whole household became believers, they started a worship service in their home. People from the village began to attend the church service. There was a prayer for sick people every week after the church service. The presence of the Holy Spirit was real in church service, and when they prayed for the sick, they were healed. Many demon-possessed people were brought to the church, and they were delivered. The church began to grow. Those who were healed or delivered were given the simple message of salvation that Jesus heals and also gives salvation from the bondage of sin. Many of them accepted Christ and went back to their villages. Those people were visited in their own houses during weekdays.

In 2015 during Christmas time I visited that place for a revival meeting. I was asked to preach in that three-day revival meeting. There were about 600 Christians and 300 non-Christians. The work of the Holy Spirit was evident in the meeting. There was healing and deliverance. Non-Christians asked for prayers, and they accepted Christ. This church, which began with the life-changing experience of Rama and her family members, has planted 15 other churches in that region in 15 years. I asked a pastor of one of those churches about the growth of the Church in the area and the impact that Christianity has made there. He told the story: This pastor's family had 50 family members. They never sent their children to school. They worked in the field and drank a lot of alcohol. They felt always oppressed by demonic forces. Many people in his home and community were possessed by demons. They used witchdoctors for deliverance and spent so much for such treatment. Once people began to believe in Christ, they were healed and delivered from evil spirits. They were taught in the church to study God's word, the Bible, and that gave orientation to the parents to send their children to school. Since they stopped drinking alcohol, they were able to save money and use it for their children's education and for other needs. The work of the Holy Spirit brought a great transformation in their society. When I was there, I met a secondary school head-teacher. He has been in the community since last 15 years. He is a Hindu Brahmin. I asked him about the change in that community since he has been there. He said that there has been a great change. Earlier he had to go to homes to ask parents to send their children to school, and they would not send them. When the church began to grow, and people became Christians now, all the children from the village go to school. Christian children are far better in studies than others. He said the gospel has changed them.

The above short case study reveals that the Holy Spirit is at work in the lives of people to bring change. A story that began with one woman brought change to an entire family and community. More than 65% of people in the church are women, and they have great potential for gospel work if we can empower them. The Holy Spirit can use women to bring change in family, society, and nation. I could recite many cases that show how the Holy Spirit has used the gospel to bring transformation in society, to both female and male.

Psychological

Though this case study shows how the Holy Spirit can change an individual and a community, the need in Nepal is still enormous, as Nepali society struggles for freedom and gender equality. There are many organizations working for gender equality and social transformation, but the overall result is still minimal. Women are not yet empowered to make decisions and stand on their own feet. They are still not able to live a life of freedom. They are discriminated against, abandoned, and dominated in society. This has a profound impact psychologically as well as practically.

Why are women not able to stand on their feet and how does their patriarchal society dominate them? Women are trapped within their abusive situations both physically and emotionally. A culture of silence makes women unable to speak about the violence they suffer at home and in society, and it leads to the severe psychological consequences of depression and anxiety disorders. Facing barriers in social, family, religious and economic life creates low self-esteem, fear, and anxiety within women who live in difficult situations. Women who experience harm and sadness or trauma because of gender differences continue to carry within themselves the injury by suppressing their pain. Feelings of rejection, guilt, dissatisfaction, and inferiority severely impact their intrapersonal and interpersonal relationships.

Human beings are created by God in his image. They have the unique character of God, without any discrimination or bias. God was concerned for all of humanity; therefore, he did not create woman as an inferior being, but rather created her in his image and gave her the same breath to live as he gave man. Even though God's purpose of creating men and women is thus clear, today women—created in God's image–are tragically considered impure and inferior in Nepal and other regions of the world. The power of decision is withheld from them, as well as the freedom to stand, in their patriarchal society. They are subordinated in the family, society, and nation of Nepal. From childhood, they are looked down upon and discriminated against by family members, neighbors, relatives, and society. Even providing education and health care for girls is not valued, because girls are not seen as important members of the family. Indeed, as discussed earlier, girls are viewed as property, and someone else's property, at that (their future husband's). Girls receive into their psyches and personalities the low value placed on them by their families and communities. They never rebel against the pervasive discrimination against them; rather they suppress those events in their unconscious mind.

Sigmund Freud developed the idea of unconscious believing; that is, the unconscious is made up of repressed and forgotten material of the individual. Carl Jung developed the idea that, along with the personal unconscious, which is filled with personal memories and sorrows, there is also another dimension to the unconscious called the 'Collective Unconscious.' According to the Meriam Webster Dictionary, "unconscious" means not knowing or perceiving, not aware. In other words, the unconscious is not marked by conscious thought, sensation or feeling.[20] It is viewed as the shadow of a 'real' conscious mind.[21]

The collective unconscious is the most powerful and influential system of the psyche and, in pathological cases, overshadows the ego and the personal unconscious.[22] Jung believed that a person has several parts, including thoughts, ideas, feelings, memories, and sensory perceptions. Some of these are remembered by the conscious mind. Others may be consciously forgotten or rendered unimportant. But others may be repressed in the unconscious due to trauma. The hurts and traumas which have been suppressed in the unconscious mind are very important for a person to release.

It is through the gift and power of the Spirit that all pain and hurts and feelings of low self-esteem can be removed. The person can receive feelings of adaptation, love, peace, and joy. Therefore, a person who receives a full experience of God and accepts the gift of the Holy Spirit can be helped to truly forgive others and make reconciliation, which is a vital part of his or her healing. The Holy Spirit can change, channel and transform our lives, so that Christ will be visible through our lives, from the inside out.

Many women in Nepal have lost their husbands or sons and daughters during ten years of Maoist war. These women are hurt, and resentment harbors inside them against the perpetrator of their harm. There is trauma lodged deep within them. How can such hurts be healed, so these women are free to live a life unfettered by resentment? This is a question that must be addressed. Resentment and revenge are so strong in Nepali society that they destroy human personalities. We as Christians have responsibilities to address these issues from God's perspective. The work of the Holy Spirit is crucial to bring healing and reconciliation within the individual, family, community, and nation.

The Holy Spirit: Towards Freedom and Equality

The Holy Spirit is helping human beings experience freedom and equality. The Spirit applies Christ's work of reconciliation through fellowship with him and gives us as Christians the assurance to know that we are children of God.[23] The mission of the Holy Spirit is to transform one into the image of God[24] and bring reconciliation in relationships between self and God, self, and others, and self with self. The Holy Spirit brings victory over bondage and allows one to experience inner healing and freedom. As Millard J. Erickson said, "Jesus taught that the Spirit's activity is essential in both conversion, which from our perspective is the beginning of the Christian life, and regeneration, which from God's perspective is its beginning."[25] The Spirit empowers, teaches, indwells, intercedes, sanctifies and helps in the continued transformation of moral and spiritual character. He works supernaturally through direct influence, renewing the sinner's capacities. The Holy Spirit convicts a person of his or her wrongdoings and convinces them to do what is right in the sight of God. Divine intervention is required for genuine change, and God through the Holy Spirit does this.

The work of the Holy Spirit in Nepal is very evident from the inception of Christianity in Nepal in the early 1950s. I have already written about Pentecostalism in Nepal elsewhere.[26] Nepalese Christianity is Pentecostal/Charismatic in nature, and it is still growing. Pentecostals in Nepal allow women ministers in the churches, and the Assemblies of God denomination has ordained women pastors. These women pastors help preach and lead the church.

The work of the Holy Spirit is evident in church and special meetings. I have been involved in such meetings since 1981, and I have seen a tremendous change in the lives of people. I remember the youth meeting we began in 1983 where about 90 young people attended, including all pastors and leaders. Because the government prohibited meetings inside Nepal at that time, we traveled about 500 km from the capital Kathmandu to participate in that meeting. Now, every year we have about 15,000 young people attending such youth meetings every year.

The work of the Holy Spirit is very evident in the lives of young people. Deliverance and the baptism of the Holy Spirit is experienced by young people. Both physical and inner healing is part of the meeting. The Holy Spirit is at work in the lives of people.

The work of the Holy Spirit needs to be given due place in our lives and churches so that we will be used of him to bring a change in our communities. The mission we are involved in is not a human enterprise. It is God's work, and God fulfills his work through his Spirit.

The Nepali church has become a community where the total healing work of the Holy Spirit is taught, sought and experienced. As seen in the case study above, the infilling work of the Holy Spirit is touching many hearts and bringing transformation. On many occasions, women who struggle within themselves due to ill feelings, pain, and misunderstanding are able to pour out their hurt after experiencing a personal encounter with the Holy Spirit. In this way, the Holy Spirit and his empowering love bring relief, inner healing, and transformation to women who experienced injuries from gender discrimination, with all the painful feelings that result.

Churches can offer holistic transformation to the lives of people even in the midst of differences. The Church as the body of Christ can offer effective healing for people who are deeply hurting and have lost hope. The Church can help and give healing to a person through worship, encouragement, helping to identify the problems, and supporting participation in the community. Healing is a pastoral function that aims to overcome some impairment by restoring a person to wholeness and by leading him/her to advance beyond his/her previous condition.[27]

According to L. K. Graham, "Healing is the process of being restored to bodily wholeness, emotional well-being, mental functioning, and spiritual aliveness."[28] The Church has been placed in the world today in order to be a healing and restoring community. If the Church does not take the responsibility to heal society through the power of the Holy Spirit, then there is no sign of its presence in the world. Therefore, let us ask the Holy Spirit to empower us so that we will be able to help others find their identity in God through the Holy Spirit and be fruitful in God's kingdom. There is a great need for churches to acknowledge and address the issue of gender differences, because Nepali churches have more females in their congregations than men, and many of these women still encounter difficult situations and have not received complete deliverance. Many have been collecting past events of discrimination, hatred, guilt, torture, and abuse, and suppressing them in their unconscious mind, which bars them from complete liberty. Therefore, the church can help these women to understand the love of God and seek the presence of Holy Spirit so that they can be renewed, revived and transformed and have a completely new life in Christ Jesus. This is a deep process.

Conclusion

This study has reported how the Holy Spirit is active in bringing transformation in individuals, families, and societies. God created human beings in His own image, both male and female, and he gave them abilities and dignities so that they live and work together. The Holy Spirit has come in order to lift up those who are downtrodden and who are seeking freedom and dignity. Women facing deprivation in various aspects of their lives need freedom and inner healing. Therefore, the church as an agent of a healing community can bring transformation in the lives of those who need a cure from their pain, low self-esteem, shame, and sense of inferiority. This occurs through the work of Holy Spirit—a counselor, comforter, redeemer, guide, and healer.

12.

Holy Sex: A Sermon

William Wilson

Abstract

The Bible contains passages that are very clear about human sexuality.[1] We will look at some of those. In addition, it is very important to clearly state that God likes sex! There are many challenges in our day to a healthy expression of sexuality, but we will see that there were many challenges to healthy sexuality during Bible times, too. God gives us his help to face those challenges; he gives clear boundaries to protect us and to protect the amazing gift of sex; and he gives instructions on the proper context for sex. We find that following his guidance leads to delight. Where we fail, we experience shame, but he invites us into the redemption that he provides through Christ.

Introduction

That is why a man leaves his father and mother and is united to his wife, and they become one flesh. Adam and his wife were both naked, and they felt no shame (Gen 2:24–25).[2]

Then the eyes of both of them were opened, and they realized they were naked; so they sewed fig leaves together and made coverings for themselves (Gen 3:7).

It is God's will that you should be sanctified: that you should avoid sexual immorality; that each of you should learn to control your own body in a way that is holy and honorable, not in passionate lust like the pagans, who do not know God; and that in this matter no one should wrong or take advantage of a brother or sister. The Lord will punish all those who commit such sins, as we told you and warned you before. For God did not call us to be impure, but to live a holy life (1 Thess 4:3–7).

Honor marriage and guard the sacredness of sexual intimacy between wife and husband. God draws a firm line against casual and illicit sex (Heb 13:4 msg).

The issue of human sexuality is one of the most volatile issues of our time, politicized and polarized in extreme ways around the globe including here in America. My heart in this communication is not to attack or denigrate anyone, and most certainly not to hurt anyone. I love our students with all my heart, and I love all those who will take in these words. It seems to me that, given the current climate around this issue, it would be impossible to speak on this subject without creating some diverse energy. Yet, because this area of a young adult's life is so challenging and so volatile, it also is impossible to talk about holy living in the twenty-first century without addressing sexuality. At Oral Roberts University (ORU), we believe in addressing human sexuality and gender issues with pastoral concern and redemptive hospitality, because our overarching goal is always healing and wellness of the whole person and the fulfilling of God's ultimate purpose for humanity.

Let me state at the beginning that God likes sex. God created sex; he believes in sex; he ordained sex. Holy sex, or sex within God's parameters, is an amazing gift from God. I also want to say that reclaiming the sanctity of sex will not be easy in our current cultural climate, but it is possible by God's grace and the authority of God's word.

A cursory reading of scripture immediately reveals that human sexuality is a powerful force—either a force for good through procreation, marital bonding, and human fulfillment; or a force for destruction through abuse, adultery, fornication, and corrupted lives. Your personal choices will determine whether your sexuality will be a force for good or a force for destruction in your life. Sexual passion is like fire: when captured, guided, and controlled, it is an awesome force for good. But when unleashed, misguided, and uncontrolled, it is a horrific force of destruction.

Challenges in Our Time

Many factors have made human sexuality a huge issue for young adults over the last two generations. One of those factors is the increasing time between puberty and marriage. People enter puberty earlier and marry later. German studies found that in 1860, the average age of the onset of puberty in girls was 16.6 years. In 1920, it was 14.6; in 1950, 13.1; 1980, 12.5; and in 2010, it had dropped to 10.5. Similar sets of figures have been reported for boys, albeit with a delay of around a year.[3] And yet, at the same time, the average age for Americans getting married has reached a historic high: 27 for women and 29 for men. This is a jump from the 1990 average marrying-age of 23 for women and 26 for men.[4]

Another factor is the sexualization of Western culture. Sexual messages surround us every day. The sexual revolution of the 1960s brought to the front pages what had been kept mostly in the bedroom, from drug ads for sexual dysfunction to unabashed reporting of topics thought taboo only 25 years previously to the intentional focused efforts by minority groups in convincing an entire generation of the normality of alternate sexual lifestyles. We are surrounded every day by messages of sexuality, and most of them are not based on God's view of sexuality. This creates significant pressure for the Christian believer against Biblical perspectives on sexuality.

There is also the growth of pornography as an industry. The word pornography, derived from the Greek *porni* ("prostitute") and *graphein* ("to write"), was originally defined as any work of art or literature depicting the life of prostitutes.[5] It is also the same root word as *porneúō*, which means "to commit fornication" (sexual immorality). Although polls show that Americans' views on pornography are drifting towards greater acceptance of it,[6] even a quick look at the meaning of "pornography" suggests its use is not harmless. Yet, CNBC has estimated that pornography is a $13 billion a year industry in the USA alone.[7]

Another challenging factor, and one that overlaps with pornography, is the proliferation of media and the internet. Media is available 24/7 to children and adults alike. The average age of people first seeing pornography online is 11.[8] The use of the internet often involves being overexposed for a long period of time, creating a significant space where messages about sexuality are confusing.

Add all these factors together with living in close community on a college campus among a few thousand young adults whose testosterone and estrogen are at their lifetime peaks, and you can understand the challenges any college student faces in this area.

Yet, it is important to note that while today's Western world is full of deceptive sexual messages, we are not the only generation of people who have been called to live holy in an overly sexualized, pornographic culture. In fact, there are many instances in scripture where this was the case as well.

Challenges in Bible Times

Corinth

Corinth was a coastal city where sailors came to port and where prostitutes from the temple on the acropolis overlooking the city made their living. Filled with sexual immorality and a place where sexual promiscuity and experimentation were normalized—that is to say, living in a sexualized culture—Corinthian believers needed help knowing how to respond.

Paul shared with these believers, "Or do you not know that wrongdoers will not inherit the kingdom of God? Do not be deceived: Neither the sexually immoral nor idolaters nor adulterers nor men who have sex with men nor thieves nor the greedy nor drunkards nor slanderers nor swindlers will inherit the kingdom of God. And that is what some of you were. But you were washed, you were sanctified, you were justified in the name of the Lord Jesus Christ and by the Spirit of our God" (1 Cor 6:9–11). Further, Paul also shared, "Flee from sexual immorality. All other sins a person commits *are outside the body, but whoever sins sexually, sins against their own body*" (1 Cor 6:18, emphasis added).

Canaanite Culture

Another highly sexualized culture was the Canaanite culture of ancient times. It was into this culture and world that the children of Israel would journey to possess the Promised Land. The land promised to Abraham was filled with sexual sin. Canaanite gods were worshiped with sex acts, bestiality was allowed, homosexuality was allowed, incest was allowed, and the religious and pleasure responses within an individual became intermingled in a way that was both addictive and destructive.

God's command to Israel was, "You must not live according to the customs of the nations I am going to drive out before you. Because they did all these things, I abhorred them. But I said to you, 'You will possess their land; I will give it to you as an inheritance, a land flowing with milk and honey.' I am the LORD your God, who has set you apart from the nations" (Lev 20:23–24). God also commanded, "You are to be holy to me because I, the LORD, am holy, and I have set you apart from the nations to be my own" (Lev 20:26).

Holy (Separate) God, Holy (Separate) People

God protects us by the walls he constructs in our life. God doesn't restrict us from certain activities because he hates us but because he loves us. His restrictions reflect the heart of a good father.

Kim Painter, in an article from a few years ago in *USA Today*, said boundaries actually help young people live better lives. Teens who had a bedtime of 10 p.m. or earlier, set by parents, got more sleep and were less likely to be depressed or consider suicide than those allowed to stay up past midnight.[9]

Other studies show that teen drivers whose parents set and enforced rules were more likely to wear seat belts and less likely to speed, get in crashes, drink and drive, or use cell phones while driving.[10] Teens whose parents set rules also smoke less, delay sex more, and do better in school, research shows.[11]

Our Heavenly Father is the best parent. He sets boundaries because he loves us—Thou Shalt Not Kill, Thou Shalt Not Steal, Thou Shalt Not Commit Adultery. In his boundaries, within the walls of *his* love, we find joy and peace. Within the protective environment of the Garden of Eden, human sexuality was a holy gift from God to Adam and Eve designed not only for procreation but also for human fulfillment and the creation of a bond between our first parents.

When Adam and Eve broke through God's boundary or wall of protection in the garden, something happened in this area and shame entered the world. So, man's failure affected man's attitudes toward sexuality. Exiting the garden, man took with him the sex drive created by God but, along with it, a now-fallen heart. This caused him to turn what was intended as a holy gift meant to glorify God into an extension of human selfishness and self-centeredness. "Whoever digs a pit may fall into it; *whoever breaks through a wall may be bitten by a snake*" (Eccl 10:8, emphasis added). This happened to Adam and Eve.

Biblical Guidelines

As God began to establish a people separated unto himself—a holy people—he established boundaries for them that would help them reclaim the holy nature of human sexuality. In Leviticus, as God's people prepared to enter the sexually polluted land of Canaan with a command to be holy as God is holy—or separated unto God's purpose—he gave them boundaries for their sexuality so they could live in a spiritual Garden of Eden in the midst of a world gone awry. Following are some of the boundaries he gave.

Sex Was to Be With a Human

"If a man has sexual relations with an animal, he is to be put to death, and you must kill the animal. If a woman approaches an animal to have sexual relations with it, kill both the woman and the animal. They are to be put to death; their blood will be on their own heads" (Lev 20:15–16).

Sex Was to Be With a Person of the Opposite Gender

"If a man has sexual relations with a man as one does with a woman, both of them have done what is detestable. They are to be put to death; their blood will be on their own heads" (Lev 20:13).

Sex Was Not to Be With a Member of Your Immediate Family Other Than Your Wife

"Do not have sexual relations with the sister of either your mother or your father, for that would dishonor a close relative; both of you would be held responsible" (Lev 20:19).

Sex Was to Be With Your Spouse

"If a man commits adultery with another man's wife—with the wife of his neighbor—both the adulterer and the adulteress are to be put to death" (Lev 20:10).

These boundaries were being set to help Israel live pure in a highly sexualized and pornographic society, like the world we live in. Though not every law or command in Leviticus was carried over into the new community of Christ-followers called the Church, these basic protections were: Jesus is clear that adultery and fornication are not within God's protective boundary. Paul is clear that sexual activity with someone of the same gender is not within God's protective boundary. And Paul is also clear in Corinthians that incest is wrong.

These boundaries protect the sanctity, or holiness, of sex within proper marriage between a man and a woman. And because of the blood of Christ who bore our shame and in obedience to God's word, we can enter into marriage without shame.

My own personal journey with sexuality was never easy, as I grew up thinking sex was something dirty, taboo, and impure. From locker room talk on the sports teams to school bus talk among friends, and from living in a community tainted with large swaths of disrespect, I thought sexuality was unclean, dirty, and nasty. Sexuality in the world I lived in in the 1960s and early '70s had been profaned *(profane* meaning to take something holy and pure and make it common or unclean). Then I was converted and started trying to make sense of it all. I started reading the Bible, including passages like those found in the Song of Solomon, and I discovered with surprise, "God talks about sex in the Bible! Without a blush!"

Delights and Redemption

"Your spring water is for you and you only, not to be passed around among strangers. Bless your fresh-flowing fountain! Enjoy the wife you married as a young man! Lovely as an angel, beautiful as a rose– don't ever quit taking delight in her body. Never take her love for granted! Why would you trade enduring intimacies for cheap thrills with a whore or for dalliance with a promiscuous stranger?" (Prov 5:17–20, MSG).

"Now, getting down to the questions you asked in your letter to me. First, is it a good thing to have sexual relations? Certainly—but only within a certain context. It's good for a man to have a wife, and for a woman to have a husband. Sexual drives are strong, but marriage is strong enough to contain them and provide for a balanced and fulfilling sexual life in a world of sexual disorder. The marriage bed must be a place of mutuality—the husband seeking to satisfy his wife, the wife seeking to satisfy her husband" (1Cor 7:1–3 MSG).

Conclusion

God wants you to enjoy the amazing gift of sex and has created boundaries to allow that for you with your spouse. Though we still live in a fallen world, God wants you and your future or present spouse to enjoy intimacy like Adam and Eve: without shame or reproach.

When Adam and Eve left the Garden of Eden, they were living in shame. God wants you to enter marriage without carrying shame. Don't take shame into your future marriage. Be cleansed and washed, establish a heart and life-culture of purity, which will allow you to delight in God's gift of sex within marriage.

It took me some time to reorient my mind, to understand that this thing called sexuality was a gift from God and that, if done within the boundaries God designs, did not bring shame but delight.

I struggled sexually as a teenager. So when I got married, I took some of that shame into marriage. I never heard messages like this that said, "Billy, get the shame taken care of before you get married." So, it took me a few years to realize that sexuality was not filthy, nasty, or profane, but instead was God's wonderful gift in marriage.

Jesus took it all; he carried it all. On the cross, Jesus took all the shame, from the beginning of time and what happened to Adam and Eve, to every abuse that's ever been perpetrated, every foul, corrupt, nasty thing, every act of bestiality or perversion or pornography. He took it all on the cross. As Christians, we believe that when we give all our shame to him, he wipes it away, and we live cleansed and free in Jesus' name. This includes in the area of sexuality. Jesus takes away all sexual shame when we give it to him.

13.

Marriage, Human Sexuality, and the Body

Timothy Tennent

Abstract

In this chapter, as in the other chapters of this book, we will look at the gift of human sexuality, followed by its brokenness, and conclude with its restoration.[1] To begin with, the gift of sexuality is embodied. In a cultural milieu that increasingly rejects the witness of the body and elevates feelings, we must allow ourselves to see that in scripture it is the opposite[1]: God starts with bodies and with material creation. The very physicality of God's design, as revealed in scripture, is part of the gift; and we are invited to live into that gift with our bodies, expressing our sexuality in marriage, as it was in the beginning, or in devoted celibacy, as Christ demonstrated for us when he walked the earth.

Against the beauty of this gift, the deceiver spoke and twisted the words of God, so that what was good was seen as not good enough, and what was complete as not complete. The original couple chose the deception and perversion. Every person on the planet has now either directly or indirectly experienced some kind of sexual brokenness. The heartache and confusion are great. And historically speaking, we are still in the middle of that.

But redemption has come, and the restoration has begun. In the Gospels, Jesus affirmed the primordial design of marriage between one man and one woman which results in life, a reflection of the Trinity. His Spirit empowers us to live into this kind of self-donating, life-giving expression of our sexuality, and so there is hope for future generations of our sons and daughters. The restoration will take time, but it has begun. And, at the end of time, all will culminate in the Marriage Feast of the Lamb, when the Son of God marries the Bride of Christ, the Church. All are invited into that vision and that reality, as we live our lives on this earth and in the world to come. We will discuss some of what this means, and how to stay the course, in his Spirit and love.

The Gift of Human Sexuality

Sacrament

Your body and my body are sacraments. One of the central realities of our time on earth as Christ followers is that the body has a sacramental presence in the world. It is only the body that makes the invisible, visible. Therefore, the body is fundamentally a *theological* category, not merely a *biological* one.

If the word "sacrament" is troubling, then perhaps saying that our physical bodies are "means of grace" is more comfortable language. That is, our physical bodies are outward and visible signs of an inward and spiritual grace. We affirm, as Protestants, that Jesus Christ only instituted two sacraments: Eucharist and Baptism. Wesleyans understand that the Holy Spirit is also the progenitor of sacraments, or "means of grace." Some notable examples would be: Reading of Scripture (John Wesley felt his heart strangely warmed after the reading of scripture at Aldersgate); Laying on of Hands to heal the sick (anointing with oil is a sign of the Holy Spirit); and Laying on of Hands to set apart for ministry (we call this ordination). These are just a few examples of special windows of grace where the Holy Spirit can touch us, empower us, and re-orient us toward God's rule and reign.

All of those sacraments (or "means of grace") are only possible through the body. The sacraments of Christ—Eucharist and Baptism—cannot be done apart from the body. It is a body that takes the Eucharist and a body that is baptized. In the sacraments of the Spirit, it is the ears that hear or the eyes which read God's word. Bodily hands are laid upon the sick and the ordinand. It is a body that is either healed or set apart for ministry. Pope John Paul II makes the point that before Christ established any sacraments, and long before the Holy Spirit established any sacraments or means of grace, there must have been, by necessity, a primordial sacrament which precedes them all—namely, the creative work of God the Father in creating bodies in general and the sacrament of marriage in particular.

Reflection of the Divine Nature

Once we recognize the Trinitarian basis for the sacraments, then we see that the Triune God invades our entire existence. There are ethical boundaries that are therefore inherent in our very creation. First, by creating us male and female God designed two different, complementary glories who come together as one, to reflect his image. Second, marriage was designed to invite us into the mystery of creation by becoming co-creators with him through the miracle of bearing children. Indeed, while honoring the special calling of celibacy, the Church understands that the building of families is at the heart of God's design. This is one of the many reasons why the Church has never declared moral equivalency of marriage between a man and a woman and a homosexual marriage. Third, God designed the family unit to reflect the mystery of the Trinity itself. Husband and wife become, through the gift of family, father and mother; and they stand before God with their children as a sign and seal of the Triune God. The family is meant to be a reflection of the Trinity with mutual gifts, mutual submission, joyful exercise of kingly and queenly authority, love, discipline, self-donation, and becoming co-creators with God.

Deep Fellowship

So through marriage we find that the communion of the Trinity takes place not only in corporate worship, but also in the daily life of a couple. Each day acts become tasks, and these tasks become acts, all deeply spiritual and so liturgical in its daily-ness that we can miss the glorious mystery of the whole thing. Because, it is in our daily lives that we find a thousand fresh ways to say to our spouse, "This is my body, given for you." This phrase, of course, is the central declaration of the Eucharistic mystery where Jesus says, "This is my body, given for you." However, this declaration is not only about Jesus giving his life for us, but it is the fundamental truth of God's whole relationship with us as his creation. He has given himself to us—completely—God's self-donation of himself. We, in turn, are called to give ourselves to one another because that is the very mystery of divine communion found only in the Triune God.

Let us look at divine communion for a moment, from the beginning. While the world was still pristine, Adam was allowed to discover his own solitude within creation. Each of the animals is brought before him to be given a name. Yet, none is found suitable. This is important because we normally only think about solitude in reference to man not having a mate—that is, man needs a woman and a woman needs a man—no other creature was found to be suitable. But, Pope John Paul points out a deeper solitude which is rooted in our very being. Man stands incomplete and alone in the universe. In a sense, Adam is "incomplete" unless he discovers the deeper communion into which God calls him and us. What is that deeper communion?

The answer to our solitude is that we are included in the mystery of God's triune nature. God does not need to create the world in order to have fellowship; it exists already within his own nature. The gift of divine communion is that we are brought into full communion with him and, secondarily, we are in communion with one another. The creation of Eve deepens our identity with God because we are invited to become co-creators with him. The sexual union of two who are "others" mirrors by design our own relationship with God who is not us, but another.

Free Will

In early Genesis, and in relationships, we also learn more of what is meant by the fact that we are *image bearers*. It means, in part, that we have been given the power to make choices. We can embrace communion with God or reject it. It could not really be any other way. You can make someone obey you, but you cannot make them love you. Thus, the tree of good and evil in the Garden is used by God to teach us what it means to be image bearers: we have choices. We are given space to love God or to reject him. Free will does not mean that we are free to create our own good and evil, but rather we are free to decide whether we will embrace what is good (the divine communion) or what is evil (rejection of that communion).

As image bearers, Adam and Eve have been granted moral weight in the universe. The word "glory" is the word for "weight" in the Old Testament. Our very physicality carries with it ethical boundaries—set at creation by God himself—the violation of which makes us "less weighty" or more "distant" from God's glory and his original design. That design is communion with Him, with one another and, indeed, with all he has made.

Original Nakedness

There is another glory, as well. The joyous creation of "male" and "female" culminates in their awakening, and we have the remarkable record of that moment in Genesis 2:25. It says, "The man and his wife were both naked and they felt no shame."

We must go back to that pre-fall Adam and Eve to capture the design of original nakedness, for it barely exists in the Western world today. The reason the man felt no shame before Eve, and Eve before Adam, is because they were one flesh. They were in the state of original unity. That was the design: "A man shall leave his mother and father and be united to his wife and the two shall become one flesh." We can joyfully recapture a glimmer of the original design through the covenant of marriage when a man and woman can stand before one another naked and without shame and say, sexually as in the rest of their life together, "This is my body, given for you." Remember those words in Ephesians 5:28, "Husbands have a duty to love their wives as their own bodies." Inside the covenant, we have the summons to be free from all shame and enter into joyful communion with the Triune God.

The Brokenness

The Fall of Humanity

The Fall is many things, but, at its core, it is the choice of man and woman to alienate ourselves from God, others and the rest of creation. Hell, as it turns out, is finally solitude—autonomy—aloneness, the rejection of community with the Triune God, with others and within the colloquy of our own inner self. That rejection mars everything.

Nakedness, Fear and Shame

For example, take nakedness. We know nakedness today only through the lens of the Fall. Therefore, nakedness for us is a sign of our shame. In the Western theological traditions, we have mostly viewed the Fall as the portal through which we have been cast into guilt as transgressors of God's law. That testimony is true. However, the actual account in Genesis names two other, perhaps even deeper, realities of the Fall—namely, fear and shame. It is fear, shame and guilt that have destroyed the original communion of persons in the primordial design, whether between man and woman, or between ourselves and the communion of the Triune God. In a post-fig-leaf world that clothes our shame, it is difficult for us to even conceptualize what it means to stand naked without shame. But it is here that we discover the true nature of our original design.

Outside of covenant, we can only know shame. Shame robs us of the self-donation that is integral to God's own nature where we fully give ourselves to the other such that we are one flesh. Sin pushes us back into our autonomous solitude, destroys the communion of persons, and heaps shame upon our bodies and ourselves. To shame your wife's body is to shame yourself and to shame the Triune God from whom all bodies come as gifts. It is sin that brings self-consciousness, or shall I say, self-orientation. Adam and Eve become aware of their nakedness and felt shame and fear.

All this is revealed through two questions God himself asks us after the Fall. The first question is, "Where are you [loss of communion with God]?" Adam answers that he and Eve had hidden themselves because, "I was afraid [fear] and I was naked [self-consciousness]." The second question is, "Who told you that you were naked?" Adam's response reveals a profound loss of communion with his wife and a newly emerging self-orientation. Eve, who was before the Fall one flesh with Adam, now becomes an object—an object upon which Adam heaps blame and guilt. "The woman you gave me..." For the first time, the husband sees his wife as object rather than as co-equal subject: she is the object of his blame. This blaming, objectifying of her occurs when he tries to deflect shame from himself in an act of self-preservation. Blaming is one way we objectify another, but it is not the only way.

Lust

Objectifying another, especially sexually, is at the heart of lust. Jesus says lust is at the heart of adultery. The seventh commandment, as understood in the Ten Commandments, is violated when a married man or woman enters into a sexual union with someone other than the one to whom they are married. To violate this within marriage is called adultery. If you are not married and you engage in a one-flesh relationship with someone who is not married, this is known as fornication. Jesus summons us all into the deeper reality of this commandment. As it turns out, there are two deeper levels that go beyond the outward physical act of adultery to which Jesus points us in this passage.

Let's first go to level one. It is lust that destroys the spousal meaning of the body. To even look at someone for sexual pleasure is wrong because it reduces God's creation, a subject, into an object by dis-embodying that person's physicality from his or her inner self. God intended a man and a woman to stand before one another in the full reciprocity of the "I"—I is subject. In the Fall, the man and woman covered the very physical markers of their distinctive human sexuality in shame. To look with lust at someone's private sexual markers is to dis-embody those physical markers from the whole person who embodies them. This is to rip someone apart. Pope John Paul II calls it the "dis-incarnation of man."

Even if we do not perform a bodily sexual act with anyone, but simply look at someone with an eye that reduces that person from a subject to an object, as in a sexual object, we have committed adultery. It is lust that turns someone into an object and dis-embodies them from the very inner life which allows us to fully participate in the visibility of the world. This is why, after the Fall, shame enters the world and men cover the physical, visible signs of masculinity, and the woman covers the physical, visible signs of femininity. These visible signs which had heretofore been integrated into their lives and bodies as a sacrament in joyful communion with God have now been separated out as objects of desire, destroying not only the union of their communion, but even the unity of their own persons.

This second level can perhaps best be raised by asking a question, "Can a man commit adultery in his heart against his own wife?" "Can a woman commit adultery in her heart in the context of her own husband?" Pope John Paul II says, and I think he is correct, that lust can destroy a marriage even within it, not just outside of it. Whenever we depersonalize someone, even our spouse, we are committing adultery. If your wife becomes just an object to satiate your sexual desires, or if your husband becomes just an object to satiate your sexual desires, you have committed adultery in your heart. There are many ways we objectify people. We can even objectify our own spouse, so that they are not God's "subject", but our "object." This is the fruit of the commodification of marriage. The body in all of its capacities, sexual and otherwise, all becomes the bodily terrain through which de-personalizing appropriation can take place.

The Kingdom, the Struggle, and the Holy Spirit

The Human Heart

Jesus creates a new threshold for us in understanding adultery. He points to the very root of the problem at the very seat of our being: the human heart. This is why Hebrews 4:12 says, "The word of God is living and active and sharper than a two-edged sword, dividing soul and spirit and discerning the thoughts and intentions of the heart." That is the great new Christian reality that creates a huge gulf between Rabbinical Judaism and the gospel, and an even larger gulf between Islam and the gospel. This is the great gospel point: Jesus Christ transforms our hearts. Nothing else will suffice and still be called Christian. The re-oriented heart, which now moves under the gravity of holy love, is the singular great potency of Christian faith and identity. And it is our re-oriented Christian heart and holy love that can bring our lives, and even our marriages, back into divine communion as intended, by the grace and power of the Holy Spirit.

The Biblical View, Compared and Contrasted

Both primordial and consummate, marriage is how the Bible begins and ends. It is one of the threads that connects the great themes of creation, redemption, and the Triune nature of God himself. We must therefore reject the notion that marriage is merely a human institution that can be shaped or defined by a majority vote as we see fit.

Other religions and worldviews falter here. A few years ago, the Supreme Court of India ruled that every person "has the right to choose their gender" because Hindus have no doctrine of creation and therefore there are no moral boundaries, they say, inherent in our creational design. Islam also, in my opinion, has a vulnerability in its doctrine of God. By rejecting the Trinity, Islam is left with a solitude God. Biblical revelation teaches that God is a communion of three distinct, eternal persons, united eternally as One. Islam rejects that in favor of the doctrine of *tawhid*—the absolute Oneness and solitude of God. That, in turn, means that the Muslim cannot "know God" in the sense of entering into the joy of God's communion, because there is no "knowing" even within Allah's own being. In Islam, the emphasis is on knowing Allah's will—that is, obeying him, not knowing and loving him and entering into fellowship with Allah.

And then there is the world's definition of marriage, which sees marriage as a shifting cultural arrangement designed to deliver happiness, companionship, sexual fulfillment and economic efficiency. Marriage in the contemporary period is a commodity. Like all commodities, you should expect returns (in this case emotional or romantic returns), or you can abandon or discard the relationship and opt for one which is better. This viewpoint has its root in the autonomous solitude which tumbled into our psyche with the Fall and lodged there.

In contrast, the Scriptures summon us to remember the deeper vision of reflecting the Trinity, the sacramental nature of the body, being image bearers in our physicality, not just our spirits, the power of self-donation, joining God as creators in the reproduction of children, and, indeed, how our very bodies prepare the world to receive the incarnation of Jesus Christ. There is a mighty chasm between these two visions, and we rightly work to recapture the original vision and design. The former is a utilitarian vision that sees marriage as a commodity; the latter is a biblical vision that sees marriage as covenant.

The Original Design, Reaffirmed

In Matthew 19:3–12 Jesus amazes the disciples by saying that even in the face of human brokenness and sin, God's original design for marriage remains intact. Jesus, in a post-Fallen world, quotes and masterfully combines Gen. 1:27 ("So God created man in his own image, in the image of God he created him; male and female he created them") and Gen. 2:24 ("Therefore a man shall leave his father and his mother and hold fast to his wife, and they shall become one flesh"). These are both pre-Fall texts. Jesus is powerfully saying that, despite the Fall and the tragic entrance of sin into the world, the original design of creation as embodied in unfallen Adam and Eve—who were created "male" and "female" and were united to become "one flesh" —remains intact as God's plan and design for us, and He will not relinquish this even in the face of sin, hardness of heart, and a whole spectrum of cultural issues which seek to cloud everything.

The Gift, Reaffirmed

It is in Genesis 4:1 that, even in a post-fallen world, the mirror of the Trinity is not fully broken in us. Adam lay with his wife and she became pregnant and gave birth to Cain. Eve says, "With the help of the Lord—Yahweh—I have brought forth a man." As we said earlier, it is marriage between a man and a woman in the mysterious communion of sexual union that unites us as "one flesh" and, in the gift of God, allows us to join him as little co-creators with God. Though science has learned how to replicate in a laboratory what naturally occurs between a man and a woman in sexual union, the lab still remains only a container which can at best incubate life, not create it, because a lab cannot create the stuff from which life comes. That stuff requires a man's body and a woman's body. Only in the sexual union of a man and a woman is the life-giving essence of God himself naturally expressed in the human race. A new life proceeds from their sacred union, further dispelling our solitude and further deepening our self-donation.

Eve came out of Adam, and a new little Adam comes forth from Eve. A child comes forth, and we now have a Trinity: an intimate unity of father, mother and child whereby we discover the mysterious spousal meaning of our bodies in all its masculinity and femininity, each given to the other, and both given to the child as a reciprocal gift of self-donation.

The world we inhabit, which only knows autonomous solitude, scorns the relational reproducibility of the body. Autonomous solitude is that inward gaze which is actually anti-sacrament; and its rejection of its own loving heterosexual reproducibility is actually, at its root, a rejection of the Trinity. Natural reproducibility is impossible in same-sex arrangements. But through the lens of autonomous solitude, the inherent problem is not recognized.

The Hope, Amidst Brokenness

I realize that, for many, thinking of one's own family causes them to say, "Wait, my family was not a picture of the Trinity, it was more of a picture from hell." The cultural landscape is littered with painful brokenness, but this is another reason why today's young adults must "go back to the beginning" and do a reboot on the whole system. The emerging generation has inherited my generation's chaos whereby marriage was actually used to promote autonomy and eschewed any notion of reciprocal self-donation. However, the Triune God keeps the constant sign before us because, even today, there are signs of hope.

I have seen many, many young adults over the years who have stood up in the midst of unspeakable wreckage and re-captured God's design, because God's design remains intact. Even in painful situations, the echo of the Trinity is there in the bearing of children. And in that family —the little Trinity—God, once again, assigns to the body the signs of love and faithfulness and conjugal loyalty.

So we see how our creation as "male" and "female" are not solely biological, functional categories, but steeped in deep mysteries and theological realities which reflect God's own nature and his original design for his creation. The sign of God's presence through human bodies will ultimately be fulfilled in the incarnation—when Jesus came in bodily form—and also expressed through the physical community of the Church.

Marriage and Singleness: Eschatological Hope

In a foreshadowing of the wedding to come between the Bride of Christ—the Church—and the Son of God, there are those who are called to celibacy and marry the church. In addition to marriage between husband and wife, there is a profound dignity in singleness.

In reference to singleness and celibacy, Jesus says, "Not everyone can accept this teaching, but only those to whom it is given" (Matt. 19:11). This clearly implies that there is a secondary gift, which, although few receive it, runs parallel with marriage; namely the sacred gift of singleness and celibacy. The word "singleness" is not the language of the New Testament; that is a modern term. If by single we mean a state of autonomous solitude, then we are not capturing a biblical view of what we call singleness. If, by single, we mean "single-minded focus" or "exclusivity of intent" or the "undivided life," then we are moving much closer to the biblical vision. Jesus points to a sacred state, which our Lord himself—and the Apostle Paul, among others—were called. This state is where a man or woman chooses (or is chosen) to not enter into the state of marriage for the sake of the kingdom.

To capture Jesus' point, we must recall what Jesus said in Mark 12:25. There, in the context of a dispute with the Sadducees (who denied the bodily resurrection) Jesus teaches that in the resurrection "they neither marry, nor are given in marriage." This is an eschatological statement with enormous ramifications. It demonstrates that marriage, as important as it is, is not an end in itself. Marriage is, after all, an image, a type, a pointer. It is an image, as we have said, of the Trinity, an image of self-donation, an image of covenant faithfulness or *hesed*; an outward image of a deeper spiritual truth. This means that marriage points to something beyond itself. St. Paul himself confirms this in Ephesians 5. He explores this world of self-donation in marriage: the wife submitting as an act of self-donation beautifully mirrored by the husband's act of self-donation in laying down his life for his wife resulting in the two subjects becoming "one flesh," again recalling the language of Genesis, "the two shall become one flesh."

But, at the apex of that passage, right after the reference to one flesh, Paul says something interesting which reflects the Mark 12:25 passage. He says, "This mystery is profound, but I am referring to…" and you expect him to say the mystery of marriage or something similar. Instead, he says, this mystery is profound, but "I am speaking of Christ and the Church." All of these texts indicate that marriage is not an end in itself, but a pointer to and, indeed, an imaging of—a reflection of—Christ and the Church. That is the eschatological reality to which we are all moving: Christ and his Church, the eternal state of our being brought into full fellowship and communion with the Triune God. In the eschaton there will be no marriage, because there will be no need for a pointer. We will all be literally engulfed into the very presence of the Triune God. There is no need for an earthly mirror when we stand before him in his heavenly glory.

We live in the "already-not yet" tension of the kingdom. That means that the rule and reign of God is already breaking in, but is not yet fully realized. So we live in this tension between the present age and the age to come. Now, some people have a particular sensitivity to the eschatological reality regarding marriage. That is, some have the gift in this age of that which will be shared by all of us in the age to come; namely, the fleshly typology of marriage is lost in the fuller reality of the Bride of Christ (the Church) married to Christ himself. In that case, a call to singleness and celibacy is a temporal anticipation of the future resurrected life. This is the "gift" Jesus refers to in our text. If you have the sacred gift of singleness and celibacy, then you have been called to live in the present age in such a way that you are already embodying the eschatological reality of the marriage supper of the Lamb that fully and joyfully unites Christ and his Church.

In the eschatological sense, we are all in our own way mirroring that future marriage. Most of us are called to mirror it through the sacrament of marriage. Others have the higher calling of mirroring it in the present as they are already married to Christ through their devotion to the church of Jesus Christ. If you are called to singleness, it is not because you are in the state of solitude, but because you have already discovered that even deeper communion to which even marriage only points as a shadow of that which is to come. This is why Paul goes so far as to say that the person who chooses marriage does *well*, but the one with the gift of celibacy and singleness does *better* in the sense that he or she actually embodies an even fuller realization of the in-breaking kingdom.

Clearly, this is a divine gift and divinely empowered through the Holy Spirit; and it is never meant to put singleness at war with marriage. This is not a zero-sum game where the only way we can honor marriage is to denigrate singleness, or by honoring the celibate life, we somehow disparage marriage. Indeed, Pope John Paul II says "the renunciation of the married state by those called to singleness is actually heightened when we are aware of not only what we are choosing, but what we are renouncing." The Church has struggled with this partly because of some of the writings of Augustine and the challenge of Manicheanism. But, these negative attitudes towards marriage were rooted in falsely equating sexual activity with the sin nature or a non-Christian view of the body—both Gnostic tendencies. However, these views actually cloud the earthly witness which both marriage and celibacy are meant to mirror, namely, the marriage of Christ and his Church.

We should also acknowledge that the choice is not merely between marriage and a life calling to celibacy and singleness or, if you prefer "the single-focused life." There is the temporary state of celibacy that everyone experiences. Many single young adults, perhaps, do not feel called whatsoever to the celibate life, but they are not yet in the married state. This is the state of temporary celibacy. It is also found even within marriage, where St. Paul says in I Cor. 7:5 that a husband and a wife by mutual agreement may enter into a period whereby they refrain from all sexual activity in order to focus on prayer and fasting. We see that though the calling of lifetime celibacy is an extraordinary and high calling for a special group, the experience of singleness and celibacy is universal. So, for example, one may not particularly sense that he or she is called to live out the eschatological realities of being married only to Christ in this life, but yet they find themselves temporarily in the single state. This is a special window of time when we can at least capture a tiny glimpse of the eschatological life by focusing single-mindedly on the kingdom in the present, even as we put our own future into God's hands. Even within marriage, as noted, we may enter into periods of temporary celibacy. So, we see that marriage and celibacy are not two separate things but one thing. Both mirror and anticipate the same reality. Both states are deeply intertwined with the other. In the Christian vision, all those called to singleness can only come into the world through marriage, and the single and celibate state prefigures the time when we will all be engulfed in the real marriage that is the mystery of Christ and his Church. Those called to marriage all experience a temporary state of singleness and celibacy both before and, at times, during marriage, and we are all moving inexorably to that day when there will be neither marriage nor giving in marriage. So marriage and celibacy are deep mysteries which are deeply entwined.

Thus it begins to become apparent how deeply the contemporary Church has been co-opted by the culture's war between singles and married, the war of the genders, and the quicksand of autonomous solitude. Because all relationships have become sexualized, deep and beautiful same-sex friendships have become eroded.

The Culture at War

We live in a culture that has become degraded and crude. We live in a culture that is shockingly deficient in love, joy, peace, patience, kindness, goodness, gentleness, faithfulness and self-control. Therefore, to bear the fruit of the Holy Spirit—both as devoted celibate and as devoted married—is to shine like bright lights in a culture filled with hatred, sadness, warfare, profanity, anxiety, impatience, faithlessness and being out of control—the anti-fruits of the Spirit—or the fruit of the flesh. We want to see the end of all bondages to sin in our community, whether it be pornography or hating your body or shaming—or gaming addictions or opioid use or drunkenness—or any other signs of brokenness that would creep into the community. We reject a truncated, post-Enlightenment form of the gospel that turns the whole enterprise into a privatized faith disconnected from the world we live in. The modern world is content with our being Christian as long as we keep it in our heads as nothing more than personal preference. The New Testament understands that holiness has implications that are personal as well as relational, societal and structural. The Church is helping to foster the in-breaking Kingdom when we live sacramentally in our marriages and in our singleness, and when our community pours out our physicality to work for justice for the poor, hope for the disenfranchised, and desperately needed reconciliation of all sorts—racial reconciliation, recovery for addicts, mercy to immigrants. The Church holds up truth in morality and righteousness in a culture that has lost its way. There is no part of creation which we do not work to see under the Lordship of Jesus Christ, as we become his co-laborers in redeeming the world! Does your heart ache for all this?

The Church must wake up to the realization that the current debate about sexuality is not married versus singles, and it is certainly not merely whether the church should "accept" or "reject" same-sex marriage. That assumes that this debate is about one issue rather than a whole vision of human identity and the sacramental nature of the body. Today we hear quite a bit about the LGBT and the LGBTQIA (Lesbian, Gay, Bisexual, Transgendered, Queer/Questioning, Intersexed and Asexual) community. The proliferation of letters beyond L and G and the growth of "choices" on Facebook clearly demonstrates that there is far more going on than a discussion of same-sex marriage. We are on the front end of something, not the end of something. Today, the debate also includes, for example bi-sexual, transgendered and intersexed persons. In other words, this is not a discussion only about sex or marriage; it is, at a deeper level, a discussion about the elimination of all gender identity, even those markers physiologically given to us through creation. This is, therefore, fundamentally about the Christian view of the body, the moral boundaries inherent in our creation, and the spiritual, sacramental nature of Christian marriage and singleness.

The Church's Response

Many of you will be the faithful bearers of re-inserting the full Christian vision of the body into the life and witness of the Church. We need not shy away from the immensity of this task. We must roll up our sleeves, build beautiful Christian families and patiently articulate the inter-connectedness of these various issues with the whole vision. We don't need a better argument, we need to embody a deeper truth in our lives. As Christians, we must recognize how deeply we have been trapped by a whole array of sexual immorality ranging from pornography to fornication. Our focus should be on the manifestation of holiness within the Church, by the indwelling of the Spirit. We have much to do in our own midst. The most important spiritual work we need to do is not within anyone "out there" but the face we meet in the mirror each morning. Let us ask God's help to make us holy so that the world will see that the Church truly is the glorious Bride of Christ. If I might draw from Homer and the wisdom of Greek mythology in reference to the Straits of Messina and the rocky shoal of Scylla and the six-headed monster of Charybdis: It is the mysterious anticipation of future realities which keeps us, whether married or single, from being destroyed by the *Scylla* of solitude and the *Charybdis* of autonomy.

Perhaps, drawing again from Homer's *Odyssey*, you may recall that Odysseus and Jason planned a strategy to resist the effects of the deadly allure of the Sirens. It involved strapping Odysseus to the mast of his ship and plugging his ears with wax. But the sound of the Sirens was too great and it penetrated the wax and only through great agony did Odysseus pass the strait. Jason, on the other hand, heeded the advice of Princes Medea, who suggested that Orpheus, the Greek God of Music, might counter the song of the Sirens with an even more compelling song, the music of heaven.

This is our task today. We must not be captivated by the song of this age which only knows the inward gaze, the war of the genders, the zero-sum game between marriage and singleness, the autonomous self, hedonistic pleasure, and thinking that Christians are only against things. We must tell a bigger story, we must cast a larger narrative; we must sing a better song.

Summary: The Beauty and the Glory

We live in a highly sexualized culture. I can think of fewer gifts to this world than those specially called men and women who have the gift of celibacy. Let us honor those called to the celibate life. It is the indwelling of the Holy Spirit that empowers them to live this beautiful, called life. Let us also honor those who build beautiful Christian marriages, for both states draw on the Spirit and image that one great marriage to which we are all moving: Christ and his Church. In your authentically Christian lives—both celibate and married—we hear a most compelling song, the song of the eschaton; the song of the transitory nature of this life; the song of the Marriage Supper of the Lamb; the song of the future bodily resurrection; the song of the New Creation which is being joyfully embodied in anticipation of the future reality and promise of our eternal communion with the Triune God. Thanks be to God.

14.

A Case Study from Malaysia: Struggling Pastor Who Pastors Strugglers

Teresa Chai and Tryphena Law

Abstract

This is a case study on the situation of homosexuality in Malaysia. Starting from a theological viewpoint on this issue, the chapter progresses to the societal climate in this primarily Muslim country and then leading to the Christian community's responses. It is also a personal testimony given by Typhena Law who is also the Director of Pursuing Liberty Under Christ (PLUC). She also provides an answer to the burning question "What harms the gift of sexuality?" More and more countries are passing legislation to legalize same-sex marriage. The American Psychological Association declares that "Gay Aren't Born That Way."[1]

Introduction

The country of Malaysia has been considered newsworthy for various reasons. One issue in the news has been the anger of LGBT groups due to the country's unbending stance against legalizing same-sex marriages. Several daily newspapers report this both locally in Malaysia and internationally. The July 29, 2013 article, "Activists: Legalizing Gay Marriages in Asia Won't Solve Malaysia's LGBT Issues," states that Malaysia's regulations against same-sex marriages exist because both "The Penal Code and Syariah[2] Criminal Enactment have criminalized certain consensual sexual activities."[3] In fact, Section 377B of the Malaysian Penal Code states that the punishment is twenty years and whipping. The preceding section of the Penal Code describes the nature of "carnal intercourse." The Syariah Criminal Offences Act (Federal Territories) 1997 (Act 559) states that the punishment of offenders who commit sodomy or lesbian relations includes fines of up to US$1,135

(Malaysian RM 5,000), imprisonment up to three years, whipping not exceeding six strokes, or any combination of these penalties.

In the same article, activist, artist and art consultant Pang Khee Teik presents a moving statement when he says, "I long for the day when people are simply given the choice to determine who they are, who they love, and who they want to tell that to, while their families and communities are allowed to support them. And that together, we are recognized through our love for each other rather than our hate."[4]

On the international scene, the October 16, 2015 *World Post* article entitled "Malaysia Staunchly Opposes LGBT Rights" states, "The country's prime minister recently compared the LGBT community to the terror group ISIS."[5] The article reports on the case against Anwar Ibrahim, the Malaysian opposition leader, for sodomy. In February 2015, Ibrahim was sentenced to five years in prison. He postulates that the accusations against him were politically motivated. Other reports in this article include more than sixty boys considered effeminate by their teachers, who were sent to "an anti-gay camp" for re-education physically and religiously. That was in 2011. In 2014 Human Rights Watch documented the abuses carried out on trans-women in Malaysia. And in June 2015, nine transgender women in Malaysia were convicted for cross-dressing.

When the United States joined the twenty countries that have legalized same-sex marriage, LGBT activists again brought the issue to the fore in Malaysia. For these activists, the issue is not just about marriage but basic human rights. They are calling for the abolishment of Penal Code 377. Hisham Hussein, chairman of an organization that works for the prevention of the spread of HIV, states that this law forces those having HIV infections to go underground rather than seek medical help.[6]

The Malaysian Church was in the limelight on this issue in 2007, when the first and only openly gay Chinese ordained pastor, Ouyang Wen Feng, returned to Malaysia from the United States and wanted to start "a gay-friendly church." He was met with opposition from both government and Evangelical church leadership. On August 12, 2007, he held a Sunday service with eighty people in attendance. Wong Kin Kong, the then-General Secretary of Malaysia's National Evangelical Christian Fellowship (NECF), made a statement to the press that Evangelical Christians do not condone sexually deviant behavior. He added, "We cannot stop him wanting to set up such a kind of church, but the evangelical churches will inform followers of our stand and advise them not to follow this teaching." Wong told Associated Press that NECF did not recognize Ouyang's ordination.[7] The registration and setting up of this church was not successful. However, the church seems to be still meeting secretly and illegally.

Another event reported by the Associated Press was the wedding banquet celebrated in 2012 by Malaysian-born Ngeo Boon Lin, a pastor, and his African-American husband Phineas Newborn III, a musical producer. This event was not widely publicized, but Ngeo and Newborn seemed to be clearly making a statement when they served heart-shaped chocolates wrapped in paper imprinted with, "God loves gays," in Chinese characters.[8]

Starting with the Bible

Does God love homosexuals? At this point in our discourse, it is important to have a biblical viewpoint on homosexuality as a framework for this question. Presented here is a "plain sense" approach to interpreting the Scriptures, as Pentecostals are known to interpret the Bible literally.

In Genesis, God established his will for humankind. He created male and female in his own image (Gen 1:27). When he saw that it was not good for Adam to be alone, he made Eve, who was a suitable wife for Adam (Gen 2:18). The man and the woman had equality and complemented each other. The woman was made using the man's rib (the words for woman and man in Hebrew are *ishah* and *ish*). Sameness and differences are seen in the creation of man and woman. Later, Genesis 2 states, "Therefore a man shall leave his father and mother and hold fast to his wife, and they shall become one flesh" (Gen 2:24). To become one flesh takes a husband and a wife being physically united. Also, "becoming one flesh" is not just a union, but a reunion. Finally, this was the way that the man and the woman would be fruitful and multiply.

Genesis 1:27 and 2:24 are re-emphasized in the New Testament by both Jesus and Paul (Matt 19:4–6, Rom 1:23–27 and I Cor 6:9). Marriage is an institution by God which has deep meaning, especially regarding the compatibility of man and woman. It is the picture of Christ and the Church as Bridegroom and Bride.

There is a prohibition of sexual intercourse outside of marriage, specifically, "You shall not commit adultery" (Exo 20:14, also in the New Testament: Matt 19:18, Rom 13:9, James 2:11). Relatedly are prohibitions to prostitution (Gen. 38:14, Lev. 19:29, 21:7, 14, much in Jeremiah and Ezekiel), incest (Lev 20:11–21; and New Testament: I Cor

5:1–2) and bestiality (Lev 18:23; 20:15–16), which are all considered sexual sins. As for same-sex intercourse, Lev 18:22 states, "You shall not lie with a male as with a woman; it is an abomination." (Lev 20:13, Gen 19; in the New Testament: Jude 7). All these actions are considered contrary to God's will and, therefore, sin.

In Genesis 19 there is the narrative of Sodom and Gomorrah. God rained down fire and brimstone upon these two cities. Thus their 'fame' is linked with sinfulness (Isa 1:9,10; Jer 23:14; Ezek 16:44–58) and the judgment of God (Deut 29:23; Isa 13:19; Jer 49:18; 50:40; Lam 4:6; Amos 4:11; Zeph 2:9). Even Jesus refers to these two cities as examples of sinfulness and judgment, warning people of the wrath of God and not to harden their hearts (Matt 10:14, 15; 11:23,24; Luke 10:10–12; 17:26–30).

What was their sin? Was it mainly the lack of hospitality, as some expound? Taking that view trivializes the gravity of the violent gang rape that was attempted. The passage in Ezekiel 16:47–50 refers to "abomination" (*to'ebah*), which is that same word used in Leviticus 18:22 and 20:13, referring to a man lying with another man as with a woman as being an abomination. "Sodom's sins were many: pride, injustice, *and* pursuing homosexual behavior."[9] These two verses in Leviticus reference homosexuality directly. As mentioned above, Lev 18:22 and 20:13 are part of the Holiness Code. The only consideration in these verses is gender: sexual activity is for male and female. There is "an absolute prohibition on homosexual behavior of every kind."[10]

When doing biblical theology, the question of continuity from the Old Testament to the New Testament arises. In the case of the prohibition on homosexuality, the command in both testaments is related to living a holy life. In Romans, Paul speaks about homosexual conduct as follows. "For this reason, God gave them up to dishonorable passions. For their women exchanged natural relations for those that are contrary to nature; and the men likewise gave up natural relations with women and were consumed with passion for one another, men committing shameless acts with men and receiving in themselves the due penalty for their error" (Rom 1:26,27). It a contrast between what is natural and what is unnatural. It is also a contrast between honorable and dishonorable. As Wayne Grudem frames it, "… [A] same-sex bond is a self-devaluing of one's own gender inasmuch as one sees the need to complement structurally one's own sex with someone of the same sex."[11]

Romans 1 makes clear that "homosexual practice is a serious sin and a violation of God's created order."[12] It is a road to depravity because it

1) exchanges the glory of God for the foolishness of idolatry; 2) replaces a truth with a lie; and 3) exchanges natural relations with unnatural ones. All this leads up to God giving those who practice it over to a depraved mind. Finally, Paul is very straightforward in his indictment: "Although they know God's righteous decree…they not only continue to do these very things, but also approve of those who practice them" (1:32).[13]

In I Cor 6:9 Paul includes homosexuality as one of the sins in his sins list. Likewise, I Tim 1:10 is part of another list, this time in relation to the law, and by its inclusion in this list, the sinfulness of homosexuality is implied (c.f. from OT: Lev18:22; 20:13). From the earliest Christian understanding of these verses, there was no doubt that any kind of homosexual behavior was totally banned.

A particular phrase in Greek led to the translation of "practice homosexuality" (*oute malakoi, oute arsenokotai*) in nine versions of the Bible. The word *arsenokotai* has the literal meaning of "bedders of men" or, "those who take males to bed." It would be logical that Paul takes his point from Lev 18 and 20. In the Septuagint, Lev 18:22 is *meta arsenos ou koimethese koiten gynaikos* ("You shall not lie down with a male as with a woman") and Lev 20:13 is *hos an koimethe meta arsenos koiten gynaikos* ("Whoever shall lie with a male as with a woman"). Paul has combined two Greek words to make one word, *arsenokotai*.

The next word is *malakos* (singular of *malakoi*) which means, "yielding to touch" and, "being passive in a same-sex relationship." This is a reference not just to a man who demonstrates soft or tender characteristics or who is deferential in relationships, but it refers to immoral sexual intimacy. "Paul would have hoped that the sanctification of a believer by Christ and the work of the indwelling Holy Spirit would remove the 'degrading passions' for same-sex intercourse and replace them with natural yearnings that would allow for normal heterosexual marriage (c.f. Rom 1:27, I Cor 7:9),"[14] or, we would add, with the embracing of celibacy. Many believers have found this to be the case, often through a process over time. That process is not passive, however. It occurs as the believer actively engages in his or her own sanctification through continual faith and pursuit of the Lord, continual receiving of the Lord's love in personal relationship with him, and the ongoing surrender to the Lord that naturally correlates with such faith and love.

When Jesus addressed people regarding the Law, it was never just about their actions but the condition of their hearts that he spoke. It was not just adultery or fornication, but lust that was on trial; not stealing, but wanting other people's property. Human beings judge what is on the outside, but God sees what is on the inside. This also applies to Christians judging without being judgmental: without a doubt, people judge people, in terms of assessing and distinguishing; but to be judgmental of the person's value, as a result, is not the end game. "The Christian directed by God's Word must avoid both an unholy *sympathy* for the homosexual and an unholy *hatred* for the homosexual."[15]

Drawing from Ed Shaw, two appendixes are helpful in summarizing, "The Plausibility of the Traditional Interpretation of Scriptures" and, "The Implausibility of the New Interpretation of Scripture." The plausibility hinges on the Bible highlighting from the very beginning creation, rebellion (sin), redemption, and perfection (eschatology). God created human beings in his image. Sexuality and sex are God's gifts to human beings. He commanded humankind to have children within the confines of marriage. Then sin entered into the scene through human beings' disobedience to God. Through this act, humanity rejected God's word, and relationships were marred, including both sexual relationships and relationship with God. Same-sex relationship perpetuates this marring. But God has a plan for salvation. This plan—or the *protevangelium*, the first gospel—is proclaimed in Gen 3:15. Jesus would carry out this rescue mission when he came to earth and, in the end, perfection will come. God will, eventually, perfectly restore this world.[16]

"The Implausibility of the New Interpretation of Scripture" refers to revisionists such as Jeffrey John, Justin Lee, James Brownson, and Matthew Vine. Driven by strong emotions, polarization, and doubt, their arguments lack objectivity. The most damaging is doubt, especially planting doubts in the minds of people about what the Bible states regarding this matter. People are moved by stories of homosexuals, and audiences want to be "politically correct." However, true exegesis ("leading out," or seeing what is in the biblical text) occurs in biblical context. Instead of this, revisionist writers rely on extra-biblical sources and perform eisegesis ("leading into," or injecting one's own opinion or experience into the text). An example of eisegesis is when revisionist authors state that the Roman centurion and his servant in Matt 8:5–13 and Luke 7:1–10 were gay lovers. There is no such indication in the text. Instead of letting Scripture interpret Scripture, revisionists "set Scripture against Scripture." For example, they take Gal 3:27–28 out of context to say there is "no longer male and female." We cannot "pick and choose from revealed truth."[17]

Pursuing Liberty Under Christ (PLUC)

It is in the context of biblical Christianity thus understood, as well as the context of Malaysia's legal system disallowing homosexual practice, that the Christian ministry Pursuing Liberty Under Christ (PLUC) operates in Malaysia. PLUC started in 2002 to assist those who are struggling with their sexual identity and who desire to be restored to God's original intention as described above, to empower them to take ownership in maintaining moral and relational wholeness through the redeeming power of God the Father and Jesus Christ by his Holy Spirit. The Scripture verse that guides this ministry is Romans 12:2, "Do not conform to the pattern of this world, but be transformed by the renewing of your mind. Then you will be able to test and approve what God's will is—his good, pleasing and perfect will."[18]

The three-fold mission of PLUC is "Relate, Advocate, and Educate." Their brochure explains their work this way:

1. Relate (Restoration): We strongly believe that freedom from same-sex attraction is possible. Thus, our unwavering mission is to connect with strugglers in their brokenness and see them restored to personal dignity and relational wholeness. We deeply respect every struggler's determination to restore their sexual identity to God's original intention and, with their families, to receive the help, hope and pastoral care they need.

2. Advocate (Awareness): In our awareness initiatives, we advocate for an inclusive environment for those trying to overcome same-sex attraction, where they are loved, respected and safe from negative perceptions and discrimination. In such an environment where truth and grace are encountered, we have seen many fruitfully journeyed with to self-awareness, healing and the freedom to form healthy relationships.

3. Educate (Enlightenment): We understand well the long-impact emotional damage that can happen in the formative years of one's life. To shed light on how to prevent this and protect our young ones, we are committed to go into schools, churches, organizations and communities to educate on the truth about same-sex attraction, common misconceptions, how sexual orientation develops, the health risks involved and how these groups can foster supportive relationships with those who struggle.

PLUC journeys-with by offering pastoral counseling to both individual strugglers and their families; and support groups, which facilitate self-discovery, personal growth and a safe environment to foster new and healthy relationships. PLUC also gives seminars to educate schools, churches, organizations, and communities; and it provides resources and materials on same-sex attraction and journeying to wholeness.

Other ministries operating in Asia that are similar to PLUC include Bagong Pagasa (Philippines), Pancaran Anugerah (Indonesia), and Choices (Singapore). Still more exist that work in the Chinese language alone, reaching an additional population. These are all listed with links from the PLUC website. The PLUC website also has a tab for resources available in English and Chinese in the form of books and DVDs.

The Executive Director of PLUC is an ordained Assemblies of God Minister, Tryphena Law. Reverend Law herself struggled with her sexual identity. She shares her testimony in a book and DVD entitled, "From Struggling Pastor to Pastoring Strugglers."[19] Law's testimony begins with her childhood.

She is the firstborn in her family. In traditional Chinese families, the parents usually prefer a male-child for their first child, because this ensures someone will carry on the family name. As a girl, Law felt she disappointed her parents from birth onward. Other factors that added to Law's poor self-image and gender confusion built upon each other and included having a strong physical build, being teased with unflattering name-calling, dressing in loose-fitting clothes, being treated by girls her age as protective (though she was as afraid as they were), and being treated by some boys her age as a buddy (though she felt sparks of attraction to one or the other of them), while her parents missed every opportunity to call her "beautiful." Thus, her girlness was left unaffirmed. Meanwhile, she compared herself with her younger sister, who was slim, had long pretty hair, and possessed the femininity which she felt she lacked.

During Law's early teenage years, two life-changing events occurred. First, she accepted the Lord Jesus Christ at a Christian fellowship meeting in her school, which was tremendously positive for her. Then, at home, after years of high tension between her parents and their arguments about his alcohol, her father threw his wife and children out of their home. This traumatic event shattered Law's ability to trust her father and, indeed, to trust any man. From that point on she became a "surrogate husband" to her mother, providing levels of emotional support and stability that were beyond the boundaries of her age and relationship.

After high school, Law went to college to become a teacher. When she had completed her teacher's training, she moved to the town where she was assigned to teach, and there dived into a lesbian lifestyle that would include many partners over the course of several years. Although her sexual lifestyle was illegal in Malaysia, it was not a conflict with her country but conflict with her faith that caused her the most consternation. As a Christian, she struggled with the dual life she lived. Yet, maintaining her dualism, she entered into a committed lesbian relationship which continued for some time. And then, to her surprise and devastation, her partner suddenly ended the relationship, saying she was engaged to be married to a man. At that point, Law planned to end her life. She would die in her car, racing it on the highway and speeding to her death. What occurred next was dramatic and inexplicable.

Taking her car key, she headed to the door of her house to go and fulfill her plan. But before she got out the door, her feet stuck to the floor, as if nailed there. She could not move. For an entire hour, she struggled to move her feet, but no amount of strength could lift them. Frustrated, she could not even die when she wanted to! And then, as if realizing it was the Lord who was holding her back, she finally surrendered and said to him, "You win." At that moment, her feet lifted, and she collapsed on the couch, exhausted. As she processed what had just happened, all she could think to do was to call someone. She called her best friend and told her all about it. Her friend advised her to call the missionaries who were visiting their town. Law followed this advice and called them. Though their phone was usually silenced at that hour, when Law called, the missionaries answered. They talked with her and helped her, and a new journey began. This was the journey that Law truly wanted to take, even though she knew it would be hard and, possibly, lifelong. This journey was in line with her core, and she knew she had had an encounter with God. She would follow him.

The missionaries walked with her for a time, even after they returned home to the U.S. As Law continued to pursue God and her desire for healing, he led her to seek counselors nearby with whom she could share her struggles. With their help, she found herself at a ministry called Choices, based in Singapore. Law was greatly helped by the counselor there. She received teaching, continued to have encounters with God as she read his Word (the Bible), and joined a support group. Through all this, she began to experience freedom and wholeness. The year was 2001. It was a milestone year in Law's restoration as a healthy heterosexual woman.

In 2002, Law met the founder of PLUC in Singapore. She was invited to join their prayer meeting and later invited to join their board. When the ministry, which was started for men, grew to include women, she was asked to co-partner in running PLUC. As she grew in her healing and in her true identity, people were drawn to her courage, honesty, authenticity, humor, strength, and gentleness. She began being able to help others who struggle with same-sex attraction and confused sexual identity. In her own words, "While I am ashamed of my past, I'm proud of God's work in my life. I'm grateful that I no longer need to live a lie—I'm living the truth!"

Law and her colleagues are not without opposition in Malaysia. Some groups charge the work of coming alongside strugglers to be "abuse" and of PLUC "being the voice of the church against gays…that defines the church instead of the Gospel of Jesus Christ."[20] However, this is the antithesis of Law, not the description of her or the ministry she leads. As one who herself needed help, Law is now a support for strugglers who reach out for help. Unlike perhaps early ex-gay groups, PLUC articulates its mission in very respectful and supportive terms. PLUC is not against; it is for. Introducing herself, Law says, "I only have one identity. My identity is not heterosexual, not homosexual. But my identity first and foremost is I am a child of God. That is the most important identity of all."[21] Thus, Law is defined by surrender not fight, and by being loved, not being enemies. She and the ministry she directs are, most of all, defined by the love and grace of the Gospel of Jesus Christ.

The Holy Spirit in Restoration

I followed up with Law in an interview that I conducted on May 1, 2017. I based my questions on one of the foci of a forum on Human Sexuality held recently in Singapore. That question was, "What harms the gift of sexuality?" I asked her to define human sexuality. She immediately referred to Gen 1:27 that God created human beings as male and female. However, the important thing is that as male and female, it is a journey to be more like him. Sexuality is often defined in terms of gender, and according to recent studies, as of this writing, there are twenty-three genders, demonstrating that things are rather fluid. It is not just that human beings are created as male or female, but we are created in the image of God and ultimately to be like Jesus. This gift of sexuality has been distorted by sin, that is, by the fall of human beings. There is now a marred image. God's ideal was equality between the sexes. Instead, in the world today, sexual violation and a ploy for domination are too often the situation.

In being pastoral in this ministry, it is all about timing. It is helping the clients see the consequences of actions and choices. The client has the free will to choose. By allowing clients to choose, they have ownership of the decision. This empowers people. For all this to happen, there must be a connection. They must feel they are in a safe relationship.

In some cases, the client allows mentoring, in others there is coaching, and for Christians, it is discipling. There is no one-size-fits-all. PLUC does not compromise on the commands and principles of the Word of God. The counselors seek to speak the truth in love to their clients. Some people may perceive this type of ministry as a compromise, but it is not. It is being patient with people who are struggling, giving them time and praying that they will come to the point of readiness and willingness to accept change as needful. It is speaking the Word in love and praying that the Holy Spirit will convict a person's heart.

Harm is inflicted against the gift of human sexuality because the forces of darkness are at work. There are those who may want to be set free but are not willing to give up things that are holding them back. These may be ungodly soul ties; they may be living in homes that do not have the same faith convictions or different spiritual values. If the clients have engaged in sexual intercourse, they must sever ties with previous partners. Often Christian strugglers are in conflict or a crisis of faith as to why there is no instant fix.

It is important that they, and we, are clear: it is a process and a journey.

15.

Spirit Baptism as a Framework for Ministry to the Struggling

Megan Grondin

Abstract

The Western Pentecostal theological discussion surrounding homosexuality has often revolved around the exegesis of specific biblical texts, resulting in an isolated conversation about homosexuality and an isolating ministry praxis. By embracing one of the distinctives of Pentecostalism, the baptism in the Holy Spirit, we can begin to construct a broader framework for ministry to gay celibate Christians in our churches. Wesley Hill, a celibate gay Christian, identifies the two main struggles of celibate gay Christians as loneliness and shame. By integrating our theology with the baptism of the Holy Spirit at the center, our theology and ministry towards gay Christians can become more inclusive and effective.

Introduction

The church's message to homosexuals has often been exclusively one that announces God's command not to engage in homosexual acts nor enter homosexual marriage. For gay people who affirm that marriage is between one man and one woman, yet still feel condemned in their homosexuality, what is our message to them? How can a church minister to those who want to obey the plain demands of scripture, yet feel caught in loneliness and shame? This chapter suggests some ways that churches can reach out to this often-overlooked group of people.

Theological discussion concerning homosexuality in broadly evangelical or more narrowly Pentecostal and charismatic circles in the Western world has often revolved around the exegesis of specific biblical texts, resulting in an isolated and isolating conversation about historic texts that are directly applied to present policies and practices. Overall, the conversation has been lacking in theologically focused thought and its possible applications to this specific challenge facing contemporary churches that would characterize themselves as "Bible believing."[1] By embracing one of the distinctives of Pentecostalism, the baptism in the Holy Spirit, we can begin to construct a framework for ministry to gay celibate Christians in our churches. Rather than stepping away from our prominent emphases, I argue that we must instead return to them, in order to truly, fully, and Christianly welcome gay Christians into our churches.[2] This framework could also be used for ministry to Christians struggling with strongholds such as pornography, alcoholism, and substance abuse, as well as those struggling with other "identities" and ways of being in the world.

Two theologically-informed voices will be central to this discussion. Frank Macchia's theology of Spirit baptism will be essential for constructing a suitable pneumatological framework. Wesley Hill, a gay celibate Christian scholar of the New Testament, will be a powerful voice that gives insight into his struggles as a gay celibate Christian and deliberations about how a Pentecostal church can respond well.

Frank Macchia explores Spirit baptism as an organizing principle for Pentecostal theology.[3] He demonstrates how Spirit baptism is truly a baptism in divine love set in the framework of the Kingdom of God, the reign of divine love and life, so that all of creation might become the dwelling place of God. This provides an eschatological understanding of Spirit baptism and the kingdom. Macchia also presents Spirit baptism as Trinitarian in nature, where the Son baptizes in the Spirit so that all might come under the loving reign of God. Through this outpouring, we participate in the life of the Trinity and the Trinity participates in our lives as well, leading to a Trinitarian and Spirit-baptized ecclesiology. The *koinonia* of the church demonstrates the life of the Trinity and embodies the very presence of God to the world. Spirit baptism, therefore, is a participatory and interactive metaphor of our involvement in God and his involvement in us.

Within this expansive context, Macchia reframes the distinctives of the Christian life—justification, sanctification, and empowerment. Rather than a forensic-legal or merits-based model of justification, Macchia reframes justification in pneumatological terms, where it is seen as the gift of righteousness in the outpouring of the Spirit that will ultimately lead to the "rightwising" and redemption of all creation. Sanctification then becomes an overlapping metaphor of justification, tying eschatological justification to the present transformation of the Christian through the Holy Spirit. Empowerment, often perceived as primarily for witness, is expanded to include enriched praise, *koinonia*, and especially a transformed capacity for love and relationships.

Wesley Hill is a celibate homosexual Christian who believes in traditional marriage and teaches in an evangelical theological seminary of the Anglican Church of North America. In his short but gripping memoir, *Washed and Waiting*, he addresses the question, how can a gay Christian be faithful to God while continuing to experience same-sex attraction?[4] Through his personal experience and theological reflection, he has found ways to deal with his feelings of loneliness and shame. These two areas are perhaps the principal struggles for homosexual Christians, and perhaps for others who have experienced sexual brokenness. Hill's insight, as well as those of several other gay celibate Christians, combined with Macchia's understanding of Spirit baptism can provide praxis guidance for churches and ministers who desire to reach this group of people.

Baptism in Divine Love vis-à-vis Loneliness

All people long for love and mutual desire, so how can gay and lesbian believers experience this in a way that does not lead to a lifestyle which, according to a plain reading of the Bible, is sin? Hill describes how God's love is the ultimate end of longing and loneliness. Sexual imagery throughout Scripture often points to divine affection and God's desire for his people. This great love is experienced through the Holy Spirit (Rom 5:5). Even with the perfection, depth, and value of God's love, Hill admits that the ache of loneliness remains. God's pneumatological substance means that we still feel the need for physical human companionship in this life, thus God's love is expressed and experienced through the Spirit-filled community. While many see marriage as the way to meet this need, first, not every marriage does; and second, marriage itself is only a temporary institution, while the church will remain in the new creation. The church, Hill says, is therefore the remedy for loneliness.[5]

Hill does not ignore, however, the difficulties with community, especially for the gay person. Because of a gay person's struggle with homosexuality, sometimes discomfort and uneasiness is sensed in the people with whom the gay person wants to be friends. Seeing this discomfort and uneasiness can cause the gay person to fear and withdraw from intimate friendships.[6] Hill acknowledges these difficulties and does not try to provide a remedy. The tension of living on this side of heaven means that loneliness still exists and will always exist.

Even though community does not remove loneliness and sometimes makes the ache worse, it does not mean that community life is an exercise in futility. Hill says, "...it merely changes the battleground."[7] Rather than fighting alone, the gay person fights while buttressed with others. Though there is pain involved and the ache remains, Hill states, "That pain is better than the pain of isolation."[8]

Dealing with loneliness, Hill says, requires a theology of brokenness. Rom 8:23 talks about the groaning of those with the first fruits of the Spirit who long for the new creation. Hill sees this "groaning" as a positive sign of fidelity that expresses discipleship.[9] In light of the glory that awaits the believer, any "disordered sexuality and the loneliness that goes with it," will only seem a momentary affliction (2 Cor 4:16–17; Rom 8:18). Hill says, "Pondering this coming glory transforms a theology of brokenness into a theology of resurrection."[10]

Throughout Hill's profound insights into the issue of loneliness for the gay celibate Christian runs a pneumatological thread. God's love is poured into our hearts through the Holy Spirit. The embodied presence and love of God is found in the Spirit-filled community. And those who have the first fruits of the Spirit groan in anticipation of the coming glory. All these elements are crucial for developing Spirit baptism as a framework for ministering to gay celibate Christians experiencing loneliness. Spirit baptism seen as God's love expressed through the Spirit-filled body of Christ and through the Holy Spirit is the ultimate end of longing and loneliness. At the same time, an eschatological framework, expressed through speaking in tongues, is necessary to allow for a theology of brokenness while awaiting resurrection.

Macchia's understanding of Spirit baptism as participation in the reign of God's love and life has significant implications for a celibate gay Christian. As creatures of God, we were created to participate in this extravagant love of God and this liberating reign of life. In this way, as Hill says, the love of God is the ultimate end to loneliness. Spirit baptism enables the believer to experience a foretaste of the great love of God that will be fully known in the future.

Yet as Hill points out, the love of God is not meant to replace human love. The Spirit-filled community is necessary to experience God's love through human relationships. Several models of community exist that could be useful in the church. Committed friendships as a practice have long existed in the history of the church. Alan Bray's study of historical friendship in the church shows how friendship was a commitment as deep as marriage and a lifelong form of kinship.[11] Bray studied different grave markers and monuments from the Middle Ages of men who were buried together as "wedded brothers," friends who swore vows of "true love and brotherhood" to become as if they were blood kin and who committed to caring for each other and each other's families.[12] Many dangers came with these friendships, such as a fear of broken obligations or a fear of unchaste relationships, but the "ardent heart" of these friendships to care for one another is obvious.

These types of friendships can be difficult to translate in our modern context, especially for gay people. Some Christians object to same-sex attracted people having these types of committed friendships, saying that it is "diet homosexuality" due to the possibility of sexual temptation.[13] However, there is still value in these types of relationships. First, most gay people learn while growing up how to have same-sex friendships that are non-sexual in nature.[14] Second, intimate same-sex friendships help to ground a homosexual person's sexual identity as a man or a woman. Third, the alternatives can be even more detrimental than the actual friendship, inciting other sins.[15]

A second model is that of intentional communities. Throughout church history, celibacy has often been lived in community, such as in monasteries, convents, and beguinages. One such contemporary movement is called the Christian "intentional community" movement.[16] Though there is a wide spectrum, these communities typically consist of lay people, whether married, single, or families, working and living together often in a counter-cultural way.

The third and most obvious model is the church. The church should play the role of an extended family and a strong support system for the gay celibate Christian. Welcoming singles into homes as part of the family gives substance to the meaning of "brothers and sisters in Christ." The church needs to be a place of honesty, a place of love, and a place of "coming out." Gay celibate Christians can be invited to feel comfortable in church sharing the joys and difficulties of living with a homosexual orientation without judgment or condemnation. Understanding we all have struggles, the church exists to create a community where growth into the image of Christ can take place in all believers. In this way, the church can be a witness of love to gay people both inside and outside the church.

While these models can be instrumental in creating community for the gay celibate Christian, communal life is not without its challenges.

One challenge facing the gay celibate Christian within community is the balance between alienation and assimilation. Relationships are not only essential to our human existence, but in many ways, they also define us. This is especially true for a gay celibate Christian. A delicate balance needs to be found between the two extremes of being completely reliant on the church for a sense of self and the risk of alienation in celibacy. Both of these things distort souls and one's inner sense of self. How can one find a reality that avoids these two extremes?

Macchia says that a sense of self that maintains distinction of self, avoids assimilation, and doesn't need acceptance of others for identification, is developed by making God and his unconditional love the center of trust. Without this, one is prone to get lost in the expectations and demands of others. With it, the proper conditions for self-realization are met and one can cultivate healthy relationships.[17] This is vital for all Christians, and it is crucial for the celibate, both gay and straight. While the love of God is mediated through the Body of Christ, it is important to remember that the center of one's existence is God's love, not the church's love. This protects against disappointment and an unhealthy sense of self and encourages healthy relationships within the church.

For the gay celibate Christian, it is important that this "center" remains God's love and is not overtaken by a gay identity. Secular culture says that homosexuality defines one's identity and, "If you are a homosexual, then you should accept yourself and not try to change." But human sexuality is not the defining attribute of one's identity. In his book *Washed and Waiting,* Hill always uses "gay" or "homosexual" as an adjective and never as a noun in order to remind his readers that "being gay isn't the most important thing about my or any other gay person's identity. I am a *Christian* before I am anything else."[18]

The gay celibate Christian may desire this community wholeheartedly, but so often the church, knowingly or unknowingly, rejects gay people. How does the Spirit help the church accept and include gay Christians? Because of the relational nature of healing, spiritual sickness is also relational in nature. Macchia says that the answer to this problem is Spirit baptism, which replaces broken relationships with restored communion.[19] In Spirit baptism, there is the inclusion of the "other." Accepting and embracing "the other" comes from the Spirit of God in a way that doesn't destroy or exploit the other. The Spirit of God transforms believers into Christ's image, "a 'de-centered self' that submits to the lordship of Christ and wills to be changed so as to admit others in, without oppressing or destroying them."[20] In this way, the Spirit transforms the will of the believer to embrace and include the other. Macchia says the goal is a "prophetic empathy for others in the Spirit."[21] He defines empathy as "a common sharing of life, a capacity to feel something of the other's agonies and ecstasies, and an ability to bear one another's burdens."[22]

Due to the stigma historically associated with homosexuality, many Christians have a difficult time expressing acceptance to homosexuals, because they believe that doing so would mean accepting their lifestyle. But Christ shows us an acceptance of the "other." In essence, *all of us* are the "other." We are so different from God; and, even more than that, we are all sinners, we all fall short. Yet God still embraced and included us. No matter what difficulties we have in loving people different from us, nothing can compare to a holy God who came to earth to die for us so that we might be included in him. Our attitude towards homosexuals should be to see them, as all people, with "grace-healed eyes," which Yancey defines as seeing "the potential in others for the same grace that God has so lavishly bestowed on us."[23] We need to have a "redemptive will to embrace" and a "prophetic empathy" in relationships, including with homosexuals, because of what God has done for us in Christ. This is true inclusion and the result of a Spirit-baptized community.

This baptism in divine love may seem contradictory to the classical understanding of Spirit baptism as a baptism of *power* for witness. How do we reconcile a baptism of power with a baptism of love? How does a baptism in divine love coincide with the Pentecostal emphasis on power?

Detrimental consequences arise when the emphasis on power overruns the emphasis on love, and this is seen nowhere better than with respect to gay Christians. Many expect God to "heal" them of their homosexual impulses through "power encounters," but this does not happen for everyone.[24] So far, an alternative way to minister has not been proposed, thus believers who experience homosexual impulses are left feeling conflicted, ashamed, and stuck. How can we minister in another way to gay and lesbian believers whose suffering with homosexuality persists? Would this approach be contradictory to one of our most prominent emphases?

An eschatological framework allows for a theology of power as well as a theology of brokenness in our pneumatology. "Power encounters" are signs of the inbreaking Kingdom of God, foreshadowing the fullness of the new creation. There have been many testimonies of homosexuals who have been dramatically freed from a homosexual lifestyle and have been happily married to a person of the opposite sex.[25] These examples of the power of the Spirit to transform lives should not be neglected or disregarded, for they are signs of the coming kingdom.

While these signs point to the fact that the kingdom is coming, not every homosexual will experience such a dramatic change in this life. Many gay people may struggle with homosexual impulses until the day they die. However, the Spirit, while we emphasize his presence in signs and wonders, is still present with us in our sufferings. Paul tells us in Rom 8:23, 26–27 that the Spirit is present with us in our sufferings and "helps" us in our weaknesses, meaning he shoulders the burden of our weaknesses.[26] Dunn says that "weaknesses" here refers not only to "external temptations" or the "inability to pray," but, "the totality of the human condition (the corruptibility of the body, the subvertedness of the flesh) which the believer is still part of and which comes to expression in prayer inability."[27] Because the gay celibate Christian has the first fruits of the Spirit, he groans in yearning for the new creation to come, and the Spirit intercedes for him with groans.

The Spirit's intercession of inexpressible groans in Rom 8:26 can be understood as speaking in tongues. Macchia sees tongues as a "broken speech for the broken body"[28] and develops a theology of glossolalia as *theologia crucis*. Often in the division between Christology and pneumatology, conversion and Spirit baptism, there is a dichotomy between the God revealed in the incarnation, life and death of Jesus, and the God of power described in Spirit baptism. The power of the Spirit is often defined among Pentecostals "more as a triumphalistic domination of the natural order through the realm of the supernatural than as Paul's 'strength in weakness' under the shadow of the cross."[29] Macchia says, "Glossolalia cannot bypass the cross as a direct, glorious experience of God."[30]

Tongues also has a communal dynamic, in which the church shares in the suffering of those who suffer. Since no one has all the spiritual gifts, Macchia discusses how the fullness of God's presence can only be experienced in koinonia. While speaking in tongues edifies the one speaking, this edification is for the body as well (Eph 4:12–13). Macchia says, "It is not a self-centered euphoria of good feelings, but a being conformed to the image of Christ so that we might move out as channels of God's grace to others."[31] The gift of interpretation of tongues shows that glossolalia is intended not just for the individual, but also for the church. Tongues is therefore both communal and individual in its experience. Macchia says it is "not only a freedom for God, but a freedom for one another."³² This freedom for one another includes the bearing of one another's burdens and yearning together for the new creation. In this way, the church participates with the gay celibate Christian in his suffering and in his yearning for the new creation.

Tongues has often been argued to be the "initial evidence" of Spirit baptism, and it is truly "evidence" that the kingdom has come. Yet it is also a sign that the new creation has not been experienced in all of its fullness. In this way, it not only expresses powerful charismatic speech but also suffering and yearning for the new creation. Speaking in tongues, therefore, can be a valuable expression for homosexual believers as they yearn for restoration and resurrection on this side of heaven.

A Spirit-Baptized Life vis-à-vis Shame

There are other challenges associated with living on this side of heaven. Intense homosexual desires that won't go away often instill shame in the heart of the celibate gay Christian. One major cause of shame seems to be a conflict of identity. The plain sense of the Bible condemns homosexual behavior, yet the gay person cannot seem to overcome same-sex attraction. How can one be gay and Christian at the same time? Several different responses have been developed to answer this conflict: the reparative response, the revisionist response, and the integrative response.

The reparative response deals with reparative therapy that looks at the "cause" of homosexual orientation and gives steps to "fix" a person's sexuality. Reparative therapy theory purports that sexual abuse or a strained relationship with a parent is the cause of a homosexual orientation, and that orientation can be reversed through counseling or therapy. While this may be true for some gay people, it is not the case for many.³³ A homosexual orientation is a complex mixture of nature and nurture that often does not have one root cause; thus, this approach does not recognize the complexity of homosexual orientation and the diversity of homosexuals themselves. By assuming that there is one root cause, we neglect those who do not fit into this "box" that we have created, and often end up causing deep harm.³⁴

The revisionist response says that the Bible does not condemn same-sex marriage, thus there is no conflict between homosexuality and the Christian faith. Though the promise of a change in homosexual orientation is alluring to many, many disappointments have arisen out of ministries holding to the reparative therapy theory. When change seems to be impossible, the only remaining choice seems to be to believe one's homosexual orientation is good and to accept attractive exegeses of texts that support this.[35] But if the Bible really does condemn homosexual behavior, as believers for centuries have thought, then there must be another way to respond to this conflict of identity and sexuality.

An integrative response says that a homosexual Christian's identity is in Christ, not in homosexuality. While a gay Christian may struggle all his life with same-sex attraction, his ultimate identity is found in Christ. Though the Bible names homosexual *behavior* as sin, same-sex *attraction* should rather be viewed as temptation. This is an important distinction to be made in order to integrate sexuality and faith for the homosexual person.[36] Same-sex attraction can be viewed as temptation, but this does not mean that a same-sex attracted person is not a Christian. After a long listing of those who will not inherit the kingdom of God, homosexual offenders included, 1 Cor 6:11 says, "And such *were* some of you. But you were washed, you were sanctified, you were justified in the name of Lord Jesus Christ and by the Spirit of our God." A homosexual *identity*, shaped by acting on homosexual dispositions, need not be a part of a gay Christian's life. Melinda Selmys says that when one becomes a Christian, there is a change of orientation, but it does not involve sexual organs or a psychological matrix; it is a change of heart, which the Bible calls "repentance."[37] Homosexuality will fade away, but an identity in Christ will not.[38] Through water baptism, a significant change in identity is made, spiritual cleansing is effected, and one is incorporated into the body of Christ.[39] However, baptism and a new identity in Christ do not promise a reversing of a homosexual orientation. While desires can be transformed, we may have to bear the cross of some of our desires until Christ returns.[40]

Even with this integrative response, a homosexual orientation can cause a sense of deep shame in a gay Christian. In his chapter, "The Divine Accolade," Wesley Hill discusses how a gay person can overcome his struggle with shame. Hill describes how, even though homosexual desires are not considered lust, they are a constant source of shame. Looking at someone and desiring that person is normal due to our inherent sexuality. Lust is defined, however, as "looking *to* desire," the second glance that is willful and intentional.[41] Looking and desiring may seem natural for the heterosexual person, but looking and desiring for the homosexual person feels illicit, since it is desiring someone of the same sex. Although this impulse is only temptation, its constant nature causes the gay Christian to feel like he is "perpetually, hopelessly unsatisfying to God."[42] This is the same experience that Christians strongly attracted to porn, alcohol, adultery, heterosexual promiscuity, gambling, or other temptations report to pastors and counselors.

The key to getting out of this vicious cycle of shame is what Hill calls "the divine accolade." As Christians, our highest joy will be when we stand before Jesus and he says, "Well done, good and faithful servant," and praises us for our lives lived in conformity to him.[43] In this way, God glorifies us. Throughout the New Testament are references to this praise and glory that the believer will receive (1 Cor 4:5; 2 Cor 10:18; Rom 2:29; John 5:44; 1 Pet 1:7). This glory is based on the forgiveness of sins, our justification, our union with Christ, and the transforming work of the Spirit in our lives (Eph 1:4, 7; Rom 2:16; 3:21–26; Gal 5:5).[44] The glory awaiting the believer has implications for this present life. Because God is pleased with us, we can be pleased with ourselves.

On the other hand, some Christians throughout history, like David Brainerd and Leo Tolstoy, believed that "the closer we get to God, the more we must sense our own remaining corruption and sinfulness."[45] However, Hill points out that the New Testament does not support this negative self-conception. The work of Christ and the work of the Holy Spirit liberates, transforms, and renews the Christian, which leads to the divine accolade when we stand before the Lord at the last day. Thus, a gay celibate Christian's journey of "struggle, failure, repentance, restoration, renewal in joy, and persevering, agonized obedience,"[46] is a sign of the Spirit's transformation and future vindication of his life.

How does this relate to Spirit baptism? Hill says that it is justification and the transforming power of the *Holy Spirit* that is the basis of the praise accorded to the homosexual Christian. The elements of a Spirit-baptized life—justification, sanctification and empowerment—are key to enabling the gay celibate Christian to overcome his shame and live a Spirit-filled life.

Macchia outlines the connection between justification and glorification in Rom 8:17–23. For Paul, sin is not mainly classified as a moral wrong, but rather as "a human condition of alienation from the glorious liberty of creation renewed by the Spirit."[47] This liberty is rooted in the "liberty of divine love" shown in Christ's incarnation, death, resurrection, and exaltation.[48] The indwelling of the Spirit directs us to this new creational liberty; in this way, glorification is through justification. However, the sufferings of this present age do not disappear because we have the Spirit; in fact, we groan for liberation *because* we have these first fruits. Yet Rom 8:18 inspires hope in those with the first fruits of the Spirit, for the suffering they experience now is no comparison to the glorious existence yet to come. Macchia says, "In this way, glorification fulfills justification (8:30)."[49]

Groaning in faith, assuming "the weakness of the flesh and the strength of the Spirit," connects to the Old Testament and Qumranic understanding of God's righteous favor being obtained through trusting in the Lord. This also relates to Hill's definition of perseverance in faith that involves "struggling and stumbling." Though the gay celibate Christian may stumble and fall in his walk, the strength of the Spirit within him reminds him of the future glory that awaits. Again, the need for an eschatological framework that allows for a "theology of brokenness" is crucial for ministry to gay celibate Christians. The Scriptures confirm that in glorification, no one will be put to shame (Rom 8:18, 30, 33; 10:10, 11). Those who suffer find hope in the fact that the Spirit is the link between justification and glorification.[50]

Sanctification provides a crucial link between justification and empowerment. It emphasizes the transformational aspect of baptism in the Spirit and implies the empowerment aspect as well. Macchia discusses how kingdom sanctification means identification with sinners, following Jesus' example. This has profound implications for Christians' use of the phrase "love the sinner, hate the sin" when discussing homosexuality with non-Christian gays. This phrase is detested among the homosexual community. Often, homosexual behavior is identical with a homosexual identity for gay people. If we say "love the sinner, hate the sin," this seems like a blatant contradiction and obvious hypocrisy to gays.[51] It also seems to put Christians in a different category than homosexuals, rather than admitting that we are all sinners in need of Jesus, and incorrectly creates an "us-versus-them" narrative. The Pharisees labeled Jesus "friend of sinners," but Jesus just saw the tax collectors and sinners as his "friends."[52] He identified with them rather than avoiding them, and in this way inaugurated the kingdom in holiness. By using the phrase "love the sinner, hate the sin," we are distancing ourselves from people, rather than identifying ourselves with them. We need to use language that is not trite and catchy, but that rather communicates we are all sinners in need of a Savior.

One manner in which sanctification is portrayed in the book of Acts is by the Gentiles joining in the holy temple of believers by the reception of the Spirit (Acts 10). The Gentiles joining the church can be likened to gay celibate Christians joining the church. Since gay celibate Christians have been "made clean," sanctified and justified through the Spirit (1 Cor 6:11), how can they be called "profane" (Acts 10:15)? Neither the shame resulting from a stigma in the church nor the shame from a negative self-conception should hinder gay celibate Christians from being fully integrated into the body of Christ by the Holy Spirit. This is the sanctifying power of the Holy Spirit; it is transformational and inclusive. Not only is sanctification transformational, but sanctification also implies empowerment, which forms the connection between justification and empowerment.

Through empowerment by the Spirit, we can meet the need Hill mentions for a more positive self-conception for the gay celibate Christian. Baptism in the Holy Spirit leads to a knowledge of the love of God, incorporation into the body, justification, sanctification, and glorification, but it also leads to power for service. While Pentecostals have often narrowly defined this power as an experience of speaking in tongues or in terms of prophetic gifting, Macchia defines this empowerment as not just naked energy for witness, but a transformed capacity for relationships. He says, "The power for witness is the power of love at work among us."[53] What would this look like for the gay celibate Christian?

First, a homosexual orientation need not be viewed as completely negative. Wesley Hill talks about Martin Hallett, a gay celibate Christian who argues that his homosexuality is a gift.[54] Though Hallett believes homosexual acts are immoral, he also believes that even his homosexual orientation can be viewed positively rather than as a handicap or an impediment. With God as the "story-teller" of our lives, sexuality can be viewed as part of that story. Through God's sovereignty, a redeemed homosexual orientation can lead to ministry, understanding of God's love and forgiveness, and various other blessings to the individual and to the church.[55] Instead of expressing his homosexual orientation through homoerotic relationships, Hallett says, "I believed I was expressing my sexuality by simply being honest with people about it."[56] A homosexual orientation also gives a person a greater sense of his or her brokenness and need for God, eventually drawing one closer to their Savior and Redeemer.[57] This fulfills the beatitude, "Blessed are the poor in spirit, for theirs is the kingdom of God" (Matt 5: 3).

Another way to view a homosexual orientation positively is through the act of sublimation. Eve Tushnet, a celibate gay Catholic, defines sublimation for the same-sex attracted individual as the redirection of eros into a more acceptable form of love, such as charity or friendship.

One way to think of sublimation is to think of the soul as a kaleidoscope. Turning it one way, desires turn into a pattern of homoerotic love. Turned another way, this love is redirected towards family or friends. In this way, the longings for love are redirected and fulfilled. Although Tushnet says this may not work for everyone, it could be helpful for some.[58]

Second, a gay celibate Christian must find that which God has created within them to be used by the power of the Spirit to minister to others. Eve Tushnet talks about vocation as "a unique call from God to love and serve others and to receive their love."[59] She does not consider celibacy as a vocation, since, "Vocation is always a positive act of love, not a refraining-from-action."[60] Possible vocations include but are not limited to friendship, intentional communities, marriage, artistic creation, and include endless possibilities.[61]

Tushnet's discussion of vocation is vital to creating a place for the gay celibate person to be active in the church. When it comes to a Pentecostal pneumatological framework, could not Macchia's idea of empowerment of the Spirit as a transformed capacity for relationships be another way of expressing Tushnet's definition of vocation?[62] Vocation for the gay celibate Christian is also an empowerment of the Spirit to serve and to love others. In this way, celibate Christians, both gay and straight, can live a fruitful, Spirit-filled life.

Seeing empowerment as vocation leads to a positive conception of the body for a gay celibate Christian. Disassociation from the body is a temptation for gay celibate Christians due to the conflict between their sexual orientation and faith. Yet service reminds Christians that bodies are created by God in his love and serving him with the body honors his creation. Instead of scolding himself for intense desires, the gay celibate Christian can refresh himself in the knowledge of and fellowship with Christ in Christ's sufferings. Instead of rejection, disgust, and even shame, positive uses of the body are prayers of gratitude for God's good creation.[63]

Shame does not have to rule the life of a gay celibate Christian. While the tension of living with a homosexual orientation and living as a Christian can be difficult, gay believers have found ways to manage the tension in a productive and fulfilling way through the Holy Spirit. One can be filled with hope through the first fruits of the Spirit and the promise of glorification through justification, while at the same time yearn with the first fruits of the Spirit for the new creation. Through the empowerment of the Holy Spirit, the gay celibate Christian can live a fulfilling life of love and service to others, and the church can join him.

Conclusion

In conclusion, Spirit baptism provides a comprehensive framework for ministry to gay celibate Christians in the church. Spirit baptism as a baptism in divine love expressed through the Holy Spirit and the church is the ultimate end of longing and loneliness for Christians, including the gay celibate Christian. Many models of community exist that the church can put more fully into place in order to provide a place of growth, love, and family to gay celibate Christians. Small groups may be a good starting point, but they often only scratch the surface. A church can encourage the formation of true friendship pacts between Christians, with agreements within the pact about the nature of the relationship, responsibilities towards one another, and accountability for one's actions. Support groups can be put into place for those who struggle with sexual temptation and can be opened to include all who struggle with any type of temptation, to reinforce the reality that we all are broken on this side of heaven. Families can open their homes to welcome all singles, not only gay and lesbian singles, to be a part of holidays, special occasions, vacations, and family nights. For churches with a large population of gay and lesbian believers, perhaps an intentional community could be birthed out of the church.

While there are many challenges to the community, especially as a gay person, the benefits and blessings of community far outweigh the challenges and risks. However, because we live on this side of heaven, an eschatological framework is necessary to allow for a theology of brokenness and yearning. The Holy Spirit as the first fruits in our hearts produces a groaning for the new creation to come, a groaning expressed through the believer by speaking in tongues. The practice of speaking in tongues can be beneficial for the gay celibate believer to express his longing and hope while he awaits the new creation. Teaching and preaching from the pulpit should also be sure to frame discussions of homosexuality and holy living through this eschatological framework.

The elements of a Spirit-baptized life—justification, sanctification, and empowerment—are vital to enabling believers, including the gay celibate Christian, to overcome shame and live a life full of the Spirit. Living with a homosexual orientation and the demands of the Gospel can cause deep inner conflict in the heart of a gay celibate Christian, and the church has not always done a good job of approaching this conflict. Reparative therapy theory has been shown to be a weak model for ministering to this need. Thus churches should be careful in how they discuss "healing" for homosexuality. On the other hand, a revisionist approach does not need to be embraced in order to minister to gay Christians. An integrative approach provides a solid path that does not dichotomize the homosexual believer's sexuality and faith, but rather integrates them into a whole.

Despite this integration, there still can be deep shame in a gay believer's heart due to the intense nature of homoerotic desires. Yet, shame does not have the last word. Justification by the Spirit is the basis for glorification, which is awaited by faith and in the midst of struggling and stumbling. Sanctification as an overlapping metaphor of the Christian life along with justification implies empowerment and love, providing the key link between living in hope and faith for eternity and living with power and love in this life. Empowerment by the Spirit is not just seen in miracles or charismatic speech but is seen in the love of God at work in and through the believer, including the gay believer. Thus, the definition of vocation as loving and serving others and receiving their love is another expression of this empowerment, for all believers. Gay celibate Christians have much to offer the church, and shame need not keep them from ministering in the power of the Spirit. Church leaders can open up roles for gay celibate Christians to minister to the church even as others minister to them. Pastors and others who lead in local congregations may encourage gay celibate Christians to serve and love in the church, for they too belong fully to the Body of Christ.

While this issue is certainly controversial in society and churches today, Spirit baptism shows us that ministry to gay celibate believers is not so different than ministry to and with any other believer. We are all in need of the great love of God, the fellowship of his body, and the life of the Spirit to walk through this life towards eternity. God desires for all of us to walk together as one body until that great and glorious day when we will leave this world behind and finally see him face to face.

16.

Women at Yoido Full Gospel Church: Pentecostalism in a Confucian Context

Julie Ma

Abstract

The Chosen Dynasty in Korea adopted Confucianism as the state religion and enforced this moral system to an extreme degree. One feature of its philosophy was a strict social hierarchy, including gender disparity. It assumed that men are more capable than and superior to women. The consequences of this are paramount even today. For example, parents in South Korean society prefer boys to girls, which creates a gender imbalance in the national demography. In such a social situation, David Yonggi Cho, the founder and now senior pastor emeritus of Yoido Full Gospel Church, made a radical decision to utilize women to lead the church's extensive cell group system. This has directly challenged the long-held social value of the inferiority of women. Although having female cell group leaders was an alternative to his original intention to appoint men to work, this act has had an enduring impact both on the church and in society. The present senior pastor, Younghoon Lee, reinforces and strengthens the largely female leadership of the cell group structure.

Introduction

Gender bias against females was a significant factor in the fall of the 500-year rule of Korea's Chosen Dynasty in 1910. The Dynasty took Confucianism as the national ideology to such an extreme extent that some of the later developments distorted the original intent.[1] One aspect of Confucian ideology was the unequal status of men and women, which led to the notion that males can achieve more and are better than females. Until recently, its impact lingered in South Korean society in the preference of boys over girls, eventually creating a gender imbalance of the national population.

The arrival of Christianity challenged this long-standing cultural value by promoting education and social roles among girls and women. This cultural challenge was significantly strengthened by the rise of Pentecostalism, which is best exemplified by the impact of Yoido Full Gospel Church founded by David Yonggi Cho. The most decisive program was Cho's radical decision to appoint women to be leaders of his popular cell group system. This was an alternative to his original intention to appoint men to cell leadership, which met with unexpected resistance from male lay leaders. The current senior pastor, Younghoon Lee, continues to utilize women as cell group leaders, and he works to strengthen the predominantly female leadership of the church's cell group system.

This study first explores the pervasive influence of Confucianism in South Korean society, particularly in the attitude of gender preference. It then addresses the question of how Cho came to decide to select the women to be leaders of the cell groups in the context of South Korean culture. Then it probes the implications of this decision to the growth of the church in various stages. It will also discuss the structure of cell leadership, cell group system, main components of a typical home cell meeting, and system's contribution to church growth.

Influence of Confucianism on Religion and Culture in South Korea

The five-century dominance of Confucianism over the Chosun Dynasty has had a deep impact on the formation of social and cultural values in Korea. Strictly speaking, Confucianism offers moral teachings that are valuable to systematically sustaining a society. On the other hand, it does not provide the role of spiritual direction as much as Buddhism does.

Moral Values of Confucianism

An essential, valuable supposition of Confucianism is to be faithful and respectful in relationships with various groups of people to minimize conflicts and to aspire to keep a balanced collaboration. Specifically, there are "the virtues of five different relationships to maintain harmony in life: the right relationship between father and son, ruler and subject, husband and wife, elder and younger, and between friends."[2] It also teaches the virtue of courtesy so that, for instance, students would speak in a polite language when speaking to their teachers. In the same way, females must talk more softly than males in public places and walk behind men.[3] The Confucian ideal assumes that "society can effectively work toward the collective good" under two conditions: 1) everyone fulfills his or her allocated duties within the societal hierarchy, and 2) the mutual responsibility of the benefactor towards the beneficiary and the beneficiary's responsibility towards the benefactor is dutifully fulfilled.[4]

For instance, the appropriate rapport between father and son is ruled by love. For the father, love is displayed by parental care. The Confucian assumption is that a wonderful father provides his son with adequate food, accommodation, clothing, schooling, and suitable ethical direction whether the son is a little boy or an adult. A son likewise is required to exhibit his love by practicing obedience, respect, and "filial piety" to his father.[5]

The Impact of Teaching of Filial Piety

In general, Confucianism has influenced the shaping of the minds and lives of South Koreans, especially in the area of "filial piety." As briefly mentioned above, the right relationship between the father and the son is built upon the son's submission and respect to the father. The son's achievement in school is considered to bring honor to the entire family. A son is a symbol of the family heredity, tasked to fulfill the ancestral rituals and to support the parents in their old age. Looking after his aged parents is the mark of a good son. The son is an embodiment of family pride.

For this reason, parental duty includes the provision of the best education to the son, even if it means a huge financial sacrifice.[6] This relationship continues after the father's death. The son must demonstrate his obligation of care and respect to his deceased father through the appropriate and dutiful performance of ceremonies of filial piety. This also serves as the son's expression of his gratitude for his father's role in bringing the son into the world and his efforts to nurture and raise him. This generational solidarity extends to further generations as the rituals demonstrate the son's gratefulness to his father for giving him life, to ancestors, e.g., his father's father, his father's grandfather, and so on.[7] This duty is the responsibility and privilege of the male descendants.

During Korea's long Chosen Dynasty, only males in a direct line of descent were permitted to lead memorial services for departed ancestors. That tradition has survived into the twenty-first century. In most South Korean families today, although a daughter keeps the family name of her father as her surname even after she marries, she normally cannot lead the memorial services for her deceased parents or grandparents. Moreover, her children will usually take her husband's family name. Therefore, without a son to carry it on, the family name will disappear within two generations. Even worse, there will be no one who can organize and lead the memorial services necessary to keep the memory of ancestors alive and to provide visual reminders that their descendants continue to appreciate all the ancestors did for them.[8]

The eldest son's responsibility is much greater than younger sons. He is expected to live with his father and mother even after being married. My husband is the eldest of five siblings. My parents-in-law longed for a time for us to live with them, even though it was impossible during our missionary years. As they were getting aged, they hoped that we would conclude our missionary service and go to live with them. But that dream was never fulfilled before they passed away.

Of course, in a society where a social security system is not fully in place; the survival of the elderly depends totally on the son's care and support. Although there are some cases where the eldest sons have left their parents behind and migrated elsewhere, they regularly send financial support to look after their parents. In such cases, the younger siblings would relocate the parents to their urban flats, even if they are small for the size of their increasing families. A massive exodus of people from large cities to rural hometowns and villages during special days, such as the Moon Festival (*chusok*), has partly to do with such family expectations and obligations. Traditionally, at the center of family reunions is the ritual to honor their deceased ancestors. The family reunion at their parent's sixtieth and seventieth birthdays is also the expression of this family tradition and obligation.[9]

Favoritism of Sons

In South Korea, some women who have only daughters invariably hope to have another child who is a son. And if the next child turns out again to be a girl, they will just try over and over again until they finally have a son. I am the eldest of five in my family. When my mother gave birth to the first child (that is me), my father was very disappointed. He did not even give me a name for fifteen days. My father's desire to have a son never diminished. Thus, my mother kept on giving birth to three more girls before having a son, who is the last.

Old folks maintain an expectation that a grown-up daughter will marry and transfer to her husband's home to be a new member of his family.

Thus, it is expected for girls to learn cooking, sewing, and caring for children as future mothers. Due to such reasons, a majority of girls stay at home to help their mother with childcare for younger siblings and house chores, including doing the laundry by pounding clothes on flat rocks beside the village stream. They will begin doing this housework when they turn only five or six. These days, this does not always apply, especially in cities.[10] Nonetheless, even today, the parents regard their role as most successful when their daughters marry a man from a decent and reputable family.

This tendency was further aggravated by a government population policy. At the start of South Korea's thrust for economic modernization, the government began a nationwide drive to stop the postwar population explosion through better family planning. Although resources were harshly restricted many years ago, the Ministry of Health and Social Affairs was capable of hiring staff for family planning in the furthest regions of the country. In the Poksu District of Kumsan County, the district headquarters appointed an employee named Mrs. Kim to encourage the residents of South Valley Hamlet to limit the number of children they wanted to have. She educated people on how to use various contraceptive devices and methods.[11] The immediate challenge was the long-held preference for sons over daughters since the sons are responsible for looking after their parents and continuing the faithful performance of family rituals to look after the deceased ancestors. Mrs. Kim's hard work was well recognized in educating the women of Poksu not only about birth control but also, and more importantly, the value of life.[12] However, she faced her own challenge. Her mother-in-law wanted her to have a son as they only had two daughters:

> Since Mr. Kim was the eldest, the mother-in-law wanted the couple to have a son to carry on the family line. She would talk about how their family had enjoyed a succession of strong, intelligent sons over many generations, but disparage her stubborn daughter-in-law, who had new-fashioned, objectionable ideas about family planning. The mother-in-law often told Mrs. Kim that she was wrong to teach about and limit families to two children. She believed that the best insurance for the future was to have sons and that the government policy was wrong.[13]

Her mother-in-law began to put pressure on her and made Mrs. Kim feel that she indeed had failed her greatest fundamental family obligation. Soon after having that thought, she was pregnant with her third child and "in due course bore a stalwart son." Finally, the Kims discontinued their efforts to have more children. However, Mrs. Kim later confessed that if the baby had been a girl, she would have attempted a fourth. "Being a good daughter-in-law turned out to be the most important thing of all, even for an award-winning family planning worker."[14]

Gender Inequality

The practice of male preference extends to the full spectrum of life. In the Korean mind and lifestyle, a superior value is placed on men over women, especially in public settings. The Confucian convention stipulates that one of the five key human relations is "the one between a husband and a wife, and that conjugal relationship is supposed to be governed by respect for gender differences in roles and responsibilities."[15] It denotes that husbands should lead their wives, and wives must be obedient to their husbands. This presumes an image of women to be frail and weak. They are to be the recipients of provision and protection from their husbands. They are confined to domestic life.[16] South Korea has one of the lowest ratios of voting women company officers among industrialized states. Male CEOs control the business realm. There are only several woman CEOs, and there are even fewer women ministers in churches in Korea.[17]

The Confucian ideology of maintaining a social status quo is seriously challenged by today's egalitarianism. Confucians promote harmony as more important than equality. In the Confucian understanding of harmony, it is attained through various members of society faithfully fulfilling their expected duties and submitting to the superiors within the hierarchy. Everyone has different works and tasks, and this accompanies "differences in status, within their families and communities."

Further,

> Confucians insisted that with human nature being what it is, such acquiescence normally would be instinctive, a spontaneous result of respect and appreciation for those who lead others, whether they are parents or community leaders. Confucian moral obligations were not seen as inhibiting normal human behavior but rather were understood as natural expressions of gratitude to those who have helped make us what we are.[18]

Today, Korean society offers many more possibilities to females than in the previous generations. Public education is provided up to high school for both boys and girls throughout the nation. Many girls continue their education in universities and graduate schools. Families sacrificially support their education. "Korean women are shedding many aspects of second-class citizenship,"[19] but they continue to be under restrictions and expectations. Their lives are primarily focused on a good marriage, and everything else is secondary to this. Although many young females are defiant of such an expectation, they are the exception rather than the rule. Though they are professors in universities and selected government officers, it is still true that ordinary family life is crucial to obtain esteem from the community. Females in high-status positions still must subject themselves to this social norm. They are identified as someone's daughter, wife, and mother.[20]

In summary, Confucian ethics have deeply shaped Korean culture, everyday life, and norms. The moral foundation for the limitations on females comes from Confucian philosophy. Restrictions on liberty for females are explained in many Confucian manuscripts and treatises by significant philosophers in the early Chosen Dynasty. For women to be respectful, they need to be humble, quietly isolated, faithful, dedicated to motherhood, and even faithful to their husbands after they die.[21]

David Yonggi Cho and Yoido Full Gospel Church

David Yonggi Cho, the founding and now senior pastor emeritus of Yoido Full Gospel Church, was born in 1936 and raised in a Buddhist home. When he was a teenager, he suffered from terminal tuberculosis. With limited access to medical services, he was left to die. One day, a girl visited him and introduced Jesus. Cho, who was in a physically feeble condition, opened his heart and accepted Christ as his personal Savior. He also experienced astonishing healing from God.[22]

In 1956, he entered into Full Gospel Bible College (for a two-year diploma program) to receive theological training. Unfortunately, in the winter of 1957, Cho had severe flu. For about two weeks, Mrs. Jashil Choi, Cho's classmate, nursed him with prayer. He soon recovered. This brought them closer to each other as ministry partners. Later Choi became Cho's mother-in-law.[23]

Three Stages of Church Growth

The initial stage of Cho's pastoral ministry began in May 1958 soon after his graduation from the Bible College. He and Choi pioneered a tent church in an outskirt of Seoul called Bulkwang-dong. Cho was the main pastor, while Choi served as his associate. Cho regularly preached on Sundays. There were only five people at his first preaching: Choi herself and her three children and a farmer's aging widow. During this pioneering period, Cho became interested in a healing ministry. He read many books on healing by Pentecostal writers, including Oral Roberts. Most books included Bible expositions, which helped Cho to understand the basis for healing. This was an important breakthrough as some "guest lecturers at the Bible College said that the age of miracles had passed with the last of the twelve apostles."[24]

Cho held summer crusades in the first year (1958). Remarkably, radical conversions and healings occurred. An old man had lost his hearing during Japanese colonization in Korea when he refused to obey their orders. Out of anger, "the Japanese had thrust a chopstick into each of the man's ears, bursting his eardrums." That cost his hearing, and he had not heard for fifteen years. During the crusade, all of a sudden he began to hear again. The next day, he brought his entire family including his grandchildren to the crusade. Numerous people converted to Christ during the crusade. The tent church kept on growing in number. As the tent church was bursting at the seams, Cho had a strong desire to move his church to a larger and better facility. He began to construct a new church building in the downtown Seodaemoon area and completed it in February 1962.[25]

The second stage began after moving his church to the new downtown location. Sam Todd, an American evangelist, held a series of revival meetings in September 1962, while the construction was still going on. A large crowd attended, and many had experiences of God's marvelous presence and miracles. The church's 1,500 seats were fully occupied.[26] In the same year, Cho was ordained by the Korean Assemblies of God, the largest Pentecostal denomination in South Korea. The church's membership reached 3,000 in 1964.

The third stage started when Cho moved his church to Yoido Island in 1973. In the Seodaemoon facility, the church grew rapidly and needed a larger space to accommodate the growing congregation. Then Cho decided to build another larger facility in Yoido Island, a newly developing financial district, away from the center of Seoul. In spite of economic struggles and some members' opposition, the church started construction and completed it in September 1973. The church grew even more rapidly after moving to the new location. In 1979, the membership reached 100,000; in November 1980, it reached 200,000; in 1985, it became 500,000, and in 1992, it grew to 700,000.[27]

Characteristics of Growth

Significant church growth took place in South Korea in the 1970s and 1980s, and at the center of this explosive growth was the example and influence of Yoido Full Gospel Church.[28] This section briefly highlights the characteristics of church growth which Cho personally enumerated.

First, Cho had a strong desire for his church to grow. Since he had grown up in a Buddhist family, he believed the local church symbolized the living God in a given community. As a local expression of the organic and living Body of Christ, he strongly believed that the church must grow. He concluded that it is the attitude of the pastor which is critical to church growth. Second, he felt that the message from the church should be positive and uplifting—that Jesus is the ultimate Provider of all our needs. The church must preach the message of hope. After the war between North and South Korea in 1950–1953, the country was devastated by the shortage of food, clothes, and shelter. But more importantly, the people had lost their hope for living. They needed to hear a message of hope for tomorrow.

Third, Cho believed that church growth would never occur without prayer. Testimonies of God's answers to prayers were widely shared in home groups, sermons, and publications. The church started all-night Friday prayer meetings and a prayer mountain with an emphasis on fasting. Fourth, he emphasized the tangible experience of the presence of the Holy Spirit. The church inspired the members to expect and gain an experience of the fullness of the Holy Spirit (or Full Gospel). Encounters with God enabled the members to grow in faith and love, which was quickly translated into evangelistic zeal. This considerably contributed to the growth of the church.

Fifth, the church developed an extensive mission engagement in local areas and overseas by providing evangelism and church planting, as well as relief for humanitarian needs and community services. Last, the dynamic cell group system also contributed to the church's growth. People who attended the church wanted to have a more intimate fellowship to develop a sense of community. Sunday services offered formal worship but rarely provided meaningful opportunities for close fellowship.[29] The last point will be elaborated below.

The Cell Group System of Yoido Full Gospel Church

The organization of a cell group system primarily led by laity did not come together easily as the teaching role in the Confucian world only comes from the social elite. The female leadership of the cell system understandably came after much struggle on the part of each party involved—Cho himself, the church, and society.

Cho's "Conversion"

As the senior pastor, Cho believed that he should take on all the ministerial responsibilities by himself. When the second era of his church, that is, the Seodaemoon era, began, he preached at two services each Sunday. However, the frequency quickly increased as the church constantly grew. In addition, he also preached at the daily dawn prayer meetings and the Wednesday evening services. He also conducted wedding and funeral services, was involved in pastoral counseling and baptized almost each week (once he baptized 300 people). He even picked up guest speakers from the airport and interpreted their sermons. While he was interpreting for a guest preacher, his legs shivered, and he fell to the floor. Deacons immediately took him to the hospital. A doctor examined him and said, "This man is completely drained!" Cho realized that he was unable to undertake all the church work by himself.[30]

Cho spent his recovery time reading the Bible and contemplating a solution for the critical shortage of church workers. He read Exodus 18:13–26 and found out that Moses faced a similar challenge. Moses was hearing all the matters people brought to him for judgment and this continued day after day. He also read Acts 2:42–46 and noted that the believers had gathered in different houses for the breaking of bread and the sharing of apostolic teaching. Thousands of early Christians had home meetings. Priscilla and Aquila had church meetings in their home, and so did Nympha and Philemon along with his family (Rom 16:3–5; 1 Cor 16:19; Col 4:15; Philemon 1–2). Cho was convinced that an effective way of church work was to share responsibilities with deacons and lay leaders. Cho soon called for a meeting among lay leaders (mostly male) and shared his findings through the scriptural readings and his plan to appoint lay leaders to organize and lead home meetings."[31] However, they were not open to Cho's plan:

> One deacon stated that he was too tired at the end of the day to lead a meeting.

Another insisted that some groups would get proud, break away, and start their own churches. A third lay leader remarked that it sounded biblical, but they had not been trained for anything like this. This plan was not part of traditional church activity. "Besides," he informed Dr. Cho, "that's what we pay you for." The meeting ended with the leaders' suggestion: "Why don't you get away and take a long vacation?"[32]

Cho came back home discouraged. His effort to have revolutionary home groups led by mostly male lay leaders failed from the start. While he was going through a time of despondency, Choi, his mother-in-law, and a group of women came to him and suggested to have female lay leaders to lead home cell groups. Cho was unwilling to consider the suggestion due to the traditional Korean bias against women. They were viewed as inferior to men, and their leadership potential was not valued. He was also mindful of particular Scripture passages.[33] Not convinced initially, Cho spent a time of prayer before making up his mind. When Cho prayed, he was reminded by the Holy Spirit about the many women who were a part of Jesus' ministry. He accounts his "conversation" with God over the issue.

"Yonggi, from whom were you born?" the Lord asked Cho.

"From woman, Lord," I responded.

"And on whose lap were you nurtured?"

"Woman, Lord."

"And who followed me throughout my ministry and helped to meet my needs?"

"Women," I said.

"Who stayed until the last minutes of my crucifixion?"

"Women."

"And who came to anoint my body in the tomb?"

"The women."

"Who were the first witnesses to my resurrection?"

"Mary Magdalene and others, women."

"To all my questions you have answered, 'Woman.' Then why are you afraid of women? During my earthly ministry, I was surrounded by dear, wonderful women. So why shouldn't my body, the Church, be surrounded and supported by women as well?"[34]

Cho conceded, "What else could I do? The Lord had made it clear to me that it was His will to use women in the Church."[35] After this conviction, Cho approached the Women's Fellowship and officially informed them of his intention to appoint women leaders. They were to lead home cell group meetings. According to Cho, their response was positive. They said, "Tell us what to do, and we will obey and do the work."[36] So the famous cell-group system was born with women leaders to lead them.

The Structure of the Cell Group System

A cell group is the smallest pastoral unit and the fundamental component of the church. A cell normally is composed of 10–12 families. By 2009, there were 14, 888 cell units which met every week in homes in various sections of the city.[37] The metropolitan area is divided into 20 large districts, 313 sub-districts, 4,374 sections.[38]

"Each home cell unit is ideally composed of between 8 to 15 households. If the number increases beyond the limit, then a new cell unit begins to form."[39] Cell groups are allocated to geographic regions. For the regions that are far from the main church, regional chapels are opened for various worship services, including early morning prayers. This also helps to effectively monitor and guide the cell system.[40] Out of these cell groups, 96% of them are led by female members. The church has 634 full-time pastors and 400 elders who manage various ministries of the church, particularly the cell group ministry. Although still called "cell" or "home group," these meetings are neither social gatherings nor home fellowship meetings. A section is formed by 25 to 90 home cell units, which is led by a pastoral member.[41]

The leader of a home cell unit conducts a weekly meeting, frequently aided by an assistant leader. The weekly meeting moves among the member homes. There are a couple of reasons for this arrangement found in the New Testament. First, believers in the book of Acts had gatherings "from house to house" (Acts 2:46), denoting that various families hosted meetings of the early church. Second, women played a unique role in the life and ministry of Jesus. Cho is convinced, "We believe that when Christians worship God in a home, that home is blessed."[42] While the members had full confidence in Cho's leadership and vision, he frequently and publicly attributed particular importance to the cell leaders. In response, cell members committed themselves to pray specifically for the host or hostess of their cell meetings. When a member, who is still young in the faith, falls ill or encounters hardship, the family is usually hesitant to host a cell group meeting in their homes. The cell leader and mature members encourage the family to open their homes so that the members would pray for the family's needs, be it healing or finances. Normally no home is supposed to host a cell group meeting more than once per month.[43]

Qualifications for the Cell Group Leader

Cell leaders are the key to the success of the given cell group ministry. For this reason, the church has established criteria for the selection of cell leaders. First, cell leaders have to have adequate knowledge of the Word of God. She or he needs to be well prepared to teach the cell members. Second, they need to share the church's passion for church growth and desire to be used of the Holy Spirit. Third, the cell leaders have to be Spirit-filled, so that they can, in turn, assist their cell members to be filled with the Holy Spirit. Fourth, they must have a vision for the cell group. They are encouraged to spend time in prayer to develop a vision for new souls to be led to Christ, which would result in the growth of the cell group. Fifth, they ought to continually strengthen their Christian faith—to not be easily discouraged and to enable cell members to grow in faith and their lives to be transformed. Sixth, cell group leaders must be role models to the members by living exemplary lives.[44]

Equipping the Cell Group Leaders

The church provides primary training to new cell leaders and continuing education to existing leaders. The church's education division organizes the primary leadership program, an eight-week cell leaders' college. Staff members of the college and regional pastors provide training based on the established curriculum on Sunday afternoons. The continuing education takes place during the semiannual conferences of sectional and cell leaders held in the spring and the fall of each year. Originally, the conference lasted for three days with inspirational messages, guidelines for cell group management and fresh new worship songs. However, in recent years, due to the large number of cell leaders, the church has reduced the conferences to a single meeting consisting of an educational lecture and a stimulating message from Cho. The same program is repeated to be able to accommodate the large number of cell leaders. For both meetings, the main sanctuary is packed to full capacity.[45]

The Responsibilities of the Cell Group Leaders

Cell leaders take on the following responsibilities: 1) to be accountable for the members of their cell units; 2) to watch a training session through videotape every Wednesday at 5:00–6:00 in the afternoon; 3) to conduct weekly home cell meetings where the leader provides a Bible study on the basis of the Wednesday session and leads a prayer time; 4) to be active, together with cell group members in inviting non-believers to cell group meetings and to church worship services; 5) to check in with their section leaders at least once a week to keep the status chart current at the church office and to submit a weekly report of their previous meetings. The report includes dates for the incoming meetings, visitation finished, significant prayer requests of any member, the amount of collection received, and the number of new believers; and finally, 6) to attend the semi-annual training conference for cell leaders.[46]

The Role of the Sectional and District Leaders

Sectional leaders are appointed from cell leaders who have served effectively for two years. They typically manage between three and eight cell groups. The expectations for the section leaders are that they: 1) serve as a connection between the pastors and the cell leaders; 2) win souls as much as they can; 3) have the financial resources to support the church; 4) have their own home large enough to host a monthly meeting with all the leaders of the section; and 5) are spiritually and emotionally mature.[47] Additional responsibilities are the following:

...the ongoing training of cell group leaders. They do this most often by modeling, especially as they go with cell leaders in ministry visits. Also, there is a monthly leaders' meeting in each section, when the group leaders of that area meet with their staff pastor in the home of the section leader for prayer and ministry. After this meeting, the staff pastor usually goes with the section leader and group leaders to make ministry visits to the homes and businesses of those in that area undergoing the most difficulty. As the staff pastor ministers and prays with these people, section and group leaders are often writing notes and learning by observing.[48]

Quite a number of the section leaders regularly speak with their home cell leaders on the phone. The frequency ranges between daily to weekly.

The section leaders then set aside one day a week to visit the cell leaders and members who face serious struggles or difficulties.[49]

District leaders are prayerfully selected among assistant pastors by the senior pastor at an annual meeting. Some are ordained, and others are licensed ministers, but all have adequate ministry experience. They are also to demonstrate sound spiritual maturity and competency in pastoral work. They are particularly responsible in three areas. First, they are to handle and counsel for delicate and sensitive issues that arise among the home cell units. Second, they are to consecrate babies and officiate wedding, funeral, and anniversary services. Third, they are to preside over Sunday morning services, speak on numerous Sunday night services, conduct dawn prayer meetings, and lead Friday all-night prayer meetings.[50]

Key Elements of a Home Cell Meeting

This section discusses several vital components of cell group meetings. The first is prayer. The members are committed to prayer, especially for each other's needs. This includes prayers for healing and financial provision. Through prayer, they practice their love, care, and concern for cell group members. Prayer is also offered for the salvation of members who are new to the group and the Christian faith. For certain critical matters, the leader and members even pray with fasting.[51] Testimonies of answered prayers are regularly shared in the cell group meetings. This is "a practice which builds even greater faith as cell unit members turn their need-directed prayer to attend others."[52] A couple once shared a moving testimony with their cell group. Due to constant clashes in their married life, they were considering a divorce. Upon learning of this challenge, the cell leader invited them to her home for prayer, but they rebuffed her. However, when the invitation was offered the second time, they accepted. Through their prayer and counsel, the couple experienced healing of their wounded relationship. Soon after, they became a husband-wife leader team over a home cell group.[53]

The second and most important element of the cell meeting is teaching the Word of God for daily Christian life and witness. The church has produced a series of seven study guides for the home cell groups. This seven-year curriculum provides a systematic study of the Bible. The content is based on more than four hundred of Cho's expository sermons mostly delivered in Wednesday evening services. Each lesson centers on one key topic of Christian life based on a scriptural passage.[54]

The layout for the weekly study guide lesson is the following:

- Today's Scripture: This is the key text for the lesson. The group reads this part of Scripture out loud collectively.
- Memory Verse: As the core of the lesson, this Scripture is read out loud in one voice by the group a few times.
- Leading questions: Commonly the leader invites a few initial questions from the reading of the day's Scripture.
- Today's Message: "Two to three pages in length, this pre-published note explains the week's topic. In most groups, the members take turns to read paragraphs of this note aloud until the entire message has been read."[55] Then the leader highlights important points of the passage, occasionally interjecting personal illustrations.
- Closing Questions: The leader invites final comments and questions as he or she brings the "material from the lesson together."
- Applications: The lesson concludes with a few suggested applications to everyday life.[56]

The last element of the cell meeting is fellowship. At this time, the members freely share personal and family affairs with other members, often over refreshments. This enhances the unity in the body of Christ.[57] The whole process of the cell group meeting contributes to the harmony of the church. This harmony is based on a firm foundation: truth, dynamic faith, spiritual vitality, care for each other's needs, and compliance to the leadership. The members are constantly taught how to exercise their faith through prayer for others. This vibrant harmony draws the members to spiritual growth in a Christ-centered and Spirit-led atmosphere. It further strengthens the members' faith and their dedication to Christ.[58]

Concluding Remarks

As discussed in this study, Confucianism has pervaded South Korean society especially in the shaping of values and social structures. The place of women has been a stark reminder of this philosophical system against gender equality.

In March 2017, the Ministry of Family and Women's Affairs published a report that South Korea ranks in the 142nd place out of 193 nations in the index of women ministers. Although the country is economically developed, the nation's progress in gender equality ranks among under-developed or developing countries. Once having a female president, it was counted among nations such as England, Germany, Italy, the Netherlands, Spain, and France, whose prime ministers were women. However, having a female president appears to be an exception in South Korea rather than a norm. The newly elected president, Jaein Moon, vowed to drastically accomplish a gender balance in his cabinet. It is a clear sign of his awareness of the deeply rooted gender bias in South Korea.[59]

It should be noted that the image of women in Asia, including South Korea, has been improving in most societies, excluding several Muslim countries. Astonishingly, women today can work in conspicuous places and occupations once exclusively available only to men. However, what we experience in current times was totally unimagined in earlier years. The recent decision of the Saudi prince to allow women to drive is a case in point.[60]

In this general context, the cell group system of Yoido Full Gospel Church was revolutionary. When Cho made a final decision to appoint women leaders over the cell groups, some women also objected to the decision. This indicates how deeply engrained was the gender-biased value system. Only the deep sense of God's vision provided Cho with the necessary perseverance and persuasion. He sustained this countercultural system through the careful training of the leaders. The church carefully maintained the qualifications of these leaders. These female leaders were Cho's ministry priority as the backbone of his church structure. As a result, the church grew in its dynamic and vibrancy, both in its spiritual life and numerical growth. After decades of experience, the system has proven to be truly empowering. Many churches throughout the world have adopted the cell-group system with necessary modifications. In South Korea, like in many social contexts, female leadership has defied the long-established gender-bias system.

17.

Postscript: A Reflection

Annamarie Hamilton

Introduction

Having read these chapters, I find myself in awe of three things in particular: the great goodness of God's heart towards his creation, including through the intricate gift of human sexuality; the great onslaught of evil against human sexuality, individually and in society; and the great restoration that is underway by God's grace and through his Spirit.

This postscript will reflect on these three things, particularly within the contexts shared by these authors. There are certainly types and depths of harm we have not mentioned; and there are many places where healing is underway, beyond the scope of this book. There is also overlap among the chapters, as, one after another, the authors elucidate teachings of scripture on this subject using time-tested methods of scholarship. The significant stories told in these chapters are a representative sample of the healing that God is doing through his Spirit and through Spirit-empowered believers around the world. This gives hope that, even when we are not aware, God is at work in the very difficult arena of sexual brokenness. This is a needed hope, for the scope of the brokenness is enormous, while the value of each human life is greater still.

The Gift: Theological Principles of Human Sexuality

As beautifully stated by many theologians, human sexuality is a gift that reflects the very image of God. In fact, so deep is this gift that "reflects" is too small a word. A mirror merely reflects an image; it does not absorb it. Yet in human beings, sexuality is infused in every cell, emotion, and experience; and the image of God, a core reality at birth, grows greater and deeper throughout the lifespan in those who seek him. "Embody" may better convey the mystery that God began when "male and female he created them, in the image of God he created them" (Gen 1:27).

The ways that our sexuality embodies God's image are several. Pope John Paul II's magnum opus *Theology of the Body*[1] articulated these ideas nearly forty years ago, and theologians including Tim Tennent, a

Wesleyan, and Christopher West, a Roman Catholic, have brought his message forward for current audiences.[2] Regarding human sexuality's gift, a few crucial thoughts from those theologians might be summarized here, in a list for clarity (see below). These are drawn mostly from Gen 1:26–28, which says, "Then God said, 'Let us make man in our image, according to our likeness....' God created man in his own image, in the image of God he created him; male and female he created them. God blessed them; and God said to them, 'Be fruitful and multiply.'"

1. Within the Godhead himself – the Holy Trinity – there exists an intimate community, which includes separateness, unity, and faithfulness.
2. God made human beings to reflect his image, including his relational nature.
3. It takes man and woman together to reflect the image of God; two men or two women do not bear his full image, according to this original design.
4. The relationship between a man and a woman is blessed, including their sexual relationship.
5. The coming together of the two separate others – man and woman – results in new life, which is both a blessing in itself and a further reflection of the nature of God: as God is Creator, the man and woman are co-creators, and the new life which comes from their union completes the picture of the Trinity.
6. This and other verses (spanning the entire Old Testament) portray the role of exclusivity in marriage, as in worship.
7. The markers of our physical body, given at birth, tell us important things about the nature of God, the nature of ourselves, and the nature of ourselves in relationship with another who is our complement (not our replica). As Tim Tennent explains the Christian view of the body (versus the gnostic) "Your heart is deceitful, but your body can be trusted."[3] This statement refers to the body's design, not its every appetite.

Much more deserves to be said on this holy subject, and it has been said elsewhere.[4] These seven points are enough to lay pertinent foundation regarding the glory and the goodness of our sexuality, from the beginning. Contained within that goodness is, implicitly, what it is not. For example, marriage is between two people, not three. Marriage is between two humans, not a human and an animal (nor another non-human, such as a robot). Marriage is between two human beings who are compatible but not the same, and we see this in the bodily interdependence of their sexuality. Marriage includes sexual expression which is designed to be capable of bringing new life. These points state what I consider to be some of the most compelling theological principles regarding sexual identity and gender, very relevant to our day.

Against the gifts in the Garden, of which sexuality is one, we know from the third chapter of Genesis that deception came (vv. 1–5), and then disobedience (v. 6), followed by shame (they covered their nakedness, v. 7), fear (they hid from God, v. 8), blame (the man blamed the woman, v. 12), and guilt (with no mention of her husband, the woman named deception and eating the forbidden fruit, v. 13). These words are tragedy. Grave tragedy. Many centuries later the Apostle Paul wrote of that earth-shattering day, "just as through one man sin entered into the world, and death through sin, and so death spread to all mankind because all sinned...." (Rom 5:12). It was never meant to be this way, with death here. Now that it was, curses followed. The curses were not the beginning of the badness, the sin was; and through that first sin, all that is badness in the world entered.

The curses are vocational and relational for the man and the woman: pain, toil, enmity, domination (Gen 3:16–17). Referenced in the curses is the cure for sin (Gen 3:15), but it would be many generations till the cure came to pass (Luke 2); and even then, sin would not be expunged from the world but overcome through faith (Phil 2:12–15, I John 5:4). Eventually, at the end of time, the heavens and earth will be made new, and all will be finally right again, within and without (Rev 21:1–5). For that time, we wait and hope. Meanwhile, after the curses, God himself provided clothing for the original man and woman in the Garden, replacing their fig leaves with animal skins (Gen 3:21)—the first example of God making sacrifice for the covering of sin, but it would not be his last (John 3:16–17)—and escorted them out of the Garden, to protect them from living forever in a now fallen world (Gen 3:22–24).

The Brokenness

Everywhere in this fallen world the pain, toil, enmity, domination, and isolation of the curse abound. The many forms of death that entered with sin ooze over our planet like oil spill and spread like wildfire. The deceiver who spoke in the Garden still hisses in the ear of believers and unbelievers alike.

Pause to look at the nature of original deception: comparing what the serpent said to Eve (see Gen 3:1–5) with what God had said to Adam (see Gen 2:16–17), we see a one-word slide of tongue—replacing God's "freely any" ("You may freely eat from any tree of the Garden") with the serpent's "not any" ("Did God really say, 'You shall not eat from any tree of the garden'")—which entirely distorts God's message. Eve in her sweet innocence engages with the snake, correcting his error of speech. And at that moment, the serpent strikes, telling his boldfaced lie ("You shall not surely die") and then stating a truth ("For God knows that in the day you eat from it your eyes will be opened, and you will be like God, knowing good and evil"). But deception states the truth in such a way that God's character of goodness and motive of love are turned upside down to the hearer.

Knowledge of good and evil? Adam and Eve already had an intimate knowledge of good! They walked with him every evening (Gen 3:8).[5] They knew face-to-face the very source and personification of all that is good, in their daily communion with God. By biting the forbidden fruit, they would add only the horrible knowledge of evil. Were they also tempted by the bait, "You shall be like God?" While still in their innocent state, how could this offer (often seen as appealing to pride or control) find a perch in their psyche? Perhaps Eve was gullible to hints of a better communion, not sensing the distortion; or for beautiful food; and for wisdom (Gen 3:6); and, for whatever reason, Adam was silent. Deceived, disobeying, and possibly with an innocent precursor to fear of missing out (FOMO), they bit. Then all hell broke loose, and Eden disappeared. Innocence and purity were gone. Evil had entered.

I hypothesize that the human frame is not fit for the knowledge of evil; our constitutions were not made for it. God can handle this knowledge, but we were not made for it. And so we wrestle with the question of evil and the presence of evil. Sometimes we blame God when evil things happen. Sometimes we are broken like dry twigs by evil: it lures us, then our appetites change, distortions draw us to great harm, and blindness prevents our escape. The very atmosphere of our existence now polluted by evil's presence, who gets to adulthood without harm and even trauma?[6] Healing depends on trusting, but whom to trust, and how, in a world filled with bent and broken mirrors? I think we were not made to know evil. But now, we do know it. Evil is part of our world.

As the deepest of all targets, human sexuality becomes evil's special prey. In this way, evil distorts the image of God on the earth. It also crushes individuals at the core of who they are. And, in a terrible final twist, the victim of sexual harm is the one stigmatized, blamed, and shamed, with reverberations that can last a lifetime. Sexual harm takes many forms. When one person dominates another sexually, or coerces, manipulates or withholds; where there is shame, self-loathing, lust;

through violence, rape, fear; obfuscation of sexual identities; barred access to education, employment and basic needs; disease; objectification; pornography, addiction, sex trafficking; adultery, incest; in all these ways and more, evil assaults humans through their sexuality. Tragically, most of these things we do to one another and to ourselves. The practitioners and scholars who have contributed to this book have first-hand knowledge of the deep heartbreak (and mind- and body-break) of harmed sexuality.

In parts of Asia and Africa, gender discrimination bars girls from attending school or makes them married before puberty. This implies a low view of girls' value, and violence against girls becomes common. In this context (and others), girls are easily raped and then shamed and outcast for any resulting pregnancy. Worldwide, sex trafficking occurs on a scale that is growing and defies recording. Even governments may be implicated in this horribly destructive practice. The Philippines is hit very hard by the scourge of child sex trafficking; yet the Pentecostal church there appears to be quiet on the issue, although they speak out on other issues. Is this crime too big, complex, and far-reaching even for the Church? It would appear that it is. In a separate but potentially related Filipino crisis, many women leave their families to become migrant workers abroad. Work migration is an excruciating decision for a mother: if she leaves the country for work, will her child(ren) be safe? If she does not, will they eat and have basic needs met? These are dilemmas of survival. Migrant workers' children are at higher risk of becoming trafficked, and the women themselves are at risk of isolation and all kinds of abuse under foreign employment. Below the lowest rung of the social ladder in many places, who is there to protect domestic foreign workers? AIDS is another ravager irrespective of boundaries. Our Zambian author lost family members to this terrible disease, and its rampage continues. And questions of gender and sexual identity proliferate worldwide, crumbling systems of every size.

The Restoration: The Holy Spirit and Spirit-Empowered Communities

"Although the world is full of suffering, it is full also of the overcoming of it," (Helen Keller).[7] We are seeing restoration in places. People are helping, including devoted people from many different vocations and groups. One group, in particular, stands out for their tirelessness and for their growing number worldwide. And especially—regardless of status, education, or wealth—for their effectiveness. That group is Christians who are empowered by the Holy Spirit. In reality, there is not a sect of Spirit-empowered Christians; they are found within every denomination of Christendom. But communities whose focus is Spirit-empowerment tend to be Pentecostal churches. It is valuable to see what they are doing, where restoration is occurring.

Stories from Korea, India, and Nepal that describe deep cultural and religious gender discrimination against girls also show the dramatic transformation that the very same, previously disadvantaged, girls and women experience when Holy Spirit-empowered ministers and churches or schools reach out to them. Through a women-led cell group movement in Korea; a loving after-school program in India; and a young woman's personal conversion followed by divine healing and the subsequent spread of her faith to an entire region in Nepal, practitioners and scholars Julie Ma (Korea), Atula and Brainerd Prince (India), and Bal and Karuna Sharma (Nepal) see the Holy Spirit healing and transforming their friends and cultures. A similar transformation occurred in the African nation of Burkina Faso when pastors' families fostered girls who escaped to them for help, and when churches founded schools which unflinchingly educated girls as well as boys, as reported by Philippe Ouedraogo. Praying and helping disadvantaged children and women by providing them with safe housing, education, mentoring, and leadership opportunities are ways the Holy Spirit, through his people, is restoring.

The pandemic of sex trafficking appears too big for the national church, as seen in the Philippines. Because the child sex trade is a *tourist* industry, it may require the global Church to band together. Filipino children, for example, are being harmed by other nations' pedophiles. How might the American, European, Latin, African and Australian Churches help address this issue, both in terms of each nation's wandering sexual predators and its own trafficked young people? Suico and Suico recommend starting by educating parishioners. They also mention several groups that are addressing the issue in the Philippines but need something to unite them. A united global Church may be required to support the many parachurch groups, to minister to victims and perpetrators alike, and to offer alternatives to the poverty and perversions that feed the sex trade. The global Church speaking out and educating, rescuing, advocating, influencing language and legislation, exposing corruption, and providing shelter and healing is needed in order to stand against and turn this massive tide of sexual brokenness. Who but the people of God, empowered by his Spirit, are up to this task, its emotional cost, and its duration?

Another face in the Filipino child sex-trafficking crisis is that of domestic workers, mostly women, many of whom are mothers and also Pentecostal Christians. Pastoral and researching-teaching team Dr. and Dr. Benavidez report what they have seen. Filipino women in financially precarious families prayerfully and carefully weigh their options before leaving home to provide income for the family. When a Pentecostal woman with children migrates, the community comprised of the children's grandparents, aunts, and church rally round the children and take care of them. This is, child by child, an answer to sex trafficking: a protective circle of care by relatives and Spirit-empowered communities. One caveat – the teenage children of migrant workers may be particularly at risk, due to their competing developmental needs. In this case, the church youth group can play a vital protective role.

Another pandemic related to human sexuality is AIDS. A case study has been occurring in Zambia, influenced by the leadership of Joshua Banda, a Bishop in the Assembly of God denomination. Two dramas are simultaneously unfolding in Zambia and other African nations. One is HIV/AIDS treatment and prevention, which is seeing much success in terms of reversal of the spread of the disease, especially when sexual behavior change is included. The Zambian Church has been a significant factor in this success, with its clear message, clinics, inexhaustible volunteers, and advocacy at high levels. The second drama is the struggle of Zambia to retain its national autonomy and cultural values in laws and policies governing marriage and homosexuality. Against this, the influence of Western nations—which tie very different values to their AIDS-prevention donations—pressures Zambia to change its laws and national character. Some have asked why the politics of "human rights" have been tied to the eradication of disease. Others have asked why groups demanding tolerance and advocating for acceptance in the West refuse to grant tolerance and acceptance to African cultures within their sovereign states.

The Church in Africa is standing against outside pressure and is defending their nations' right to claim their own culture and laws. They experience Western, strings-attached AIDS donations to be another wave of European colonialism, this time as a wealth-based invasion of sexual values that are deeply at odds with African sensibilities. Bishop Banda and others present sociocultural and medical empirical evidence that supports the benefits and African-ness of Zambian policies for AIDS prevention, including behavioral components. The good news for Africa is that these policies are working and the spread of this deadly disease is slowing. For nations as for individuals, sexual issues are identity issues.

Practitioner Atula Walling Prince articulates sexual identity questions in her work with children in India, where there is pronounced gender disparity and abandonment. "What does it mean to be biologically female? What consequences are there for being born female? Who am I? How am I supposed to live as a woman in society, what role and expectations are expected of me as a woman?"[8] Women around the world ask these questions. (I propose that men do too, in modified form.) In Hindu society, the answer to each of those questions relies completely on a man. This puts girls at great risk, and it diminishes their value as co-equal heirs in the image of God. Restoring a fuller vision of femininity, Atula and her colleagues engage with girls in their interests and stories, and they tell the stories of history-changing biblical women. Importantly, the workers lovingly minister from within their own stories and charismata, without directing the impact. The Holy Spirit does his work, weaving ancient stories through the imaginations of living girls, and they are empowered. Atula's young friends report that they like being a girl. This is miraculous. The divine image is being restored in these places.

Questions of gender and sexual identity occur everywhere around the globe. The shape of the conversation changes from place to place, depending on laws and culture, but the questions are being asked everywhere, and limits are being pushed. One wonders what is behind this epidemic of confusion. Has the human race always struggled to know sexual identity and orientation at the rate that is occurring now? My sense is that it has not. Would the conversation be so widespread or controversial if homosexuality and gender change had been prolific throughout the centuries? And—crass, perhaps, but pertinent—would human societies have survived this long if many of its pillars (married, heterosexual, procreating couples) had been changing their orientations and commitments, rather than providing stable shelter for children from generation to generation? I think human society cannot long sustain widespread instability at its core. The breadth of what is now occurring in this arena around the globe is surely a phenomenon in human history. What is causing it? Michael McClymond of Saint Louis University sheds light on the theoretical, theological, philosophical and political aspects of transgenderism, including stories from transitioners and detransitioners. His insights are prescient and deeply compassionate.

There is also the long-term, stable gay. This is a struggle all its own. Western society presses for public support of all kinds of sexual expression; but for many, this only intensifies the struggle. For gay Christians, Megan Grondin, drawing from Wesley Hill and Frank Macchia, describes how church communities can include and support celibate gay persons in their midst, helping to stand against the isolation, loneliness, and shame they experience. Shame and loneliness crouch near the core of many, if not all, human hearts. A theology of brokenness and the sweet power and love of the Spirit bring comfort and healing, in community. Tryphena Law, Malaysian Assembly of God pastor, describes her own experience with this as she journeyed into and back out of a homosexual lifestyle in Malaysia. With gentleness, candor, and courage she now helps other strugglers through PLUC, Pursuing Liberty Under Christ, and Spirit-filled community increases. The Holy Spirit is empowering his people for healing.

Recommendations for Prayer and Additional Strategic Focus

In addition to praying for heroic people who are already helping to heal the broken, it is wise to take stock and look for places that merit additional strategic work and also see where gaps exist. Grouping sexual brokenness by type, we might see four broad categories: sex trafficking and rape; gender discrimination; sexual/gender identity/change and queer theory; and domestic alignments for both married and singles.

Sex Trafficking and Rape

Pastors Suico and Suico have recommended educating populations regarding the occurrence of sex trafficking and all its facets. Campaigns to educate more people should be encouraged. In this way, people are empowered to take a stand against trafficking and the systems that allow it. The particular information and style of presentation will be unique to each culture, but globally, education campaigns are warranted similar to those that occurred early in the AIDS pandemic. One small example is basic safety, including internet safety: churches can partner with police departments to educate parishioners on safety, including the safe use and monitoring of technology. Risky internet use is one way predators lure at-risk teens into sex trafficking, online victimization, meetings that turn into rape, or into gangs. Rape victims are often sexually revictimized.[9] In gangs, lured teenagers are often enslaved into the sex trade for the purpose of generating income for the gang, with a "sustainable commodity" more profitable than drugs.[10] Internet protection is just one example of the type of education needed to help protect young people from becoming victims. Each culture's content needs to be appropriate to educate for its setting, but one universal goal would be to raise awareness of the magnitude and pervasiveness of sex trafficking. It occurs right under our nose.

I earlier recommended the global Church unite to make sex trafficking a strategic focus of prayer and effort, especially recognizing that because this evil intentionally crosses geopolitical borders, the Church must also. Spirit-empowered communities encircling children—literally, providing childcare—to protect at-risk youth from sex trafficking should be highly encouraged and caused to increase. The suggested educational campaign can include celebrating the enormous positive difference these protecting, care-giving churches are already making and build on that strength.

While churches are teaching and nurturing, Christians can make a very significant impact by lobbying for effective laws and law enforcement. Sweden provides an excellent example. Sex trafficking is on the rise throughout the world, but Sweden is a notable exception. In Sweden the laws have been reversed: sex is no longer illegal to sell, rather it is illegal to buy. Sweden recognized that people who sell their bodies are desperate and either don't have options or were previously victimized, or both. It makes no sense to criminalize and fine these people. However, people who purchase sex have some means to do so, and they come from all walks of life. Criminalizing the buying of sex, rather than the selling of it, is more logical and more humane, and Sweden's example shows that it is effective. Significantly, it also reverses the usual pattern of stigmatizing and blaming the victim. Sex trafficking and prostitution have been practically eliminated in Sweden since these laws have become written and enforced. In addition, "john schools" were established to rehabilitate the habitual consumer. This combination has been highly effective for restoring that society from the brokenness of commercial sex.[11] Is advocacy for laws of this nature, including their enforcement, something Spirit-empowered communities can do in countries around the world? This could change the planet and millions of individual lives.

Gender Discrimination

The case studies that demonstrate restoration in the area of gender discrimination can be lifted up as models. The way women serve as leaders in Korean cell groups deserves to be studied and replicated, because it seems they have found the balance that brings real freedom and empowerment, avoiding both rigidity, which excludes women from leadership, and reverse discrimination, which elevates women at the expense of men. The Koreans' reversal of gender bias within the Pentecostal church has everything to do with spiritual maturity, as well as need. Duplicating the balance they have achieved draws from—and promotes—spiritual maturity.

Other case studies show the absolutely transformative power of the Gospel and healing. The preaching and youth rallies that are now occurring in Nepal are remarkable. The transformation of an entire region, after a woman's conversion and healing, is a miracle like the woman at the well who met Jesus (John 4). We must remember and not neglect the simple preaching of the Bible, sharing our faith with our neighbor, and praying for the sick, all through the Spirit.

The stories from Atula Walling's after-school program are inspiring, as well. The personal attention each child receives, the guidance and companionship for learning new skills, and the Bible stories of significant women have changed that culture. In Burkina Faso the same thing is happening, girl by girl and school by school. These successes demonstrate the difference that grassroots efforts can achieve. In particular, I am struck by the impact that warm attention and well-told Bible stories can make. This is very promising!

Sexual/Gender Identity/Change and Queer Theory

This category is complex. As Dr. McClymond mentioned, support and kindness are to be the Church's normal way of treating every neighbor, including those with different views or experiences of sexuality. Only in this way can person to person dialogue occur, for helping and healing everyone involved. Also, there is strong and recurring evidence that research findings incongruent with LGBTQ+ postulates are being suppressed in Western culture.[12] The mingling of politics, agendas, the media, and science confuses the conversation and the way forward, not to mention many people's lives. In another context, we would call this suppression propaganda. In the U.S. it is billed as compassion. However, actual compassion is forestalled if all the evidence cannot be discussed. Spirit-empowered communities can pray and can treat our neighbors with kindness and respect because it's right, and because we love each other, and because the conversation depends on it.

Domestic Alignments for Marrieds and Singles

Each of us is our own "case study" in sexuality. In marriage, each spouse has a responsibility to be aware and honest regarding his or her own pleasure and needs, as well as attentive to their spouse's. This process is not always easy, nor is it physically static. It involves discovery, communication, and change throughout the lifespan. It also requires attention to other parts of the marriage, because we know that desire, arousal, and pleasure are all linked but do not occur in the same way for men and women.[13] Further, an intimate emotional bond is a crucial component in a full and authentic sexual experience.[14] The emotional bond encompasses the whole of the marriage. The spiritual bond is closely linked, as well.[15] As married people live out their sexual lives—which is to say, the *whole* of their lives—attention to their inner experience as individuals and to their intimate experience as a couple, in every dimension, is part of their shared sexuality. This is a holy bond, mirroring worship. And so we are back to where we started: human sexuality is a gift, reflective of the divine nature, and lived out in the flesh with the chosen and treasured other, sacramentally.

I find my personal restoration in the divine image is enhanced as I meditate on God's lovingkindness, his nearness, purposes, and gifts, including sexuality. I find my communion deepened with him and with my spouse when I refresh myself in a theology of the body, articulated by Pope John Paul, Timothy Tennent, and others. Living in a noisy culture centered far differently than that theology, the song of restoration diminishes unless I remind myself frequently, humming along. The Holy Spirit helps me do this, for he sings it in my ear and he beckons me to refresh myself in him. Reading the scriptures and these authors reminds me, too. We live lives of cherishing.

For singles, alignment with one's own core values takes a slightly different expression, and even journey, than for those married. For the Christian single, finding one's footing in the myriad of worldview choices now available, especially about sexuality, may be like choosing a patch of ice on which to stand in the Arctic Ocean. Big, little, floating, or the tip of an iceberg, they look a lot alike from the surface, though some have more grounding than others.

Recognizing that Christians hold a variety of worldviews, especially in terms of sexual and gender issues, let us acknowledge that for centuries of human history most people agreed that there were two sexes and that those two sexes were distinguished by their external physical markers. Let us further agree that for centuries, Christians have heard or read the Bible at face value and so—although application has varied widely throughout the epochs—the general view for most of human history has been that Genesis indicates marriage is between one man and one woman, it is intended to be lifelong, and the general design is that most people will get married. This is not the only Christian view, but it has been the dominant Judeo-Christian view for most of human history. In that context, the Christian single now comes to a maturing twenty-first century.

The current century not only surrounds the young adult single Christian with billions of worldviews (while raising suspicion of her parents'), it also engulfs her in the unprecedented sexual brokenness of rampant sex trafficking everywhere (except Sweden), with whatever that says about her society and about her; pornography immersion and how that inoculates the brain against normal arousal and pursuit;[16] a gender-dysphoria epidemic, blurring every trans with "normal" in the new worldviews, further diluting pursuit and connection; and brokenness and isolation in many of the relationships which previously would have provided a safe space for growth and healing. Into this mix, the Christian single comes of age. The *Theology of the Body* speaks a rich vision for singles called to a celibate life. But what about the single who longs for an intimate spousal relationship, in a world where human sexuality lies scattered in shards or blurred to obscurity?

The Holy Spirit is here, too. In every brokenness, the Holy Spirit is near and ready to comfort and to help. We believe this not because we can always see it, but because he said it and we know him. There is a hissing that says he is not near, he is not able, he is not good, he has abandoned our youth. To this hiss, I say no. God is good. I see his restoration in some places in the world. I believe it even when I do not see it. I nestle into the goodness of God; I do not need to bite into forbidden things to believe that I have the good right here within my grasp. Holding onto his goodness like a good father's hand, I—we, the community of Spirit-empowered believers—reach out to young friends and old, and beckon them to take our other hand, to step onto this anchored iceberg of believing and belonging. We will sing and dance, kindle a fire and warm ourselves together here, enjoying the pleasures of friendship, hot drinks, Northern Lights, knowing and being known, together, until the coming of the Lamb.

Notes

Introduction

[1] Harold D. Hunter and Neil Ormerod (eds.), *The Many Faces of Global Pentecostalism* (Cleveland, TN: CPT Press, 2013).
[2] Vinson Synan, ed., *Spirit-Empowered Christianity in the 21st Century: Insights, Analysis, and Future Trends* (2011); and four-volume series edited by Vinson Synan and Amos Yong, *Global Renewal Christianity: Past, Present, and Future* (Lake Mary, FL: Charisma House), covering Asia and Oceania (2016), Latin America (2016), Europe and North America (2017) and Africa (2016).
[3] Vinson Synan, ed., *The Truth about Grace: Spirit-Empowered Perspectives* (Lake Mary, FL: Charisma House, 2018).
[4] Mark Hall and Brainerd Prince/Atula Walling in *Spiritus: ORU Journal of Theology* 3:1 (2018).

Chapter 1

[1] See, for instance, Robert Menzies' discussion of "Spiritual Gifts: Essential Principles," in William W. Menzies and Robert P. Menzies, *Spirit and Power: Foundations of the Pentecostal Experience* (Grand Rapids, MI: Zondervan, 2000), 179–188; Wonsuk Ma, "The Tragedy of Spirit-Empowered Heroes: A Close Look at Samson and Saul," *Spiritus: ORU Journal of Theology* 2 (2017), 23–38. See also Wonsuk Ma, "The Charismatic Spirit of God," in Julie C. Ma and Wonsuk Ma, *Mission in the Spirit: Towards a Pentecostal/Charismatic Missiology* (Oxford: Regnum Books, 2010), 29–39.
[2] See Phyllis A. Bird, "Genesis 1–3 as a Source for A Contemporary Theology of Sexuality," in *Missing Persons and Mistaken Identities* (Minneapolis: Fortress Press, 1997), especially her chapter on 155–173. See also John K. Tarwater, *Marriage as Covenant: Considering God's Design at Creation and the Contemporary Moral Consequences* (Lanham, MD: University Press of America, 2006), 53–75; Richard M. Davidson, *Flame of Yahweh: Sexuality in the Old Testament* (Peabody, MA: Hendrickson, 2007), 15–80.
[3] James B. Hurtley, *Man and Woman in Biblical Perspective* (Grand Rapids, MI: Zondervan, 1981), 31.
[4] Richard Averbeck, "A Literary Day, Inter-Textual, and Contextual Reading

of Genesis 1–2," in J. Daryl Charles, ed., *Reading Genesis 1–2* (Peabody, MA: Hendrickson, 2013), 25.

[5] Kenneth A. Mathews, *Genesis 1–11:26* (Nashville, TN: Broadman & Holman, 1996), 172.

[6] See Victor P. Hamilton, "זכר *zākār*," *New International Dictionary of Old Testament Theology and Exegesis*, Willem VanGemeren, ed. (Grand Rapids, MI: Zondervan, 1997), 1, no. 1107.

[7] Bill T. Arnold, *Encountering the Book of Genesis* (Grand Rapids, MI: Baker, 1998), 35.

[8] Davidson, *Flame of Yahweh*, 18.

[9] Mathews, *Genesis 1–11:26*, 173.

[10] J. Andrew Dearman, "Marriage in the Old Testament," in Robert L. Brawley, ed., *Biblical Ethics and Homosexuality* (Louisville, KY: Westminster John Knox, 1996), 55.

[11] Rebecca Merrill Groothuis, *The Feminist Bogeywoman: Questions and Answers about Evangelical Feminism* (Grand Rapids, MI: Baker, 1995), 27.

[12] John E. Hartley, *Genesis* (Peabody, MA: Hendrickson, 2000), 49.

[13] Davidson, *Flame of Yahweh*, 50.

[14] Dearman, "Marriage in the Old Testament," 55.

[15] Davidson, *Flame of Yahweh*, 50.

[16] Hartley, *Genesis*, 61.

[17] See Davidson, *Flame of Yahweh*, 29.

[18] Donald G. Bloesch, *Is the Bible Sexist: Beyond Feminism and Patriarchalism* (Westchester, IL: Crossway, 1982), 25.

[19] Allen P. Ross, *Creation and Blessings: A Guide to the Study and Exposition of Genesis* (Grand Rapids, MI: Baker, 1988), 126.

[20] Allan M. Harman, "עזר (*'ezer I*)," *New International Dictionary of Old Testament Theology and Exegesis*, 3, no. 379.

[21] Bird, *Missing Persons and Mistaken Identities*, 165.

[22] Tarwater, *Marriage as Covenant*, 62 observes that the phrase "bone of my bones and flesh of my flesh" in v. 23 is a figure of speech signifying kinship. For example, when Abimelech returned to his mother's house in Shechem, he attempted to persuade the people to follow him by reminding them of his kinship stating, "Remember that I am your own flesh and blood" (Jud 9:2).

[23] Tarwater, *Marriage as Covenant*, 62.

[24] Mathews, *Genesis 1–11:26*, 214.

[25] James Brownson, *Bible, Gender, Sexuality: Reframing the Church's Debate on Same-Sex Relationships* (Grand Rapids, MI: Eerdmans, 2013), 87.

[26] Gordon Wenham, *Genesis 1–15* (Waco, TX: Word, 1987), 70–71.

[27] Tarwater, *Marriage as Covenant*, 60.

[28] Wenham, *Genesis 1–15*, 71.

[29] Mathews, *Genesis 1–11:26*, 223.

[30] Mathews, *Genesis 1–11:26*, 223.

[31] Tremper Longmann, III, "What Genesis 1–2 Teaches (and What it Doesn't)," in J. Daryl Charles, ed., *Reading Genesis 1–2*, 112.

[32] Brownson, *Bible, Gender, Sexuality*, 87.

[33] J. Andrew Dearman, "Marriage in the Old Testament," 55.

[34] See John Calvin, *Genesis* (Wheaton, IL: Crossway, 2001), 40.

[35] Tarwater, *Marriage as Covenant*, 101. While the word "covenant" is not used in Gen 1 and 2, Tarwater argues, "By Scripture consistently identifying sexual intercourse with the sign of marriage, and by the author of Genesis making explicit reference to the one flesh union ["They will become one flesh" (Gen 2:24)], being naked ["They were both naked, the man and his wife, and were not ashamed" (Gen 2:25)], and Adam "knowing" his wife ["Now Adam know Eve his wife, and she conceived" (Gen 4:1)], sufficient evidence exists for recognizing the presence of the general feature sign of the covenant in the marriage of Adam and Eve." See Tarwater, *Marriage as Covenant*, 63–64.

[36] Raymond Collins, "The Bible and Sexuality," *Biblical Theology Bulletin* 7 (1977), 154.

[37] Davidson, *Flame of Yahweh*, 51.

[38] David G. Firth, "The Spirit and Leadership: Testimony, Empowerment and Purpose" in David G. Firth and Paul D. Wegner, eds., *Presence, Power and Promise: The Role of the Spirit of God in the Old Testament* (Downers Grove, IL: IVP, 2011), 261.

[39] Firth, "The Spirit and Leadership," 262.

[40] John Rea, *The Holy Spirit in the Bible: All the Major Passages about the Spirit* (Lake Mary, FL: Creation, 1990), 40.

[41] Walter Brueggemann, *Genesis* (Atlanta, GA: John Knox, 1982), 333.

[42] Davidson, *Flame of Yahweh*, 306.

[43] Wenham, *Genesis 16–50* (Dallas: Word, 1994), 375.

[44] Davidson, *Flame of Yahweh*, 345.

[45] Hamilton, *The Book of Genesis: Chapters 18–55*, 463.

[46] Hartley, *Genesis*, 321.

[47] Ma, "The Tragedy of Spirit-Empowered Heroes," 24; Firth, "The Spirit and Leadership," 274–277.

[48] Daniel I. Block, *Judges, Ruth: An Exegetical and Theological Exposition of Holy Scripture* (Nashville, TN: Broadman & Holman, 1999), 403.

[49] Block, *Judges*, 424 notes that the verb pā'am "occurs in the *niphal*, 'to be disturbed,' in Gen 41:8; Ps 77:5; Dan 2:3, and in the *hithpael* form 'to feel disturbed' in Dan 2:1, and "the *qal* form of the verb 'to stir, impel' is unattested elsewhere, and its meaning here is uncertain."

[50] See Ma, "The Tragedy of Spirit-Empowered Heroes," 27.

[51] Block, *Judges*, 424.

[52] E. John Hamlin, *Judges: At Risk in the Promised Land* (Grand Rapids, MI: Eerdmans, 1990), 133.

[53] R. E. Harlow, *Winning and Losing: Studies in Joshua, Judges, Ruth* (Ontario,

Canada: Everyday Publications, 1967), 90.

54 Tetsuo Sasaki, *The Concept of War in the Book of Judges* (Tokyo: Gakujutsu Tosho Shupan-sha, 2001), 96.

55 Tami J. Schneider, *Judges* (Collegeville, MN: A Michael Glazier, 2000), 216.

56 Lawson Younger, *Judges/Ruth* (Grand Rapids, MI: Zondervan, 2002), 314.

57 Athena E. Gorospe and Charles Ringma, *Judges* (Carlisle, UK: Langham Publishing, 2016), 197.

58 Davidson, *Flame of Yahweh*, 309.

59 Block *Judges*, 471.

60 Schneider, *Judges*, 218.

61 Gerhard von Rad, *Old Testament Theology*, (Edinburgh: Oliver and Boyd, 1962), 1:334.

62 Daniel I. Block, "Empowered by the Spirit of God: The Holy Spirit in the Historiographic Writings of the Old Testament," *Southern Baptist Journal of Theology* 1 (1997), 53.

63 Lloyd R. Neve, *The Spirit of God in the Old Testament* (Tokyo: Seibunsha, 1972), 27. See also David M. Howard, "The Transfer of Power from Saul to David in 1 Sam 16:13–14," *Journal of the Evangelical Theological Society* 32:4 (Dec. 1989), 479, 480.

64 Block, "Empowered by the Spirit of God," 51. See also David Toshio Tsumura, *The First Book of Samuel* (Grand Rapids, MI: Eerdmans, 2007), 424.

65 Howard, "The Transfer of Power from Saul to David," 475.

66 Neve, *The Spirit of God in the Old Testament*, 23. See also Block, "Empowered by the Spirit of God," 53.

67 Wilf Hildebrandt, *An Old Testament Theology of the Spirit of God* (Peabody, MA: Hendrickson, 1995), 126.

68 Robert D. Bergen, *1, 2 Samuel* (Nashville, TN: Broadman & Holman, 1996), 181.

69 Davidson, *The Flame of Yahweh*, 532.

70 Amanda W. Benckhuysen, "Reading the Bible with Rembrandt: A Fresh Look at Bathsheba in 2 Samuel 11," *Calvin Theological Journal* 50 (2015), 248.

71 Bergen, *1, 2 Samuel*, 467.

72 Davidson, *The Flame of Yahweh*, 527.

73 Wenham, *Genesis 16–50*, 375.

74 Benckhuysen, "Reading the Bible with Rembrandt," 248.

75 Davidson, *The Flame of Yahweh*, 527.

76 Davidson, *The Flame of Yahweh*, 527.

Chapter 2

1 Paul Nathan Alexander, "Presidential Address 2013: Raced, Gendered,

Faithed, and Sexed," *Pneuma* 35 (2013), 319.

[2]Alexander, "Presidential Address," 343–344.

[3]Alexander, "Presidential Address," 344.

[4]The pursuit of a distinctive Pentecostal (or Spirit-empowered) hermeneutic has been a key feature of much twentieth and twenty-first century Pentecostal scholarship, ranging all the way from Gordon D. Fee's "genre hermeneutic" ("Hermeneutics and Historical Precedent—A Major Problem in Pentecostal Hermeneutics," in *Perspectives on the New Pentecostalism*, ed. Russell P. Spittler [Grand Rapids, MI: Baker, 1976], 118–132; "Acts—The Problem of Historical Precedent," in *How to Read the Bible For All Its Worth: A Guide to Understanding the Bible*, by Gordon D. Fee and Douglas Stuart [Grand Rapids, MI: Baker, 1982], 87–102; and Gordon D. Fee, "Baptism in the Holy Spirit: The Issue of Separability and Subsequence" *Pneuma* 7:2 [1985]: 87–99) to Howard M. Ervin's "pneumatic and epistemological hermeneutic" (Howard M. Ervin, "Hermeneutics: A Pentecostal Option," *Pneuma* 3:2 [1981], 11–25. Reprinted with slight alterations under the same title in *Essays on Apostolic Themes: Studies in Honor of: Howard M. Ervin*, ed. Paul Elbert [Peabody, Mass.: Hendrickson Publishers, 1985], 23–35.) to William W. Menzies' "holistic hermeneutic" ("The Methodology of Pentecostal Theology: An Essay on Hermeneutics," in *Essays on Apostolic Themes*, 1–14). A good article outlining the development of the Pentecostal hermeneutic is by Roger Stronstad ("Trends in Pentecostal Studies," *Enrichment Journal*, 2018, n.p., http://enrichmentjournal.ag.org/top/month_holyspirit.cfm [23 March 2018]). More recently, Craig Keener has proposed a more traditional approach of Word and Spirit in connection to the Pentecostal experience (*Spirit Hermeneutics: Reading Scripture in Light of Pentecost* [Grand Rapids: Eerdmans, 2016]) along with more interactive models like Kenneth J. Archer (*A Pentecostal Hermeneutic: Spirit, Scripture, and Community* [New York: T & T Clark International, 2004]) and Amos Yong (*Spirit-Word-Community: Theological Hermeneutics in Trinitarian Perspective* [Eugene, OR: Wipf & Stock, 2002]), who both emphasize a triadic engagement of the Word, the Spirit, and the community.

[5]Gordon D. Fee and Douglas Stuart, *How to Read the Bible for All Its Worth*, 3rd ed. (Grand Rapids: Zondervan, 2003), 18.

[6]J. D. Charles cites thirteen New Testament virtue lists: 2 Corinthians 6:6–8; Galatians 5:22–23; Ephesians 4:32; 5:9; Philippians 4:8; Colossians 3:12; 1 Timothy 4:12; 6:11; 2 Timothy 2:22; 3:10; James 3:17; 1 Peter 3:8; and 2 Peter 1:5–7, omitting 1 Corinthians 13, because "it concerns the theological virtues and contains particular features of the ethical catalog." J. D. Charles, "Virtue and Vice Lists," *Dictionary of New Testament Background: A Compendium of Contemporary Biblical Scholarship*, ed. Stanley E. Porter and Craig A. Evans, ed. (Downers Grove, IL: InterVarsity Press, 2000), 5.

[7]J. D. Charles ("Virtue and Vice Lists," 5) cites twenty-three New Testament vice lists, twenty-one found in epistles: Matthew 15:19; Mark 7:21–22; Romans

1:29–31; 13:13; 1 Corinthians 5:10–11; 6:9–10; 2 Corinthians 6:9–10; 12:20–21; Galatians 5:19–21; Ephesians 4:31; 5:3–5; Colossians 3:5, 8; 1 Timothy 1:9–10; 2 Timothy 3:2–5; Titus 3:3; James 3:15; 1 Peter 2:1; 4:3, 15; Revelation 9:21; 21:8; 22:15.

[8] Charles, "Virtue and Vice Lists," 6.

[9] Anthony C. Thiselton, *The First Epistle to the Corinthians: A Commentary on the Greek Text*, The New International Greek Testament Commentary (Grand Rapids: Eerdmans, 2000), 410.

[10] Douglas Moo, *The Epistle to the Romans*, The New International Commentary on the New Testament (Grand Rapids: Eerdmans, 1996), 118.

[11] Thiselton, *First Epistle to the Corinthians*, 410.

[12] New American Bible, Rev. ed., italics added.

[13] Formerly known as the "Manual of Discipline," italics added.

[14] All Scripture is taken from the New American Standard Bible unless otherwise noted.

[15] "First Epistle of Clement to the Corinthians," trans. J. B. Lightfoot, *Christian Apologetics and Research Ministry*, 1990, n.p., https://carm.org/first-epistle-clement-corinthians (12 March 2018), italics added.

[16] "Didache: The Teaching of the Twelve," trans. Kirsopp Lake, *Early Christian Writings*, n.d., n.p. http://www.earlychristianwritings.com/text/didache-lake.html (12 March 2018), italics added.

[17] Thiselton, *First Epistle to the Corinthians*, 410.

[18] Thiselton, *First Epistle to the Corinthians*, 412.

[19] Thiselton, *First Epistle to the Corinthians*, 442; author's italics.

[20] Brian Rosner, *Paul, Scripture, and Ethics: A Study of 1 Corinthians 5–7* (New York: Brill, 1994), 121.

[21] Richard N. Longenecker, *The Epistle to the Romans: A Commentary on the Greek Text*, The New International Greek Testament Commentary (Grand Rapids: Eerdmans, 2016), 217. Translations in parentheses are from Longenecker.

[22] All Greek references are from *The Greek New Testament*, 4th rev. ed., Barbara and Kurt Aland, Johannes Karavidopoulos, Carlos M. Martini, and Bruce M. Metzger (Stuttgart: Deutsche Bibelgesellschaft, 1994).

[23] Walter Bauer, W. F. Arndt, F. W. Gingrich, and F. W. Danker, *A Greek-English Lexicon of the New Testament and Other Early Christian Literature*, 3rd ed. (Chicago: University of Chicago Press, 2000), 1089; hereafter cited as BDAG; author's italics.

[24] BDAG, 1070.

[25] The KJV, NKJV, and MEVtranslate the phrase like this.

[26] E. F. Rogers, "Same-Sex Marriage as an Ascetic Practice in the Light of Romans 1 and Ephesians 5," *Modern Believing* 55, no.2 (2014), 115–125.

[27] Moo, *Romans*, 116. Some of Moo's notes have been incorporated into the quotation above.

[28] Moo, *Romans*, 116–117.

[29] Longenecker, *The Epistle to the Romans*, 215.
[30] Both the RSV and ESV are consistent in translating this phrase like this.
[31] Moo, *Romans*, 110–111, 118.
[32] C. E. B. Cranfield, *A Critical and Exegetical Commentary on the Epistle to the Romans*, vol. 1, The International Critical Commentary on the Holy Scriptures of the Old and New Testaments (Edinburgh: T & T Clark, 1975), 33.
[33] John Chrysostom, *Homilies on the Epistle to the Romans, Nicene and Post Nicene Fathers*, vol. 11, ed. Philip Schaff (Grand Rapids: Eerdmans, 1989), 354.
[34] Frederic Godet, *Commentary on St. Paul's Epistle to the Romans* (New York: Funk & Wagnalls, 1883), 107.
[35] Moo, *Romans*, 111.
[36] Everett F. Harrison and Donald A. Hagner, "Romans," *Romans-Galatians*, The Expositor's Bible Commentary, vol. 11 (Grand Rapids: Zondervan, 2008), 49–50.
[37] Thomas R. Schreiner, *Romans*, Baker Exegetical Commentary on the New Testament (Grand Rapids: Baker Academic, 1998), 92.
[38] Moo, *Romans*, 113.
[39] Schreiner, *Romans*, 92.
[40] Longenecker, *Romans*, 216–217.
[41] Alexander James Lucas, "Romans 1:18–2:11 and the Substructure of Psalm 106 (105): Evocations of the Calf?" (Ph.D. diss., Loyola University, Chicago, 2012), pp. 79, 84, 228–231, http://ecommons.luc.edu/luc_diss/419.
[42] Longenecker, *Romans*, 218.
[43] Joseph A. Fitzmyer, *Romans* (New Haven: Yale University Press, 1993), 271.
[44] R. H. Charles, *The Apocrypha and Pseudepigrapha of the Old Testament*, vol. 2 (New York: Oxford University Press, 1913), archive.org. Richard Longenecker points out that "The Testament of Napthali" "is probably a Jewish writing that was later redacted by first-century Jewish Christians" (218).
[45] Thiselton, *First Epistle to the Corinthians*, 452.
[46] Schreiner, *Romans*, 94.
[47] David Garland, *1 Corinthians*, Baker Exegetical Commentary on the New Testament (Grand Rapids: Baker Academic, 2003), 211.
[48] BDAG, 613.
[49] Garland, *1 Corinthians*, 214.
[50] Philo, *Special Laws*, 3.7.37.
[51] Gordon Fee, *The First Epistle to the Corinthians*, The New International Commentary on the New Testament (Grand Rapids: Eerdmans, 1987), 243–244.
[52] Fee, *The First Epistle to the Corinthians*, 244.
[53] Garland, *1 Corinthians*, 211.
[54] H. G. Liddell, R. Scott, H. S. Jones R, McKenzie, *A Greek and English Lexicon, A Simplified Edition*, ed. Didier Fontaine, 1940, www.areopage.net, 105.
[55] BDAG, 135.
[56] BDAG, 135.

[57] George W. Knight III, *The Pastoral Epistles: A Commentary on the Greek Text*, The New International Greek Testament Commentary (Grand Rapids: Eerdmans, 1992), 86.

[58] Philip H. Towner, *The Letters of Timothy and Titus*, The New International Commentary on the New Testament (Grand Rapids: Eerdmans, 2006), 127–128.

[59] New International Version note to 1 Corinthians 6:9.

[60] John Boswell, *Christianity, Social Tolerance, and Homosexuality: Gay People in Western Europe from the Beginning of the Christian Era to the Fourteenth Century* (Chicago: University of Chicago Press, 1980), 92.

[61] Boswell, *Christianity, Social Tolerance, and Homosexuality*, 106–107.

[62] Robin Scroggs, *The New Testament and Homosexuality: Contextual Background for Contemporary Debate* (Philadelphia: Fortress Press, 1983), 108.

[63] Dale B. Martin, "Arsenokoitês and Malakos: Meaning and Consequences," in *Biblical Ethics and Homosexuality: Listening to Scripture*, ed. Robert Lawson Brawley (Louisville, KY: Westminster John Knox Press, 1996), 118–119, 124, 128–129.

[64] Robert A. J. Gagnon, *The Bible and Homosexual Practice: Text and Hermeneutics* (Nashville: Abingdon Press, 2001), 306.

[65] Fee, *The First Epistle to the Corinthians*, 244.

[66] Garland, *1 Corinthians*, 212–213.

[67] H. G. Liddell, R. Scott, H. S. Jones R, McKenzie, *A Greek-English Lexicon* (Oxford: Oxford University Press, 1990), 967.

[68] Liddell and Scott, *A Greek-English Lexicon*, 970.

[69] "The Greek Old Testament (Septuagint)," *The Greek Word*, n.d., n.p., http://www.ellopos.net/elpenor/greek-texts/septuagint/chapter.asp?book=3&page=18 (12 March 2018).

[70] "The Greek Old Testament (Septuagint)," *The Greek Word*, n.d., n.p., http://www.ellopos.net/elpenor/greek-texts/septuagint/chapter.asp?book=3&page=20 (12 March 2018).

[71] Garland, *1 Corinthians*, 213.

[72] Garland, *1 Corinthians*, 213.

[73] Towner, *Timothy and Titus*, 128.

[74] Andreas Kostenberger, "1 Timothy," *Ephesians -Philemon*, The Expositor's Bible Commentary, vol. 12, rev. ed. (Grand Rapids: Zondervan, 2006), 503–504.

[75] Longenecker, *Romans*, 217.

[76] BDAG, 946.

[77] BDAG, 946.

[78] Thiselton, *First Epistle to the Corinthians*, 447.

[79] Gagnon, *The Bible and Homosexual Practice*, 338.

Chapter 3

[1] I recognise that the interpretation of the few Scripture passages that deal with this issue is precisely what is at issue. However, it is fair to say that in the minds of most 'ordinary' Christians who hold to the Bible's enduring authority, its teaching is not obscure on this issue. Furthermore, this is also and unequivocally the case for every ancient author whose views are surveyed here.

[2] This period is usually taken to extend from the end of the Apostolic age (c. AD) 100 to the mid-fifth century (the Council of Chalcedon). For this, see Alister E. McGrath, *Historical Theology: An Introduction to the History of Christian Thought*, 2 ed. (Malden, MA: Wiley-Blackwell, 2012), 17.

[3] I recognize that this is not uncontroversial. Dale B. Martin, *Sex and the Single Savior: Gender and Sexuality in Biblical Interpretation* (Louisville, KY: Westminster John Knox, 2006), 38–47 is an excellent example of a number of authors who attempt to dismiss the plain meaning of the words *aresenokoites* and *malakos* in the NT vice lists.

[4] Citations have been sourced from J. Allenbach and Andre Pautler, *Biblia Patristica: Index Des Citations Et Allusions Bibliques Dans La Littérature Patristique*, ed. Centre d'analyse et de documentation patristiques (France), 7 vols. (Paris: Editions du Centre national de la recherche scientifique, 1975). It should be noted that only those citations deemed significant have been presented here so the list should be taken as indicative rather than exhaustive.

[5] Irenaeus, *Adversus haereses* 4.27.4 in *Irénée de Lyon: Contre les heresies*, ed. and trans. A. Rousseau and L. Doutreleau, SC 100.1–100.2, 152–153, 210–211, 263–264, 293–294 (Paris: Cerf, 1965–1982), 100.2: 748–749, lines 150–159. For the sake of efficiency, the Ante Nicene Fathers translation has been used here (and following) available online: Irenaeus, "Against All Heresies," trans. Philip Schaff, *Christian Classics Ethereal Library*, accessed May 26, 2017, http://www.ccel.org/ccel/schaff/anf01.ix.vi.xxviii.html#fnf_ix.vi.xxviii-p19.2.

[6] Note that online ANF version has a textual error here (*not* effeminate instead of *nor*. The syntax of the Latin and Greek, both of which are attested, clarifies that 'nor' is intended) which I have presumed to emend.

[7] The English translation here predictably follows the King James Version. The Greek text of Irenaeus is quoted accurately from the NT οὔτε μαλακοὶ οὔτε ἀρσενοκοῖται; the Latin (also attested) follows the Vulgate here: *neque molles, neque masculorum concubitores.*

[8] Irenaeus, *Adv. haer.* 4.27.4, lines 162–167, SC 100.2, 748–750.

[9] Irenaeus, *Adv. haer.* 4.27.4, lines 172–175, SC 100.2, 750.

[10] Irenaeus, *Adv. haer.* 4.37.4, lines 73–93, SC 100.2, 928–932.

[11] Irenaeus, *Adv. haer.* 5.11.1, lines 36–38, SC 153, 136–137.

[12] The English here is clearly derived from the Latin text, *sed pristinam vanitatis conversationem*, however, the Latin appears to be a mis-translation of the Greek

(also attested in this section) which reads τὴν προτέραν τῆς ματαιότητος ἀναστροφήν, which perhaps is better translated "the former vain reversal." In other words, conversion restores a believer to the state that God intended. For Latin see lines 56 and 57, SC 153, 138, 140. For Greek see line 155 on p. 139 of the same.

[13]Irenaeus, *Adv. haer.* 5.11.1–2, SC 132–140.

[14]Tertullian, *De Anime* 22.4, Corpus Christianorum Series Latina vol. 2. (Tornhout, Belgium: Brepols, 1954), 813–14, lines 24–34. The translation used (here and following) is from ANF available online at Tertullian, "On the Soul," *Tertullian.org: ANF Vol. 3 "On the Soul,"* accessed May 26, 2017, http://www.tertullian.org/anf/anf03/anf03-22.htm#P2793_946788.

[15]Tertullian, *De Anime* 22.6–77, 814, lines 34–42.

[16]Tertullian, *De Pudicitia* 16.5, CCSL 2, 1312, lines 16–19.

[17]'Ιησοῦς (Jesus) is of course Joshua's name in the LXX, the Old Testament with which Origen was most familiar.

[18]Origen, *Homilies on Joshua* 15.5. This translation is from Origen, *Homilies on Joshua*, ed. Cynthia White, trans. Barbara Bruce, vol. 105, *The Fathers of the Church* (Washington, DC: Catholic University of America Press, 2002), 146. It is attested in Latin in Migne's PG vol. 12.

[19]Origen, *Homilies on Joshua* 15.5, Ibid., 105:147.

[20]See Origen, *Homilies on Leviticus, 1–16,* trans. Gary Wayne Barkley, vol. 83, *Fathers of the Church,* 82 where Origen simply appends the latter half of 1 Cor 6:11 as an alternate ending onto the end of Titus 3:5.

[21]Origen, *Homilies on Joshua* 15.5 in Origen, *Homilies on Joshua*, 105:147.

[22]Origen, *Homilies on Joshua* 6, in Origen, 105:73.

[23]Cyril of Jerusalem, *Catechesis* 3.8 in Cyril of Jerusalem, *The Works of Saint Cyril of Jerusalem, Volume 1 (The Fathers of the Church, Volume 61)*, ed. Anthony A. Stephenson, trans. Leo P. McCauley, vol. 61, Fathers of the Church (CUA Press, 2010), 113–114. The Greek text can be found in. Migne's PG 33.

[24]Cyril, *Catechesis*, 61, 114.

[25]Cyril, *Catechesis*, 61, 114.

[26]John Chrysostom, *Homily 5* in John Chrysostom, *The Homilies of S. John Chrysostom, of St. Paul the Apostle to Timothy, Titus, and Philemon,* trans. Anonymous members of the English Church, A Library of Fathers of the Holy Catholic Church, Anterior to the Division of the East and West (Oxford: John Henry Parker, 1858), 317.

[27]Chrysostom, *Homily 5*, in Chrysostom, *Homilies on the Epistles*, 319.

[28]Chrysostom, *Homily 5*, in Chrysostom, *Homilies on the Epistles*, 320. He makes reference here to Plato's view in the *Republic*, that women should be sent out to war alongside men. This he sees as a subversion of natural boundaries in the same way as men having intercourse with other men instead of women.

[29]Here and the above quote, Chrysostom, *Homily 5* in Chrysostom, *Homilies on the Epistles*, 320–321.

[30] John Chrysostom, *Homilies on 1 Corinthians*, Homily 16 in John Chrysostom, *The Homilies of S. John Chrysostom, Archbishop of Constantinople, on the First Epistle of St. Paul the Apostle to the Corinthians: Hom. 1–24. Pt. 2. Hom. 25–44*, vol. IV, A Library of Fathers of the Holy Catholic Church, Anterior to the Division of the East and West (Oxford: Parker, 1839), 218.

[31] Note that Chrysostom's comments here, while not limited to homosexual sin, certainly include it in "all things that have been enumerated."

[32] Ambrose himself briefly cites 1 Cor 6:11, though it barely warrants a mention in the present context. Like Epiphanius, Ambrose makes the citation in his treatise *On the Holy Spirit* 3.4.23–24: "As the Apostle also set forth, saying: But you were washed, but you were sanctified, but you were justified in the Name of our Lord Jesus Christ, and in the Spirit of our God. You see, then, that the Father works in the Son, and that the Son works in the Spirit." (this translation from Ambrose of Milan, "CHURCH FATHERS: On the Holy Spirit, Book III (Ambrose)," accessed May 26, 2017, ttp://www.newadvent.org/fathers/34023.htm.). While Epiphanius's emphasis is to demonstrate the co-activity of Christ and the Spirit, Ambrose seeks to explore full-blown Trinitarian activity as seen in the work of the Holy Spirit.

[33] The English translation is unhelpful here. It seems inexplicably to have been 'sanitised.' The Latin text simply follows the Vulgate rendering of 1 Cor. 6:9 (as one would expect) already referenced above *neque molles, neque masculorum concubitores* ("neither the effeminate, nor men who have sex with men"). It is important for the present enquiry to note that the commentator does not understand this in the somewhat less direct sense that the translator renders, but has in view male homosexual sex.

[34] Ambrosiaster, *Commentaries on Romans and 1 and 2 Corinthians*, 1 Cor 6:9–11, PL 17, 224 in Ambrosiaster, *Commentaries on Romans and 1–2 Corinthians*, trans. Gerald L. Bray, First printing edition., Ancient Christian Texts (Downers Grove, Ill: IVP Academic, 2009), 145–146.

[35] See Augustine of Hippo, *Sermons 151–183*, ed. John E. Rotelle, trans. Edmund Hill, The Works of Saint Augustine: A Translation for the 21st Century III/5 (Brooklyn, NY: New City Press, 1992), 143 fn 1. Note that it seems the editor makes an error here. Clearly the chapter is 6, not 9.

[36] Augustine, *Sermons* 161.3.

[37] Augustine, *Sermons* 161.11.

[38] Augustine, *Sermons* 161.1–2.

[39] Augustine, *Sermons* 162.3.

[40] Elsewhere in the Fathers, in particular in commentary on Romans 1:26, 27 (as one would expect) the reality of homosexual sin being contrary to nature is likewise noted.

Chapter 4

[1] Katy Steinmetz, "Oxford English Dictionary Adds 'Merica, Gender-Fluid and Squee,'" *Time* [magazine], 11 September 2016; http://time.com/4485727/oed-merica-gender-fluid-squee-new-words.

[2] Ryan T. Anderson, *When Harry Became Sally: Responding to the Transgender Moment* (New York: Encounter Books, 2018), 1.

[3] Russell Goldman, "Here's a list of 58 Gender Options for Facebook Users," *ABC News*, 13 February 2014. http://abcnews.go.com/blogs/headlines/2014/02/heres-a-list-of-58-gender-options-for-facebook-users/. Agender; Androgyne; Androgynous; Bigender; Cis; Cisgender; Cis Female; Cis Male; Cis Man; Cis Woman; Cisgender Female; Cisgender Male; Cisgender Man; Cisgender Woman; Female to Male; FTM; Gender Fluid; Gender Nonconforming; Gender Questioning; Gender Variant; Genderqueer; Intersex; Male to Female; MTF; Neither; Neutrois; Non-binary; Other; Pangender; Trans; Trans*; Trans Female; Trans* Female; Trans Male; Trans* Male; Trans Man; Trans* Man; Trans Person; Trans* Person; Trans Woman; Trans* Woman; Transfeminine; Transgender; Transgender Female; Transgender Male; Transgender Man; Transgender Person; Transgender Woman; Transmasculine; Transsexual; Transsexual Female; Transsexual Male; Transsexual Man; Transsexual Person; Transsexual Woman; and Two-Spirit."

[4] According to Ashley McGuire, in *Sex Scandal: The Drive to Abolish Male and Female* (Washington, DC: Regnery, 2017), Wesleyan University in Connecticut has already expanded its acronym to include these variant sexual practices. There the accepted acronym is "LGBTTQQFAGPBDSM," which means, "lesbian, gay, bisexual, transgender, transsexual, queer, questioning, flexural, asexual, genderf**k, polyamorous, bondage/discipline, dominance/submission, sadism/masochism" (52). These fourteen identities nonetheless exclude several that are recognized elsewhere. Rogers Brubaker, in *Trans: Gender and Race in an Age of Unsettled Identities* (Princeton, NJ: Princeton University Press, 2016), uses the acronym: "LGBTQQIAAP2S," which may be translated to mean lesbian, gay, bisexual, transgender, queer, questioning, intersex, asexual, ally, pansexual, two-spirit (42). Four identities in Brubaker's acronym—intersex, asexual, ally, pansexual, two-spirit—would need to be added to Wesleyan University's list, to give a grand total of eighteen identities. As indicated above (n. 3), Facebook includes far more gender identities than these eighteen options.

[5] Joseph-Marie Verlinde, *L'ideologie du gender: comme identité reçue ou choisie?* (Mesnil Saint-Loup: Éditions le Libre Ouvert, 2012), 37, 50.

[6] Anderson, *When Harry Became Sally*, 13.

[7] In Sweden—where some of the first sex reassignment surgeries took place—those who wish legally to change their gender do not have to undergo

surgery. "Sweden to Modernize Law on Changing Gender." https://www.thelocal.se/20170316/sweden-to-modernize-law-on-changing-gender

[8] https://genderneutralpronoun.wordpress.com/tag/ze-and-zir/

[9] Eugene Volokh, "You can be fined for not calling people 'ze' or 'hir,' if that's the pronoun they demand that you use, *Washington Post*, 17 May 2016; https://www.washingtonpost.com/news/volokh-conspiracy/wp/2016/05/17/you-can-be-fined-for-not-calling-people-ze-or-hir-if-thats-the-pronoun-they-demand-that-you-use.

[10] Mary Katherine Ham and Guy Benson, *End of Discussion: How the Left's Outrage Industry Shuts Down Debate* (New York: Crown Forum, 2015), 239, 236n.8.

[11] Anderson, *When Harry Became Sally*, 34–35; PFLAG, *Our Trans Loved Ones* [2008, 2015], 9; www.pflag.org/ourtranslovedones

[12] The concept of the "memory hole" appears in George Orwell's novel *Nineteen Eighty-Four* (1949), where the Ministry of Truth systematically removes all *past documents* that might contradict the Party's *present interpretation* of the past. On finding archival documents that challenge the party line, Winston Smith cuts out newspaper articles, and tosses them into the "memory hole," where they are incinerated and forever forgotten. In the novel, Oceania had once been allied with Eastasia, but the records were changed to conceal this fact. Orwell wrote: "The past was alterable. The past never had been altered. Oceania was at war with Eastasia. Oceania had always been at war with Eastasia." In the case of a transgender life-history, something like this seems to be going on, whereby the record of the past is altered to conform it to the present interpretation of the life-history.

[13] The transgender author, Virginia Ramey Mollenkott, *Omnigender: A Trans-Religious Approach* (Cleveland, OH: Pilgrim Press, 2001), mentioned a 1999 poll taken by *The Advocate*—a national gay magazine—asking whether transgender people should be included as part of the gay rights movement. Only forty-six percent said "yes," while forty-eight percent said "no" (38–39). This suggests that the link between "LGB" and "T" may not be as close as many activists suggest. The "LGB" groups are concerned with sexual orientation and expression, while the "T" are concerned with gender identity, and so it is perhaps not surprising that a disparity exists. During the 1990s and at least into the early 2000s, if not more recently, gay and lesbian persons—along with most heterosexuals—resisted claims to recognition by transgender persons.

[14] Northwestern University researcher J. Michael Bailey, author of *The Man Who Would be Queen: The Science of Gender-Bending and Transsexualism* (Washington, DC: Joseph Henry Press, 2003), estimates that some 70–80% of transgender persons born as males are *autogynephilic*—i.e., anatomical males who are sexually aroused by the thought of being a female. The autogynephilic male may not intend to make a full transition and live as a woman, but

experiences sexual fulfillment when dressing as a woman, seeing himself as female, and receiving male attention in presenting himself as female. See Ray Blanchard, "Clinical Observations and Systematic Studies of Autogynephilia," *Journal of Sex and Marital Therapy* 17 (1991), 235–251.

[15] John Riley, "Alternative Scottish Pride Event Reverses Decisions Not to Book Drag Acts," 27 July 2015; https://www.metroweekly.com/2015/07/alternative-scottish-pride-event-reverses-decision-not-to-book-drag-acts/. While the tension between transsexuals and drag queens or cross-dressers seems to be relatively new, the tension between drag queens and others in the lesbian and gay community goes back a long way. Viviane Namaste speaks of how the Lesbian and Gay Pride Parade in 1992 sought to ban drag queens from participating. Both the drag queens—and those wearing leather—were considered to be going beyond "respectable" community standards. The advertisement for a Toronto lesbian and gay film festival in 1993 was written so as to stress the exoticism of the transgender characters in the films: "Bearded ladies, chicks with dicks and drag queens are among the queer sightings in Gender Bender, an evening [that]…explores cross-dressing, transsexualism, transvestism, androgyny, and other sexual anomalies." Transgender persons were incensed at being described as "sexual anomalies" (Viviane K. Namaste, *Invisible Lives: The Erasure of Transsexual and Transgendered People*; Chicago: University of Chicago, 2000; 11–12). One gets the impression here of a certain LGB voyeurism vis-à-vis transgender persons.

[16] Some who hold to the "trans-exclusive" position are lesbians, yet all holding this position might accurately be described as feminists. Some of the key texts include: Janice G. Raymond, *The Transsexual Empire: The Making of the She-Male*, rev. ed. (New York: Teacher's College Press, 1994); and Sheila Jeffreys, *Gender Hurts: A Feminist Analysis of the Politics of Transgenderism* (Abingdon, UK: Routledge, 2014).

[17] Chad Felix Greene, "Lesbians Accused Of Hate Crimes For Objecting To Transgenderism At London Pride Festival," 10 July 2018; http://thefederalist.com/2018/07/10/lesbians-accused-hate-crimes-objecting-transgenderism-london-pride-festival/.

[18] Princeton Professor Robert George detects in transgender ideology the scent of gnosticism, involving a body-self dualism, and he comments, "The idea that human beings are non-bodily persons inhabiting non-personal bodies never quite goes away." But one must ask who or what exactly is the "real self," as something distinct from the body? This leads Robert George into a philosophical paradox: "It is clearly *false* to say that this biological male is *already* perceived as a woman. He wants to be perceived this way. Yet the pre-operative claim that he is 'really a woman' is the premise of his plea for surgery. So it has to be prior. What, then, does it refer to? The answer cannot be his inner sense. For that would still have to be an inner sense *of something*—but there seems to be no 'something' for it to be the sense *of*" (p. 106; citing Robert P.

George, "Gnostic Liberalism," *First Things*, Dec. 2016; www.firstthings.com/article/2016/12/gnostic-liberalism).

[19] Anderson, *When Harry Became Sally*, 3–4.

[20] Jonathan Ames, ed., *Sexual Metamorphosis: An Anthology of Transsexual Memoirs* (New York: Vintage, 2005) is an autobiographical collection of interest and with literary qualities, but these accounts focus rather narrowly on experiences directly linked to the process of transition and its aftermath. With the exception of Jan Morris's account—"Conundrum" (77–97)—the early life experiences crucial for understanding decisions to transition—and sometimes to detransition—are largely absent from this collection.

[21] See John Money, "Hermaphroditism, Gender, and Precocity in Hyperadrenocorticism: Psychologic Findings," *Bulletin of the Johns Hopkins Hospital* 95 (1955) 253–264. www.ncbi.nlm.nih.gov/pubmed/14378807.

[22] Rogers Brubaker explains in *Trans: Gender and Race in an Age of Unsettled Identities* (Princeton, NJ: Princeton University Press, 2016) that German and Austrian thinkers of the late 1800s and early 1900s proposed an idea of "universal bisexuality" (99–100). Here "bisexuality" did not refer to sexual behavior but to the notion that all human beings contain a mixture of masculine and feminine traits. In the psychological theories of Carl Gustav Jung (1875–1961), the female psyche contains a male principle (*animus*) and the male contains a female principle (*anima*). This version of "bisexuality" is not quite the same as "androgyny," i.e., a transcending of male-female polarity rather than inclusion of both. Nor is it the same as what is today called "gender fluidity," though all three of these ideas have certain affinities.

[23] Verlinde, *L'ideologie du gender*, 16–17.

[24] Verlinde, *L'ideologie du gender*, 20–21; translation mine.

[25] Eve Kosofsky Sedgwick, *Tendencies*, Series Q (Durham, NC: Duke University Press, 1993), 8.

[26] Paul Kengor, *Takedown: From Communists to Progressives, How the Left has Sabotaged Family and Marriage* (Washington, DC: WND Books, 2015), 2–3.

[27] Walt Heyer, "Public Schools Force Kids Into Transgender Wars"; http://thefederalist.com/2015/12/02/public-schools-force-kids-into-transgender-wars/; 2 December 2015.

[28] Lawrence S. Meyer and Paul R. McHugh, "Sexuality and Gender: Findings from the Biological, Psychological, and Social Sciences," *The New Atlantis: A Journal of Technology and Society* 50 (Fall 2016), 1.

[29] Meyer and McHugh, "Sexuality and Gender," 7–8.

[30] Anderson, *When Harry Became Sally*, 2, 5.

[31] Allie Shah, "Gay teens have higher pregnancy rates than their straight peers"; http://www.startribune.com/gay-teens-have-higher-pregnancy-rates-than-their-straight-peers/320842991/; 6 August 2015.

[32] Glenn T. Stanton, "…LGBTQ sexual orientation is not a fixed identity, but

rather something that fluctuates"; http://thefederalist.com/2017/08/07/lesbian-teens-two-seven-times-many-babies-heterosexual-peers/; 7 August 2017; citing Lisa M. Diamond, *Sexual Fluidity: Understanding Women's Love and Desire* (Cambridge, MA: Harvard University Press, 2008). Diamond over a decade's time charted the relationships of almost one hundred women who at some point had experienced same-sex attraction. She documented how these women shifted from male to female lovers, and then back again.

[33] Meyer and McHugh, "Sexuality and Gender," 8–9.

[34] Walt Heyer, "Public Schools Force Kids Into Transgender Wars"

[35] David Batty, "Sex Changes Are Not Effective, Say Researchers"; https://www.theguardian.com/society/2004/jul/30/health.mentalhealth; 30 July 2004.

[36] Paul McHugh, "Transgenderism: A Pathogenic Meme within Bioethics, Culture, Science, Sexuality": http://www.thepublicdiscourse.com/2015/06/15145/; 10 June 2015.

[37] Anderson, *When Harry Became Sally*, 18–19; citing Paul R. McHugh, "Transgenderism: A Pathogenic Meme," *Public Discourse*, 10 June 2015.

[38] Jesse Singal, "When Children Say They Are Trans," https://www.theatlantic.com/magazine/archive/2018/07/when-a-child-says-shes-trans/561749/

[39] See Judith Butler, "Recovery and Invention: The Projects of Desire in Hegel, Kojeve, Hyppolite, and Sartre" (PhD dissertation, Yale University, 1984).

[40] Among Judith Butler's many books are: *Subjects of Desire: Hegelian Reflections in Twentieth-Century France* (1987), *Gender Trouble: Feminism and the Subversion of Identity* (1990), *Bodies That Matter: On the Discursive Limits of "Sex"* (1993), *Excitable Speech: A Politics of the Performative* (1997), *The Psychic Life of Power: Theories in Subjection* (1997), *Precarious Life: The Powers of Mourning and Violence* (2004), *Undoing Gender* (2004), *Giving an Account of Oneself* (2005), *Frames of War: When is Life Grievable?* (2009), *Parting Ways: Jewishness and the Critique of Zionism* (2012), and *Dispossession: The Performative in the Political* (2013).

[41] The discussion here of Judith Butler draws from Gabrielle Kuby, *The Global Sexual Revolution: Destruction of Freedom in the Name of Freedom*, trans. James Patrick Kirchner (Kettering, OH: Angelico Press / Lifesite, 2015), 44–48.

[42] Judith Butler, *Gender Trouble: Feminism and the Subversion of Identity* (New York: Routledge, 1999), 8.

[43] Judith Butler, *Bodies that Matter: On the Discursive Limits of "Sex"* (New York: Routledge, 1993), 21.

[44] Kuby, *The Global Sexual Revolution*, 46; citing Judith Butler, *Unbehagen der Geschlechter*, trans. Kathrina Menke (Frankfurt am Main: Suhrkamp,1991), 209.

[45] Kuby, *The Global Sexual Revoluation*, 46; citing Butler, *Unbehagen*, 115, 118.

[46] Kuby, *The Global Sexual Revolution*, 46; citing *Unbehagen*, 209.

[47] Kuby, *The Global Sexual Revolution*, 47.

[48] Viviane K. Namaste, *Invisible Lives: The Erasure of Transsexual and Transgendered People* (Chicago: University of Chicago, 2000).

[49] Namaste, *Invisible Lives*, 1.

[50] Namaste, *Invisible Lives*, 2, 9–10.

[51] Namaste, *Invisible Lives*, 10; citing Judith Butler, *Gender Trouble*, 175.

[52] Namaste, *Invisible Lives*, 10–11.

[53] Namaste, *Invisible Lives*, 11.

[54] Namaste, *Invisible Lives*, 14.

[55] In Butler, *Bodies That Matter*, 121–142.

[56] Namaste, *Invisible Lives*, 13; citing Butler, *Bodies That Matter*, 131.

[57] Namaste, *Invisible Lives*, 13, emph. added. As another example of inadequate theorizing, Namaste cites the work of Marjorie Garber on the cultural and literary representation of cross-dressing. See Marjorie Garber, *Vested Interests: Cross-Dressing and Cultural Anxiety* (New York: Routledge, 1992). Garber's analysis spans a wide variety of cultural texts—from the Kabuki theater, to the Renaissance stage, and the rock performances of David Bowie (14). She is interested in showing how the "transvestite" represents a "crisis of category" regarding the male-female binary. The transvestite is for her just a "rhetorical device that points to the crisis of category" (14–15). "What is missing from her research is a conceptualization of transvestite identity as a real, lived, viable experience" (14). For Namaste, Butler, and Garber both engage in superficial readings that gloss over the diversity that exists within the trans community (15).

[58] Namaste, *Invisible Lives*, 16, 19.

[59] Namaste, *Invisible Lives*, 20, 22, 23. An essay Namaste cites that supports her argument is Donald Morton, "The Politics of Queer Theory in the (Post) Modern Moment," *Genders* 17 (1993) 121–150. Christian believers who are skeptical of contemporary gender theory will find a surprising ally in the atheistic professor of psychology at Harvard University, Steve Pinker, who in his book *The Blank Slate* (2002), rejects the claim that there is no such thing as human nature. Here Christian theology and biological science are not opposed to one another, but both stand together or fall together. In this study, Pinker provides an abundance of hard evidence—much of it gathered by female scientists—showing that there are not only external, physical differences between boys and girls, and men and women, but many differences in brain function and psychological orientation as well. A social theory like that of Judith Butler, which dismisses biological evidence with a wave of the hand and would seek to construct a new society in defiance of sound science, is a recipe for personal and political disaster.

[60] Anderson, *When Harry Became Sally*, 56.

[61] Anderson, *When Harry Became Sally*, 53–55.

[62] Anderson, *When Harry Became Sally*, 53, 55, 56.

[63] Anderson, *When Harry Became Sally*, 56, 58.
[64] Anderson, *When Harry Became Sally*, 59, 61, 60, 74.
[65] Anderson, *When Harry Became Sally*, 73–75.
[66] Anderson, *When Harry Became Sally*, 62–63.
[67] Anderson, *When Harry Became Sally*, 63–64.
[68] Anderson, *When Harry Became Sally*, 64–65.
[69] Anderson, *When Harry Became Sally*, 65.
[70] Anderson, *When Harry Became Sally*, 64–66.
[71] Anderson, *When Harry Became Sally*, 69.
[72] Anderson, *When Harry Became Sally*, 69.
[73] Anderson, *When Harry Became Sally*, 70.
[74] Anderson, *When Harry Became Sally*, 69–71.
[75] Denise Shick, "When My Father Told Me He Wanted to Be a Woman," *Public Discourse*, 27 March 2015.
[76] The term *kathoey* has acquired certain negative connotations among some Thai speakers, and so some use the alternate phrase *sao braphat song* to refer to the same people. In this essay the better-known term *kathoey* will be used.
[77] LeeRay Costa and Andrew Matzner, *Male Bodies, Women's Souls: Personal Narratives of Thailand's Transgendered Youth* (New York: The Haworth Press, 2007). This volume is not simply an edited collection, since it includes both personal narratives and detailed analysis of the narratives.
[78] Costa and Matzner, *Male Bodies, Women's Souls*, viii.
[79] Costa and Matzner, *Male Bodies, Women's Souls*, 139. Gay males in Thailand, in turn, do not care for *kathoey* who seek to pass as women (111).
[80] Costa and Matzner, *Male Bodies, Women's Souls*, 136. Costa and Matzner note that the sexual pairing of the *kathoey* with the Thai heterosexual male challenges the accustomed Western conceptualizations of "heterosexuality" and "homosexuality": "How might researchers understand sexual intimacies involving two male bodies if one partner feels she is a woman and expresses herself according to local, culturally defined rules of femininity? Should such desire be defined in terms of homoeroticism, transgenderism, or something else? And what of the 'real man' who is in a relationship with a [*kathoey*]? How does he articulate his own desires, both to himself and to others?" (135). Costa and Matzner draw a cross-cultural contrast with the Brazilian *travesti* (transgender prostitutes) who desire partners who are men (*homens*) and not gays (*viados*). In this respect, they are like *kathoey*. Yet unlike kathoey, the *travesti* do not want to become women and do not think of themselves as women (137). Citing D. Kuklick, "The Gender of Brazilian Transgendered Prostitutes," *American Anthropologist* 99 (1997), 576–577.
[81] The journalist Rakkit Rattachumpoth writes: "No Thai homosexual or transgender person feels that they are living in a gay or homosexual paradise. On the contrary, many feel that their lives are miserable, if not a living hell, where they are threatened by public denunciation, job discrimination, malicious

gossip, and indirect interference in both private and working spaces." Costa and Matzner, *Male Bodies, Women's Souls*, 29–30; citing Rattachumpoth, "Foreword," in P. Jackson and G. Sullivan, eds., *Lady Boys, Tom Boys, Rent Boys: Male and Female Homosexualities in Comtemporary Thailand* (Binghamton, NY: Haworth Press, 1999), xi–xviii, citing xii.

[82] Costa and Matzner, *Male Bodies, Women's Souls*, 30–31.

[83] Costa and Matzner, *Male Bodies, Women's Souls*, 138–139.

[84] Costa and Matzner, *Male Bodies, Women's Souls*, 143.

[85] Costa and Matzner, *Male Bodies, Women's Souls*, 25.

[86] Costa and Matzner, *Male Bodies, Women's Souls*, 144.

[87] Costa and Matzner, *Male Bodies, Women's Souls*, 120–121. Dini writes, "I began taking birth control pills just like my *kathoey* friends at school had recommended so that I could get whiter skin and breasts" (56).

[88] Costa and Matzner, *Male Bodies, Women's Souls*, 73, 77.

[89] Costa and Matzner, *Male Bodies, Women's Souls*, 83.

[90] Costa and Matzner, *Male Bodies, Women's Souls*, 105, 107, 112.

[91] Costa and Matzner, *Male Bodies, Women's Souls*, 100–101.

[92] Costa and Matzner, *Male Bodies, Women's Souls*, 68.

[93] Costa and Matzner, *Male Bodies, Women's Souls*, 93–94, 98.

[94] Costa and Matzner, *Male Bodies, Women's Souls*, 64.

[95] Costa and Matzner, *Male Bodies, Women's Souls*, 54.

[96] Costa and Matzner, *Male Bodies, Women's Souls*, 121.

[97] Costa and Matzner, *Male Bodies, Women's Souls*, 153.

[98] Anderson, *When Harry Became Sally*, 3. Viviane Namaste, in *Invisible Lives*, corroborates Anderson's point with regard to transgender persons: "Many transsexuals…do not align themselves with American lesbian/gay politics" (2).

[99] Mark Regnerus, in his insightful essay, "The Mission Creep of Dignity" (12 January 2015: http://www.thepublicdiscourse.com/2015/01/14253) distinguishes what he calls "Dignity 1.0" from "Dignity 2.0" in this way: "Dignity 1.0, the older conception shared by Christians, natural law theorists and others, refers to the idea that humans have 'inherent worth of immeasurable value that is deserving of certain morally appropriate responses.'" Yet this is not the idea of "dignity" that prevails generally in LGBTQ+ activism: "The basis for Dignity 2.0 in the West does not rest on external standards, on traditional restraints such as kinship, neighborhood, religion, or nation, which are all stable sources of the self. Rather, it is based upon the dis-integrated, shifting 'me,' subject to renegotiation, reinvention, and reconstruction, reinforced by expansive conditions and regulations." Dignity 2.0, in short, means rendering to others whatever tokens or measures of respect that they think that you owe to them. No wonder then that Regnerus comments, "It's exhausting—though profitable to attorneys. And Facebook. But it also explains my confusion: there are rival forms of dignity, and the version you employ matters a great deal."

[100] "California Assembly Passes a Bill to Ban 'Conversion Therapy,'" 19 April 2018; https://www.eqca.org/california-assembly-passes-bill-to-ban-conversion-therapy/; Conor Friedersdorf wrote an editorial opposing the bill, "Conversion Therapy for Gays is Awful, but so is California's Bill to Ban it," 27 April 2018. http://www.latimes.com/opinion/op-ed/la-oe-friedersdorf-gay-conversion-20180427-story.html

[101] Anderson, *When Harry Became Sally*, 35; PFLAG, *Our Trans Loved Ones*, 19.

[102] Anderson, *When Harry Became Sally*, 44; citing Human Rights Campaign, *Schools in Transition: A Guide for Supporting Transgender Students in K–12 Schools*, 34; assets.hrc.org/files/assets/resources/Schools-In-Tradition.pdf.

[103] Fourier's writings in French appeared from 1808 to 1818, but the proposals for free love were shocking at that time, and so his writings were not widely diffused until the 1960s. See Jonathan Beecher and Richard Bienvenu, eds. *The Utopian Vision of Charles Fourier: Selected Texts on Work, Love, and Passionate Attraction* (Boston: Beacon Press, 1971). Frank E. Manuel and Fritzie P. Manuel, eds., in *French Utopias: An Anthology of Ideal Societies* (New York: Schocken Books, 1971 [1966]) excerpt Fourier's work *The System of Passionate Attraction* in their anthology (299–328). Among the various French writers, "only the Marquis de Sade and Fourier would open wide the floodgates of promiscuous sexual encounters to those who desired them" ("Introduction," 13). "Of all the utopians, only Fourier seriously attacks the family structure as the basic unit of social life. The others direct themselves toward strengthening the relationship, ennobling it, purifying it of dross" ("Introduction," 13).

[104] Manuel and Manuel, "Introduction," in *French Utopias*, 15.

[105] Kuby, *The Global Sexual Revolution*, 22.

[106] Kengor, *Takedown*, 20–21; citing Richard Weikart, "Marx, Engels, and the Abolition of the Family," *History of European Ideas* 18 (1994) 657–672, citing 668–669.

[107] Kengor, *Takedown*, 26–28.

[108] Kuby, *The Global Sexual Revolution*, 22.

[109] Kengor, *Takedown*, 86.

[110] Kengor, *Takedown*, 27; citing Friedrich Engels, *The Origin of the Family, Private Property and the State* (New York: International, 1942), 67.

[111] Kengor, *Takedown*, 86–87, 32–33.

[112] Kengor, *Takedown*, 34–36.

[113] Kengor, *Takedown*, 39–40.

[114] Kuby, *The Global Sexual Revolution*, 23.

[115] Kengor, *Takedown*, 87.

[116] Kuby, *The Global Sexual Revolution*, 37–38.

[117] Kuby, *The Global Sexual Revolution*, 38–39.

[118] Kengor, *Takedown*, 135.

[119] Kengor, *Takedown*, 147–148, 144–145, 158–160.

[120] Mary Ann Tolbert, "Foreword: What Word Shall We Take Back?," in Robert Goss and Mona West, eds., *Take Back the Word: A Queer Reading of the Bible* (Cleveland, OH: The Pilgrim Press, 2000), vii–xi, citing vii. A later and more comprehensive work is Deryn Guest, Robert E. Goss, Mona West, and Thomas Bohache, eds., *The Queer Bible Commentary* (London: SCM, 2006).

[121] Tolbert, "Foreword," ix.

[122] Tolbert, "Foreword," x.

[123] Robert E. Goss and Mona West, "Introduction," in Goss and West, eds., *Take Back the Word*, 3–9, citing 6–7.

[124] Virginia Ramey Mollenkott, "Reading the Bible from Low and Outside: Lesbiantransgay People as God's Tricksters," in Goss and West, eds., *Take Back the Word*, 13–22, citing 13.

[125] Goss and West, "Introduction," 7.

[126] In breaking from heterosexual normativity, Christopher King is less categorical than are Goss and West. King admits that "the Song of Songs celebrates the love, desire, and sexual life of a man and a woman," and yet he insists that it "celebrates socially transgressive eros." Citing Christopher King, "A Love as Fierce as Death: Reclaiming the Song of Songs for Queer Lovers," in Goss and West, eds., *Take Back the Word*, 126–142, citing 141.

[127] Here I pass over the discussion—not germane to this paper—on the proper rendering of the Hebrew in Song 1:5, and whether it should be construed as *adversative* ("black but lovely"; the Vulgate has *nigra sum, sed formosa*) or else as *conjunctive* ("black and lovely"; per some recent interpreters).

[128] Lee Edelman, *No Future: Queer Theory and the Death Drive* (Durham, NC: Duke University Press, 2004); book description at https://www.dukeupress.edu/no-future; accessed 13 December 2016.

[129] See the discussion at http://www.vhemt.org; accessed 14 December 2016; and the essay by James S. Ormrod, "'Making Room for the Tigers and the Polar Bears': Biography, Phantasy and Ideology in the Voluntary Human Extinction Movement," *Psychoanalysis, Culture and Society* 16 (2011), 142–161.

[130] Marcella Althaus-Reid, *Indecent Theology: Theological Perversions in Sex, Gender and Politics* (New York: Routledge, 2001), 200.

[131] Marcella Althaus-Reid, *The Queer God* (New York: Routledge, 2003), cited from https://en.wikipedia.org/wiki/Queer_theology; accessed 10 Dec. 2016.

[132] Kuby, *The Global Sexual Revolution*, 77.

[133] Pope Benedict XVI, cited in Kuby *The Global Sexual Revolution*, 267–268.

[134] Joseph-Marie Verlinde, *L'ideologie du gender: comme identité reçue ou choisie?*

[135] For Pope Francis's comments in context, see: https://cruxnow.com/global-church/2016/10/01/pope-calls-gender-theory-global-war-family/

[136] Available online at: stjosaphateparchy.com/encyclical-concerning-the-danger-of-gender-ideology.

[137] Pete Baklinski, "Gender ideology is 'destructive,' 'anti-human' and must be opposed: Ukrainian Greek Catholic Church," *Life Site News*, 22 December 2016; https://www.lifesitenews.com/news/gender-ideology-is-destructive-anti-human-and-must-be-opposed-ukrainian-gre.

[138] Kuby, *The Global Sexual Revolution*, 8–9.

[139] Robert Spaemann, "Foreword," in Kuby, *The Global Sexual Revolution*, 1–2, citing 1.

[140] Owen Strachan and Gavin Peacock, *The Grand Design: Male and Female He Made Them* (Fearn, Ross-shire, UK: Christian Focus, 2016), 13–14.

[141] Strachan and Peacock, *The Grand Design*, 14.

[142] Anderson, *When Harry Became Sally*, 18; citing Paul R. McHugh, "Surgical Sex," *First Things*, https://www.firstthings.com/article/2004/11/surgical-sex.

[143] Baklinski, "Gender ideology."

[144] Anderson, *When Harry Became Sally*, 5–6.

[145] Lisa Littman, "Parent Reports of Adolescents and Young Adults Perceived to Show Signs of a Rapid Onset of Gender Dysphoria," Plos One 13 (16 August 2018); https://doi.org/10.1371/journal.pone.0202330; citing 1, 33, 35; Lisa Littman, "Correction: Parent Reports of Adolescents and Young Adults Perceived to Show Signs of a Rapid Onset of Gender Dysphoria," Plos One 14 (19 March 2019); https://doi.org/10.1371/journal.pone.0213157; citing 2; Mark Regnerus, "Queering Science," First Things, December 2018; https://www.firstthings.com/article/2018/12/queering-science

Chapter 5

[1] Paul Tillich, "Reason and Revelation, Being and God," *Systematic Theology*, vol. 1 (Chicago: University of Chicago Press, 1973), 60.

[2] Tillich, *Systematic Theology*, 1:61.

[3] Adrian Thatcher, "Introduction," in *The Oxford Handbook of Theology, Sexuality, and Gender*, Adrian Thatcher, ed. (Oxford: Oxford University Press, 2017), 4–5.

[4] Robby Waddell, Professor of New Testament, Southeastern University, wrote in a private correspondence, "There is not very much on human sexuality/embodiment from a Pentecostal perspective." E-mail correspondence to Dr. Bill Prevette and authors (4 May 2017).

[5] William K. Kay and Stephen J. Hunt, "Pentecostal Churches and Homosexuality," in *The Oxford Handbook of Theology, Sexuality, and Gender*, 357.

[6] Kay and Hunt, "Pentecostal Churches and Homosexuality," 358.

[7] Michael Wilkinson and Peter Althouse, "Call for Papers, Annual Review of the Sociology of Religion, Volume 8: Pentecostals and the Body, 2015," n.d.,

n.p., http://www.religiousstudiesproject.com/wp-content/uploads/2015/06/ARSR_Call_for_Papers_2017.pdf (7 May 2017).

[8] Paul Ricoeur, *Time and Narrative*, trans. Kathleen Blamey and David Pellauer, vol. 3 (Chicago: University of Chicago Press, 1988), 246.

[9] Paul Ricoeur, *Oneself as Another*, trans. Kathleen Blamey (Chicago: University of Chicago Press, 1992), 141.

[10] Ricoeur, *Oneself as Another*, 116.

[11] Ricoeur, *Oneself as Another*, 121. Italics original.

[12] Simon Brodbeck and Brian Black, "Introduction," in *Gender and Narrative in the Mahabharata*, Simon Brodbeck and Brian Black, eds. (London: Routledge, 2007), 10–11.

[13] Brodbeck and Black, "Introduction," 11.

[14] Thatcher, "Introduction," 5.

[15] Vasudha Narayanan, "Gender in a Devotional Universe," in *The Blackwell Companion to Hinduism*, Gavin Flood, ed. (New York: John Wiley and Sons, 2008), 569.

[16] Narayanan, "Gender in a Devotional Universe," 578.

[17] Brodbeck and Black, "Introduction," 16.

[18] Brodbeck and Black, "Introduction," 17.

[19] Brodbeck and Black, "Introduction," 18.

[20] Elizabeth Stuart, "The Theological Study of Sexuality," in *The Oxford Handbook of Theology, Sexuality and Gender*, 18.

[21] Janet Martin Soskice, *The Kindness of God: Metaphor, Gender and Religious Language* (Oxford: Oxford University Press, 2007), 49.

[22] Tina Beattie, "The Theological Study of Gender," in *The Oxford Handbook of Theology, Sexuality and Gender*, 41.

[23] Amos Yong, *Hospitality and the Other: Pentecost, Christian Practices and the Neighbour* (New York: New York University, 2008), 36.

[24] Yong, *Hospitality and the Other*, 36. See Eddie Gibbs and Ryan K. Bolger, *Emerging Churches: Creating Christian Community in Postmodern Cultures* (Grand Rapids: Zondervan, 2005).

[25] Priyanka Dasguptal, "12-year-old Mother Takes Transfer from School," *The Times of India*, 5 May 2017, n.p., http://timesofindia.indiatimes.com/city/kolkata/12-year-old-mom-takes-transfer-from-school/articleshow/58523785.cms (6 May 2017).

Chapter 6

[1] Elizabeth M. King and M. Anne Hill, eds., *Women's Education in Developing Countries: Barriers, Benefits, and Policies* (Baltimore, MD: Johns Hopkins University Press, 1993), 26.

[2] Colin Brock and Nadine Cammish, "Factors Affecting Female Participation

in Education in Seven Developing Countries," 2nd ed., *Education Papers* 9 (London: Dept. for International Development, 1997), 21; accessed from https://files.eric.ed.gov/fulltext/ED411432.pdf on 2/23/2019.

[3] An alternative report by the MBDHP on Burkina Faso's 4th and 5th combined periodic reports submitted to the Committee on the Elimination of Discrimination against Women at the 33 session (5–22 July 2005) New York.

[4] Jean-Victor Ouédraogo, *Sidwaya* no. 5877 of Thursday 19 April 2007.

[5] Jean-Victory Ouédraogo, www.sidwaya.bf/dossier_communre rurale de Kain, 19 April 2007.

[6] Jean-Victor Ouédraogo in the *Sidwaya Daily* 19 April 2007 no. 5877 on commune rurale de Kain, le calvaire quotidien des populations' (Internet edition No5894, accessed on 10 May 2007).

[7] News given on the national Radio Burkina 27 January 2005, http://www.radio.bf/ index.php.

[8] Brock and Cammish, "Female Participation in Education."

[9] Pastor Tapsoaba Flavien, Treasurer General of the FEME, face-to-face interview, 8 February 2006.

[10] Wife of village pastor in the Center North, interview, 11 March 2006.

[11] Mrs. E. Sawadogo, pastor's wife, face-to-face interview, 2006.

[12] Philippe Ouédraogo, "Transforming Communities through Education," in *Good News from Africa: Community Transformation through the Church*, ed. Brian E. Woolnough (Oxford: Regnum Books, 2013), 82.

[13] Interview with Pastor Simporé, former secretary-general of the Evangelical Educators of Burkina Faso, March 2006 in Ouagadougou.

[14] Pastor Pierre Dupret and his wife, as French missionaries, were called on by the American missionaries for help, seeing that the country was a French colony.

[15] Abel Zongo is the director of the Association of Evangelical Schools of the Assemblies of God.

[16] Lakoue Ibrango, a former school advisor, and Headmaster of the evangelical school in Ouahigouya, the capital of the northern province of Yatenga. With over 40 years of experience in teaching in the same school, he taught the author in the middle class in 1968–69. Interview conducted in the school at Ouahigouya, March 2006.

[17] Pastor Gouba, also a witness and a teacher in the evangelical school since 1953, noticed that Pastor Dupret integrated girls and boys in the school.

[18] Gouba, a teacher at the second national evangelical school with Pastor Dupret, the first being the late Pastor Kéré Gédéon. Gouba celebrated 50 years of marriage and concluded that mixed evangelical education can promote harmonious families when both partners went to school and benefited from Christian education.

[19] Pastor Sibiri Simporé, face-to-face interview, 20 March 2006.

[20] Pastor Douna Hamidou, President of SIM churches in Burkina Faso, face-to-face interview, June 2007.

21 Pastor Hamidou, interview, June 2007.
22 Pastor Hamidou, interview, June 2007.
23 Pastor Innocent Kientega, director of AOG technical school, face-to-face interview, 21 Feb 2005.
24 Pastor Gouba Tobado, face-to-face interview, 22 February 2006.
25 Mrs. Antoinnette Ouédraogo, pastor's wife and public school worker, interview, 9 Feb 2005.
26 Mrs. Clémence Ilboudo, Secretary General at the Ministry of Women's Promotion, interview 6 Feb 2009 in Ouagadougou.
27 Mrs. Clémence Ilboudo, interview.
28 N'Dri Assie, "Educational Selection and Social Inequality in Africa" (PhD. Dissertation, University of Chicago, 1983).
29 Mrs. Clémence Ilboudo, interview.
30 Jokebed Damoaliga, teacher at National Health Teacher Training School, and member of Christian Medical Fellowship in Ouagadougou, face-to-face interview 9 Feb. 2005.
31 Interview with Mrs. Priscilla Zongo at the Burkina Faso residence in Washington on Saturday 28 May 2005.
32 Philippe Ouédraogo, *Female Education and Mission: A Burkina Faso Experience*, with Forward by Prime Minister Tertius Zongo (Oxford: Regnum Books, 2014).

Chapter 7

[1] This paper is largely based on two unpublished academic papers written by the authors: "Sexual Exploitation of Children in the Philippines and the Role of Evangelical Churches" (Lulu Suico: MA Theology and Development, OCMS/ University of Leeds, 2002), and "Institutional and Individualistic Dimensions of Transformational Development: The Case of Pentecostal Churches in the Philippines (Joseph Suico: PhD, OCMS/University of Wales, 2003), with updated statistics and documentation.
[2] https://digitallibrary.un.org/record/222024.
[3] According to the GSI, India, China, Pakistan, Indonesia, Bangladesh, and Thailand are in the top 10 countries with the highest number of trafficking victims in the world. India tops the list with 14 million victims of trafficking, China comes in second at 3.2 million, and Pakistan is third with 2.1 million trafficking victims. India and Pakistan are also in the top 10 countries in the world with the highest prevalence of human trafficking.
[4] https://www.ilo.org/global/about-the-ilo/newsroom/news/WCMS_007994/lang--en/index.htm, accessed 3/2/2019.

[5] Ana Quintana, Sarah Torre and Olivia Enos, "Strengthening the End Modern Slavery Initiative (EMSI)," 7 April 2016, www.heritage.org. 2017.

[6] http://ibon.org/2018/06/time-for-govt-to-come-up-with-realistic-poverty-threshold-ibon/, accessed 3/2/2019.

[7] Gini Coefficient according to Michael Todaro [see footnote 9] is "an aggregate numerical measure of income inequality ranging from 0 (perfect equality) to 1 (perfect inequality)."

[8] "Attacking Poverty: World Development Report" (New York: Oxford University Press, 2000).

[9] *National Census and Statistics,* 1995 cited in CPP, 2000.

[10] FG Tantoco, "Philippines: Street Children," *Children Worldwide* 20, no. 2–3 (1993), 35.

[11] Jason Gutierrez, "Manila in All-Out War vs. Child Abuse," *United Press International,* 4 Oct. 1996, www.upi.com/Archives.

[12] Niriniaina Ralambomamy, trans. Carolyn Yohn, "Sexual Exploitation of Children in the Philippines," Humanium, 9 May 2017, www.humanium.org.

[13] Olivia Enos, "A Better Way to Fight Modern Slavery," 6 June 2016, https://www.heritage.org/global-politics/commentary/better-way-fight-modern-slavery.

[14] Uli Schmetzer, "U.S. Naval Base in Philippines Means Ships, Sex," 7 Sept. 1989, *Chicago Tribune,* www.chicagotribune.com.

[15] Kevin Ireland, "Sexual Exploitation of Children and International Travel and Tourism," *Child Abuse Review* 2, no. 4 (1993), 270.

[16] "Combatting Child Prostitution and Domestic Sexual Abuse: The history of the Work of Preda," accessed 3/2/2019, https://www.preda.org/about-preda-foundation/preda-history/.

[17] Stanley Palisada, "Child Pornography Dot Com," *The News Today, Online Edition,* 24 Aug 2009, http://www.thenewstoday.info/2009/08/24/child.pornography.dot.com.dot.ph.html.

[18] Ireland, "Sexual Exploitation of Children," 270.

[19] Ireland, "Sexual Exploitation of Children," 270.

[20] Sara Terry, "How One Town in the Philippines Fights Back against Child Prostitution," 2 July 1987, *Christian Science Monitor,* https://www.csmonitor.com/1987/0702/zbtot3.html.

[21] Uli Schmetzer, "Philippine Town Haven for Touring Pedophiles," 9 April 1992, *Chicago Tribune,* www.chicagotribune.com.

[22] Maria Ressa, "Child Sex Trade Plagues Filipino Resort," 31 Aug 1996, *CNN Interactive, World News Story Page,* http://www.cnn.com/WORLD/9608/31/pedophile/index.html.

[23] https://www.dswd.gov.ph/

[24] Leif Corlim, "Undercover Journalists Trawl Manila's Seedy Red Light District," 16 May 2013, *CNN World: The Fighter, a CNN Freedom Project Documentary,* http://www.cnn.com/2013/05/06/world/asia/.

[25] https://www.dswd.gov.ph/
[26] "UN Urges Action on Millions of Asian Trafficking Victims," 29 March 2000, PREDA Foundation, https://www.preda.org/2000/03/.
[27] Peter Lau, "GMA Signs Anti-Child Labor Law," posted Feb 2004, https://www.scribd.com/document/6822562/child-labor, accessed 3/4/2019.
[28] Michael Todaro, *Economic Development* (Harlow, England: Addison-Wesley, 2000), 618.
[29] Phyllis Kilbourne and Marjorie McDermid, eds., *Sexually Exploited Children: Working to Protect and Heal*, (Monrovia, CA: MARC, 1998).
[30] Ravi Kanbur et al., "World Development Report 2000/2001: attacking poverty," (Sept. 2000), documents.worldbank.org.
[31] Todaro, *Economic Development*, 348.
[32] Vitit Muntarbhorn, "Report of the Special Rapporteur on the Sale of Children, Child Prostitution, and Child Pornography," United Nations Economic and Social Council, Commission on Human rights, 52nd Session, Agenda Item 20 (New York: UN), E/CN.4/1996/100 (1996), 2.
[33] Muntarbhorn, "Report …on the Sale of Children," 3.
[34] Chris and Phileena Heuertz in *Sexually Exploited Children*, Kilbourne and McDermid, eds., 85.
[35] Heuertz and Heuertz in *Sexually Exploited Children*, 85.
[36] Robert Linthicum in *Sexually Exploited Children*, Kilbourne and McDermid, eds., 21.
[37] PEOPLE OF THE PHILIPPINES, *plaintiff-appellee*, vs., Romeo G. Jalosjos, *accused-appellant* [G.R. Nos. 132875-76, 16 Nov 2001], http://sc.judiciary.gov.ph/jurisprudence, accessed 3/6/2019.
[38] Sophia Dedace, "Convicted Rapist Jalosjos Freed after 13 Years in Prison," GMA [Greater Manila Area] News Online, 19 March 2009, https://www.gmanetwork.com/news/news/nation.
[39] Caroline O. Moser, "Confronting Crisis: A Summary of Household Responses to Poverty and Vulnerability in Four Poor Urban Communities," *ESSD Environmentally & Socially Sustainable Development Work in Progress: Environmentally Sustainable Development Studies and Monographs Series*, 7 (Washington DC: World Bank Group, 1996), 10.
[40] Josefina Gutierrez, interview, Quezon City, 1997.
[41] Moser, "Confronting Crisis," 10.
[42] Lisa Grace S. Bersales and Romeo S. Recide, *Survey on Overseas Filipinos 2016: A Report on the Overseas Filipino Workers* (Quezon City: Philippine Statistics Authority), ix, https://psa.gov.ph, accessed 3/6/2019.
[43] Muntarbhorn, "Report …on the Sale of Children," 2.
[44] Ireland, "Sexual Exploitation of Children…and Tourism," 22.
[45] Ireland, "Sexual Exploitation of Children…and Tourism," 22.
[46] Narvasen cited in Ireland, "Sexual Exploitation of Children…and Tourism," 37.

[47] Ron O'Grady, *Tourism in the Third World: Christian Reflections* (Maryknoll, NY: Orbis Books, 1982), 39.
[48] Fr. Shay Cullen, "Saving Filipino Children from Traveling Pedophiles," 15 Oct 2017, *The Manila Times*, https://www.manilatimes.net/saving-filipino-children-traveling-pedophiles/356517/.
[49] Judith Ennew, *The Sexual Exploitation of Children* (New York: St. Martins Press, 1986), 110.
[50] Ennew, *Sexual Exploitation of Children*, 110.
[51] Ennew, *Sexual Exploitation of Children*, 114.
[52] Ennew, *Sexual Exploitation of Children*, 114.
[53] Julia O'Connell Davidson, *Prostitution, Power and Freedom* (Ann Arbor, MI: University of Michigan Press, 1998), 178.
[54] Ireland, "Sexual Exploitation of Children…and Tourism," 43; Ron O'Grady, *Tourism*, 43.
[55] Ron O'Grady, *Tourism*, 43.
[56] O'Connell Davidson, *Prostitution, Power and Freedom*, 28.
[57] Ron O'Grady, *Tourism*, 36–37.
[58] Ennew, *Sexual Exploitation of Children*, 106.
[59] UNICEF, 2000.
[60] Ron O'Grady, *Tourism*, 37.
[61] Ireland, "Sexual Exploitation of Children…and Tourism," 43.
[62] Jon Melegrito, "U.S. House Hearing: PH Making Only Slow Progress vs. Trafficking," 22 March 2018, globalnation.inquirer.net, accessed at https://www.preda.org, 3/6/2019.
[63] Peter Kreuzer, "Philippine Governance: Merging Politics and Crime," PRIF Reports No. 93 (Frankfurt: Peace Research Institute Frankfurt, 2009), https://www.researchgate.net/publication/228921337, accessed 3/6/2019.
[64] O'Connell Davidson, *Prostitution, Power and Freedom*, 73.
[65] Christopher Wright, *Living as the People of God* (Westmont, IL: InterVarsity Press, 1983), 194.
[66] Wright, *Living as the People of God*, 196.
[67] Patrick Parkinson, *Child Sexual Abuse and the Churches* (London: Hodder and Stoughton, 1997), 26–27.
[68] Parkinson, *Child Sexual Abuse*, 194.
[69] Lausanne Conference for World Evangelization, 1989, 47.
[70] Michael Eastman in Parkinson, *Child Sexual Abuse and the Churches*, 25.
[71] Carl E. Amerding, "The Child at Risk: A Biblical View," *Transformation* 14, no. 2 (April/June 1997), 25, https://www.jstor.org/stable.
[72] Murray W. Dempster, "Eschatology, Spirit Baptism, and Inclusiveness: An Exploration into the Hallmarks of a Pentecostal Social Ethic," in *Perspectives in Pentecostal Eschatology: World without End*, eds. Peter Althouse and Robby Waddell (Cambridge: James Clarke & Co., 1999), 152.
[73] "Brussels Statement on Evangelization and Social Concern," *Transformation:*

An International Journal of Holistic Mission Studies 16, no. 2 (April 1999), 43, https://doi.org/10.1177/026537889901600202.

[74] Ron Sider, *Evangelism & Social Action* (London: Hodder & Stoughton, 1993), 183.

[75] Bryant L. Myers, *Walking with the Poor* (New York: Orbis, 1999), 134.

[76] Myers, *Walking with the Poor*, 134.

[77] Melba Maggay, *Transforming Society* (Quezon City: Institute for Studies in Asian Church and Culture, 1996), 61.

[78] Maggay, *Transforming Society*, 8.

[79] Heuertz and Heuertz in *Sexually Exploited Children*, 91

[80] Viju Abraham, "Mobilizing the Church for Action," in *Sexually Exploited Children*, 300.

[81] Joyce Bundellu, "Rescuing Children of Sex Workers," in *Sexually Exploited Children*, 81.

[82] Deryke Belshaw, "Socio-economic Theology and Ethical Choice in Contemporary Development Policy: an Outline of Biblical Approaches to Social Justice and Poverty Alleviation," *Transformation* 14, no. 1 (1997), 7.

[83] Allen Anderson, "Pentecostal Approaches to Faith and Healing," *International Review of Mission XCI*, no. 363 (Oct 2002), 533.

[84] Michael Wourms, *J.I.L. Love Story* (El Cajon, CA: Christian Services Publishing, 1992); Oscar Baldemor, "The Spread of Fire: A Study of Ten Growing Churches in Metro-Manila" (Master's Thesis, Fuller Theological Seminary, 1990), 103–108.

[85] In contrast, the Assemblies of God has a Malaysian school for evangelists, the founder and director of which, to the present, is a missionary from the U.S.

[86] An important articulation of theological doctrine by Pentecostal scholars is the *Globalization of Pentecostalism*, eds. Murray Dempster, Bryon Klaus and Douglas Petersen (Eugene, OR: Wipf and Stock, 1999).

[87] Michael Haralambos & Martin Holborn, *Sociology Themes and Perspectives* (London: HarperCollins, 1995), 459.

[88] Kyle McDonnell, "Ideology of Pentecostal Conversion," *Journal of Ecumenical Studies* 5 (Winter, 1968), 117.

[89] McDonnell, "Ideology of Pentecostal Conversion," 117.

[90] Dempster, Klaus and Peterson, *Globalization of Pentecostalism*, 88.

[91] Juan Sepulveda, "Reflections on the Pentecostal Contribution to the Mission of the Church in Latin America," *The Journal of Pentecostal Theology* 1 (Oct 1992), 101–102; Doug Petersen, "Pentecostals: Who Are They?" in *Mission as Transformation: A Theology of the Whole Gospel*, eds. Vinay Samuel and Chris Sugden (Oxford: Regnum, 1999), 96.

[92] Donald Dayton, *Theological Roots of Pentecostalism* (Grand Rapids: Francis Asbury Press, 1987), 9.

[93] See also Robert M. Anderson, *The Vision of the Disinherited* (New York:

Oxford University Press, 1979).

[94] Dayton, *Theological Roots.*

[95] Petersen, "Pentecostals: Who Are They?" 98–99.

[96] See also Carver T. Yu, *Being and Relation: A Theological Critique of Western Dualism and Individualism* (Edinburgh: Scottish Academic Press, 1987).

[97] Juan Sepulveda, "Pentecostal Theology in the Context of the Struggle for Life," in *Faith Born in the Struggle for Life,* Dow Kirkpatrick, ed. (Grand Rapids: Eerdmans, 1988), 299.

[98] Sepulveda, "Pentecostal Theology," 299.

[99] Sepulveda, "Pentecostal Theology," ix.

[100] For example, the Philippine Assemblies of God did not have an official position or response regarding the two significant political events (EDSA 1 and 2) that took place in 1986 and 2001 respectively. In recent times, there has been no reaction at all to issues like "Extra-Judicial Killing," and the restoration of the death penalty (2016, 2017).

[101] George Marsden, *Fundamentalism and American Culture: The Shaping of Twentieth-Century Evangelicalism: 1870–1925* (New York: Oxford University Press, 1980), 86.

[102] For a more thorough treatment of this, see Vinson Synan, *Aspects of Pentecostal-Charismatic Origins* (Plainfield, NJ: Logos International, 1975).

[103] Ron Sider, *Evangelism and Social Action: Uniting the Church to heal a Lost and Broken World* (London: Hodder and Stoughton, 1993), 34.

[104] See for example, *The Report of the International Dialogue 1990–1997 Between the Roman Catholic Church and Some Classical Pentecostal Churches and Leaders* (1999).

[105] David Martin, *Tongues of Fire* (Cambridge, MA: Basil Blackwell, Inc., 1990), 265.

[106] Vincent Synan, *The Holiness-Pentecostal Movement in the United States* (Grand Rapids, MI: Eerdmans, 1971), 185.

[107] EDSA stands for "Epifanio de los Santos Avenue" the location where the People's Revolution in 1986 took place.

[108] Paul Freston, *Evangelicals and Politics in Asia, Africa and Latin America* (Cambridge: Cambridge University Press, 2001), 70.

[109] Doug Petersen, *Not By Might Nor By Power* (Oxford: Regnum Books, 1996), 135.

[110] *The Report ... of the International Dialogue,* 119.

[111] Jorge Maldono, "Building 'Fundamentalism' from the Family in Latin America," in *Fundamentalisms and Society: Reclaiming the Sciences, the Family, and Education,* eds. Martin E. Marty and R. Scott Appleby (Chicago: University of Chicago Press, 1993), 218.

[112] Martin, *Tongues of Fire,* 13.

[113] An example of this is the 1986 EDSA Revolution where Cardinal Sin and other church leaders called for people to support the soldiers who turned against

the dictatorial government of Marcos.

[114]Orlando Costas, quoted by Murray Dempster, in *"Social Concern in the Context of Jesus' Kingdom, Mission and Ministry, Transformation: Social Concern in the Context of Jesus' Kingdom, Mission and Ministry* 16, no. 2 (1999), 43–53.

Chapter 8

[1]Ivan Wolffers, Irene Fernandez, Sharuna Verghis, and Martijn Vink, "Sexual Behaviour and Vulnerability of Migrant Workers for HIV Infection," *Culture, Health and Sexuality* 4, no. 4 (2002), 459–473.

[2]Martin Ruhs, "The Potential of Temporary Migration Programs in Future International Migration Policy," *International Labor Review* 145, nos. 1–2 (2006), 7–36.

[3]Shirly Hune, "Migrant Women in the Context of the International Convention on the Protection of the Rights of All Migrant Workers and Members of Their Families," *International Migration Review* 25, no. 4 (1991), 800–817; and International Labor Organization (ILO), *Domestic Workers Across the World: Global and Regional Statistics and the Extent of Legal Protection* (Geneva, Switzerland: ILO, 2012).

[4]Asha D'Souza, *Moving Towards Decent Work for Domestic Workers: An Overview of the ILO's Work* (Geneva, Switzerland: ILO, 2010), 9.

[5]Coordination of Action Research and Mobility (CARAM), *The Forgotten Space: Mobility and HIV Vulnerability in the Asia Pacific* (Kuala Lumpur, Malaysia: CARAM-Asia, 2002).

[6]Philippine Overseas Employment Administration (POEA), *POEA Annual Report 2009* (Mandaluyong City, the Philippines: United Nations [UN], 2009); *International Migrant Stock: The 2008 Revision*, http: //esa.un.org/migration (accessed 6 Feb 2019).

[7]Leah Briones, *Empowering Migrant Women: Why Agency and Rights Are Not Enough* (Surrey, UK: Ashgate Press, 2009).

[8]ILO, *Domestic Workers Across the World*.

[9]Carlos Delclos, Fernando Benavides, Ana M.Garcia, et. al, ITSAL [Immigration, Work and Health] Project (2010); Emily Ahonen, Maria Jose Lopez-Jacob, Maria Luisa Vazquez, et. al., "Invisible Work, Unseen Hazards: The Health of Women Immigrant Household Service Workers in Spain," *American Journal of Industrial Medicine* 53, no. 4 (2009), 405–416; Bridget Anderson, *Doing the Dirty Work? The Global Politics of Domestic Labor* (New York: Zed Books, 2000); Christine B. N. Chin, *In Service and Servitude: Foreign Female Domestic Workers and the Malaysian "Modernity" Project* (New York: Columbia University Press, 1998); Nicole Constable, "At Home

but Not at Home: Filipina Narratives of Ambivalent Returns," *Cultural Anthropology* 14, no. 2 (1999), 203–228; Nicole Constable, "Filipina Workers in Hong Kong Homes: Household Rules and Relations," in Barbara Ehrenreich and Arlie Russell Hochschild, eds., *Global Woman: Nannies, Maids, and Sex Workers in the New Economy* (New York: Henry Holt and Co., 2003), 115–141; Eleanor A. Holroyd, Alex Molassiotis, and Ruth E. Taylor-Pilliae, "Filipino Domestic Workers in Hong Kong: Health Related Behaviors, Health Locus of Control and Social Support," *Women and Health* 33, nos. 1–2 (2001), 181–205; Rhacel S. Parrenas, "Mothering from a Distance: Emotions, Gender, and Intergenerational Relations in Filipino Transnational Families," *Feminist Studies* 27, no. 2 (2001), 361–390.

[10] SM El-Hilu, et al., "Psychiatric Morbidity among Foreign Housemaids in Kuwait," *International Journal of Social Psychiatry* 36 (1990), 291–299; Phyllis W. L. Lau, Judy G. Y. Cheng, Dickson L. Y. Chow, et al., "Acute Psychiatric Disorders in Foreign Domestic Workers in Hong Kong: A Pilot Study," *International Journal of Social Psychiatry* 55, no. 6 (2009), 569–576; Muhammed Ajmal Zahid, Abdullahi Fido, Rashed Alowaish, et al., "Psychiatric Morbidity Among Housemaids in Kuwait. III: Vulnerability Factors," *International Journal of Social Psychiatry* 49 (2003), 87–96.

[11] Dennis Saleebey, "Power in the People: Strengths and Hope," *Advances in Social Work* 1, no. 2 (2000), 127–136.

[12] Michael Rutter, "Resilience: Some Conceptual Considerations," *Journal of Adolescent Health* 14 (1993), 626–631.

[13] Friedrich Losel and Thomas Bliesener, "Resilience in Adolescence: A Study on the Generalizability of Protective Factors," in Klaus Hurrelman, and Friedrich Losel, eds., *Health Hazards in Adolescence* (New York: Walter de Gruyter, 1990), 90–110.

[14] Karen J. Aroian and Anne E. Norris, "Resilience, Stress, and Depression among Russian Immigrants to Israel," *Western Journal of Nursing Research* 22, no. 1 (2000), 54–67.

[15] Daniel Fu Keung Wong, and He Xue Song, "The Resilience of Migrant Workers in Shanghai China: The Roles of Migration Stress and Meaning of Migration," *International Journal of Social Psychiatry* 54, no. 2 (2008), 131–143.

[16] James Joseph Keezhangatte, "Transnational Migration, Resilience and Family Relationships: Indian Household Workers in Hong Kong" (2006, Thesis), University of Hong Kong, Pokfulam, Hong Kong SAR. Retrieved from http://dx.doi.org/10.5353/th_b3576038.

[17] Jeffrey P. Bjorck, William Cuthbertson, John W. Thurman, and Yung Soon Lee, "Ethnicity, Coping, and Distress among Korean Americans, Filipino Americans, and Caucasian Americans," *The Journal of Social Psychology* 141, no. 4 (2001), 421–442; Gemma Tulud Cruz, "Faith on the Edge: Religion and Women in the Context of Migration," *Feminist Theology* 15, no. 1 (2006), 9–25;

Michael S. Ritsner, Ilan Modai and Alexander M. Ponizovski, "The Stress-support Patterns and Psychological Distress of Immigrants," *Stress and Health* 16, no. 3 (2000), 139–147; Francis Sanchez and Albert Gaw, "Mental Health Care of Filipino Americans," *Psychiatric Services* 58, no. 6 (2007), 810–815.

[18] Juliet Corbin and Anselm Strauss, *Basics of Qualitative Research: Techniques and Procedures for Developing Grounded Theory* (London: SAGE, 2008).

[19] Respondent Angelyn.

[20] Respondent Gina.

[21] Respondent Rowena.

[22] Respondent Faye.

[23] Respondent Grace.

[24] Respondent Teresita.

[25] Respondent Aileen.

[26] Respondent Teresita.

[27] Respondent Grace.

[28] Respondent Faye.

[29] Respondent Rowena.

[30] Respondent Angelyn.

[31] Respondent Ginalyn.

[32] Respondent Grace.

[33] Cruz, "Faith on the Edge."

[34] Jonas Nakonz and Angela Wai Yan Shik, "And All Your Problems Are Gone: Religious Coping Strategies among Philippine Migrant Workers in Hong Kong," *Mental Health, Religion and Culture* 12, no. 1 (2009), 25–38.

[35] Nakonz and Shik, "And All Your Problems Are Gone."

[36] Nakonz and Shik, "And All Your Problems Are Gone."

[37] Susan Folkman, "Personal Control and Stress and Coping Processes: A Theoretical Analysis,"
Journal of Personality and Social Psychology 46, no. 4 (1984), 839–852; Susan Folkman, Richard S. Lazarus, Christine Dunkel-Schetter, et. al, "Dynamics of a Stressful Encounter: Cognitive Appraisal, Coping, and Encounter Outcomes," *Journal of Personality and Social Psychology* 50, no. 5 (1986), 992–1003; Carolyn J. Forsythe and Bruce E. Compas, "Interaction of Cognitive Appraisals of Stressful Events and Coping: Testing the Goodness of Fit Hypothesis," *Cognitive Therapy and Research* 11, no. 4 (1987), 473–485; John Mirowsky and Catherine E. Ross, *Social causes of Psychological Distress* (New York: Aldine de Gruyter, 1989); Peggy A. Thoits, "Patterns in Coping with Controllable and Uncontrollable Events," in E. Mark Cummings, Anita L. Greene and Katherine H. Karrakar, eds., *Life-span Developmental Psychology: Perspectives on Stress and Coping* (Hillsdale, NJ: Psychology Press, 1991), 235–258; R. Jay Turner and Patricia Roszell, "Psychosocial Resources and the Stress Process," in William R. Avison and Ian H. Gotlib, eds., *Stress and Mental Health: Contemporary Issues and Prospects for the Future* (New York: Plenum, 1994),

179–210.

[38] Lisa F. Berkman, "Assessing the Physical Health Effects of Social Networks and Social Support," *Annual Review of Public Health* 5, no. 1 (1984), 413–432; Sheldon Cohen and Thomas Ashby Wills, "Stress, Social Support, and the Buffering Hypothesis," *Psychological Bulletin* 98, no. 2 (1985), 310–357; James S. House, Karl R. Landis and Debra Umberson, "Social Relationships and Health, *Science* 241 (1988), 540–545; Ronald C. Kessler and Jane D. McLeod, "Social Support and Mental Health in Community Samples," in Sheldon Cohen and S. Leonard Syme, eds., *Social Support and Health* (San Diego, CA: Academic Press, 1985), 219–240; Karen S. Rook, "The Negative Side of Social Interaction: Impact on Psychological Well-Being," *Journal of Personality and Social Psychology* 46, no. 5 (1992), 1097–1108.

[39] Francis Sanchez and Albert Gaw, "Mental Health Care of Filipino Americans," *Psychiatric Services* 58, no. 6 (2007), 810–815.

[40] Respondent Grace.

Chapter 9

[1] John S. Mbiti, *African Religions and Philosophy* (London: Heinemann, 1969), 1.

[2] Herling-Ruark was a then-research fellow at Harvard Institute for Public Health.

[3] H. E. Erastus Mwencha, Deputy Chairperson of African Union, Keynote Opening Address, African Biblical Leadership Initiative (ABLI), Kampala. Uganda. 03 August 2012.

[4] Edward C. Green and Allison H. Ruark, "Interrogating a Rights-Based Approach to HIV Prevention" (a paper presented at the Fellowship of Confessing Anglicans Consultation on Human Rights, Abuja, Nigeria, 2011), based on a chapter in their book, *AIDS, Behaviour and Culture: Understanding Evidence-based Prevention* (Walnut Creek, CA: Left Coast Press, 2011).

[5] Objections by Islamic Republic of Iran & Arab Republic of Syria; support for the original motion led by Brazil and Mexico.

[6] Green and Ruark, "Interrogating a Rights-Based Approach to HIV Prevention."

[7] Ban Ki-Moon, Secretary-General of United Nations, Speech to the Zambian National Parliament, February 24, 2012 (emphasis added).

[8] Karel Vasak, "Human Rights: A Thirty-Year Struggle: The Sustained Efforts to Give Force of Law to the Universal Declaration of Human Rights," *UNESCO Courier* 30, no. 11 (1977), 29–32.

[9] Vasak, "Human Rights."

[10] His divisions follow the three watchwords of the French Revolution: Liberty,

Equality, Fraternity. The three generations are reflected in some of the rubrics of the Charter of Fundamental Rights of the European Union. The Universal Declaration of Human Rights includes rights that are thought of as second generation as well as first generation ones, but it does not make the distinction in itself (the rights listed in it are not in specific order).

[11] Daniel Kaufmann, "Human Rights and Governance: The Empirical Challenge," in *Human Rights and Development: Towards Mutual Reinforcement*, eds. Philip Alston and Mary Robinson (Oxford: Oxford University Press, 2005).

[12] Kaufmann, "Human Rights and Government."

[13] Age limit was eventually raised to 19 as per amended Constitution signed into law in January 2016.

[14] Printed document presented to President Mogae, September 2010.

[15] Adriaan S. van Klinken, "The Homosexual as an Antithesis of Biblical Manhood? Heteronormativity and Masculinity Politics in Pentecostal Sermons in Zambia," *Journal of Gender and Religion in Africa* 2 (December 2011).

[16] "Countries that ban homosexuality risk losing aid, David Cameron warns," 30 October, 2011, http://www.guardian.co.uk/politics/2011/oct/30/ban-homosexuality-lose-aid-cameron?newsfeed=true.

[17] "Countries that ban homosexuality risk losing aid."

[18] "Countries that ban homosexuality risk losing aid."

[19] "Countries that ban homosexuality risk losing aid."

[20] "Countries that ban homosexuality risk losing aid."

[21] "Countries that ban homosexuality risk losing aid."

[22] "Hillary Clinton declares, 'Gay rights are human rights,'" 07 December 2011, http://www.bbc.co.uk/news/world-us-canada-16062937.

[23] Jabin Botsford, "Conservative Christians Working on HIV/AIDS See Burden of Sexual Liberalism," 25 July 2012, http://www.faithstreet.com/onfaith/2012/07/25/conservative-christians-working-on-hivAIDS-see-burden-of-sexual-liberalism/10197.

[24] "DOH groundBREAKERS," accessed 01 February 2019.

[25] Kylie Thomas, "A Better Life for Some: The loveLife Campaign and HIV/AIDS in South Africa," *Agenda: Empowering Women for Gender Equity* 62 (2004), 29-32.

[26] Personal interview with AIDS practitioner, 2013.

[27] Rena Singer, "Is loveLife Making Them Love Life?" 24 August 2005, Mail & Guardian: Africa's Best Read, https://mg.co.za/article/2005-08-24-is-lovelife-making-them-love-life.

[28] "That's Why We're Promoting loveLife," accessed 17 March 2015, http://www.lovelife.ch/en/campaign/archive/the-models/.

[29] Green and Ruark, *AIDS, Behavior, and Culture: Understanding Evidence-Based Prevention*.

[30] "Abstinence and the purity propaganda can harm Youth," accessed 18 March

2015, www.libchrist.com/index.html.

[31] Polyamory is the philosophy or state of being in love or romantically or even sexually involved with more than one person at the same time. This is usually with the full knowledge or consent of other partners involved.

[32] Christopher Sugden, concept note during consultation on *Human rights and Sexuality* unpublished].

[33] Sugden, consultation.

[34] Martin Meredith, *The State of Africa: A History of Fifty Years of Independence* (London: Free Press, 2005).

[35] Green and Ruark, "Interrogating a Rights-Based Approach to HIV Prevention."

Chapter 10

[1] Donald Miller and Tetsunao Yamamori, *Global Pentecostalism: The New Face of Christian Social Engagement* (Oakland, CA: University of California Press, 2007).

[2] David C. Atkins and Deborah E. Kessel, "Religiousness and Infidelity: Attendance, but not Faith and Prayer, Predict Marital Fidelity," *Journal of Marriage and Family* 70, no. 2 (2008), 407–418.

[3] Eleanor Gouws, Karen A. Stanecki, Rob Lyerla and Peter D. Ghuys, "The Epidemiology of HIV Infection among Young People Aged 15–24 Years in Southern Africa," *AIDS* (2008), 5–16.

[4] Doug Kirby, "Changes in Sexual Behavior Leading to the Decline in the Prevalence of HIV in Uganda: Confirmation from Multiple Sources of Evidence," *Sexually Transmitted Infections* 84, no. 2 (2008).

[5] Joshua Banda and David Anderson, "Politicians Must Reconcile, Forgive Each Other," *Times of Zambia* (2 March 2004), accessed Feb 9, 2019.

[6] Joshua Kembo, "Changes in Sexual Behavior and Practice and HIV Prevalence Indicators among Young People Aged 15–24 Years in Zambia: An In-depth Analysis of the 2001–2002 and 2007 Zambia Demographic and Health Surveys," *Sahara Journal* 10, nos. 3–4 (2013), accessed Nov 2015, 150–162.

[7] Kembo, "Changes in Sexual Behavior and Practice and HIV Prevalence Indicators."

[8] Kembo, "Changes in Sexual Behavior and Practice and HIV Prevalence Indicators."

[9] Kembo, "Changes in Sexual Behavior and Practice and HIV Prevalence Indicators."

[10] Joshua Kembo, "Risk Factors Associated with HIV Infection among Young Persons Aged 15–24 Years: Evidence from an In-depth Analysis of the 2005–06 Zimbabwe Demographic and Health Survey," *Sahara Journal* 9, no. 2 (2012),

54–63; Phillimon Ndubani, "Young Men's Sexuality and Sexually Transmitted Infections in Zambia," thesis, Karolinska Institute, 25 October 2002.

[11] Kembo, "Risk Factors" and Ndubani, "Young Men's Sexuality."

[12] Kembo, "Risk Factors" and Ndubani, "Young Men's Sexuality."

[13] Edward C. Green et al., "Uganda's HIV Prevention Success: The Role of Sexual Behavior Change and the National Response," *Aids and Behavior* 10, no. 4 (2006), 335–346.

[14] Green, "Uganda's HIV Prevention Success."

[15] Kim Longfeld, Megan Klein and John Berman, "Criteria for Trust and How Trust Affects Sexual Decision-Making among Youth" (October 2002), https://www.researchgate.net/publication/237262624_Criteria_for_Trust_and_How_Trust_Affects_Sexual_Decision-Making_among_Youth.

[16] Joshua H.K. Banda, "MCP- The Experience of the Church in MCP: The Evangelical Perspective," in Jane Wambui Rosenow, ed., *Multiple and Concurrent Sexual Partnerships: A Consultation with Senior Religious Leaders from East and Southern Africa* (Pan African Christian AIDS Network PACANet], 2011), 71.

[17] Vinod Mishra and Simona Bignami-Van Assche, "Concurrent Sexual Partnerships and HIV Infection: Evidence from National Population-Based Surveys," *DHS Working Papers* 62 (Calverton, MD: Macro International, 2009).

[18] Mishra and Assche, "Concurrent Sexual Partnerships and HIV."

[19] J. D. Shelton, "Partner Reduction Remains the Predominant Explanation," Letter in *BMJ* 9 March 2005, http://bmj.bmjjournals.com/cgi/eletters/330/7490/496-a#99730.

[20] James D. Shelton, et al., "Partner Reduction Is Crucial for Balanced 'ABC' Approach to HIV Prevention," *BMJ* 328:7444 (2004), 891–893. Accessed 22 November 2015.

[21] Green, "Uganda's HIV Prevention Success."

[22] Green, "Uganda's HIV Prevention Success."

[23] www.google.com/webhp?sourceid=chrome-instant&ion=1&espv=2&es_th=1&ie=UTF-8#q=protestant%20work%20ethic&es_th=1 Accessed 14th May, 2014 & 17th March, 2015.

[24] Peter Althouse, *Pneuma Review* (20 July 2005), review of David Martin, *Pentecostalism: The World Their Parish* (Oxford: Blackwell Publishers Ltd., 2002).

[25] Martin, *Pentecostalism*.

[26] Pneumatology: The branch of Christian theology concerned with the Holy Spirit. Also, the term comes from two Greek words, namely, *pneuma* meaning, "wind," "breath," or "spirit" (used of the Holy Spirit) and logos meaning, "word," "matter," or "thing." As it is used in Christian systematic theology, "pneumatology" refers to the study of the biblical doctrine of the Holy Spirit. Generally, this includes such topics as the personality of the Spirit, the deity

of the Spirit, and the work of the Spirit throughout Scripture (https://bible.org/seriespage/4-pneumatology-holy-spirit).

[27] Robert Jamieson, A.R. Fausset and David Brown, *Commentary Critical and Explanatory on the Whole Bible* (Oak Harbor, WA: Logos Research Systems, Inc., 1997).

[28] Robert Woodberry, "The Missionary Roots of Liberal Democracy," *American Political Science Review* 106, no. 2 (May 2012), https://doi.org/10.1017/S0003055412000093.

[29] Green, "Uganda's HIV Prevention Success."

[30] UNAIDS Guidance on terminologies, 2015 (See Appendix).

[31] Joshua HK Banda, *Impacts of Congregation-based HIV/AIDS Programs in Lusaka, Zambia: How Abstinence and Marital Fidelity Efforts Function in Overall Strategies Addressing HIV/AIDS*, Ph.D. Thesis (Middlesex, UK: Oxford Center for Mission Studies, 2017).

[32] National AIDS Strategic Framework, Revised (R-NASF) 2014–16.

[33] Edward C. Green, et. al, "The Time Has Come for Common Ground on Preventing Sexual Transmission of HIV," *Lancet* 364:9449 (Nov 27-Dec 3, 2004), http://dx.doi.org/10.1016/S0140-6736(04)17487-4.

[34] Edward C. Green and Allison H. Ruark, "Paradigm Shift and Controversy in AIDS Prevention," *Journal of Medicine and the Person*, 4, no. 1 (2006), 23–33.

[35] Richard Allen Green, "Africa among World's Most Religious People, Study Finds," *CNNWorld+* (15 April 2010), http://www.cnn.com/2010/WORLD/africa/04/15/africa.religion/index.html.

[36] Luis Lugo and Alan Cooperman, "Tolerance and Tension: Islam and Christianity in Sub-Saharan Africa" (15 April 2010), http://www.pewforum.org/2010/04/15/executive-summary.

[37] Green, "Uganda's HIV Prevention Success."

[38] Green and Ruark, "Paradigm Shift and Controversy."

[39] Green and Ruark, "Paradigm Shift and Controversy."

Chapter 11

[1] Samira Luitel, "The Social World of Nepalese Women," *Occasional Papers in Sociology and Anthropology* 7 (2001), 109.

[2] Bishnu Raj Upreti & Ashlid Kolas, "Women in Nepal's Transition," *PRIO Policy Brief* 11 (2016), 25 March 2017, www.prio.org.

[3] *Women and Sexuality in Nepal: A Study Report* (Kathmandu: Forum for Women, Law and Development, 2007), 2.

[4] *Women and Sexuality in Nepal*, 3.

[5] *Women and Sexuality in Nepal*, 5.

[6] Luitel, "The Social World of Nepalese Women," 102.

[7]"The Women-An Introduction," *WEL Nepal: Women's Education and Literacy in Nepal,* http://www.welnepal.org/women.html (20 April 2017).

[8]Sally Engle Merry, "Women, Violence, and the Human Rights System," Marjorie Agosin, ed., *Women, Gender, and Human Rights: A Global Perspective* (Jaipur: Rawat Publications, 2003), 88.

[9]L. E. Saltzman, et al., *Intimate Partner Violence Surveillance Uniform Definitions and Recommended Data Elements* (Atlanta, GA: Centers for Disease Control and Prevention, National Center for Injury Prevention and Control, 1999).

[10]Simkhada, "Why Are So Many Nepali Women Killing Themselves," *Journal of Manmohan Memorial Institute of Health Sciences* 1, no. 4 (2015), 44.

[11]"Field Bulletin on Chaupadi," *United Nations Resident and Humanitarian Coordinator's Office* 1 (April 2011), 1–2.

[12]Pashupati Shumshere J.B. Rana, *Contemporary Nepal* (Bangalore: Vikas Publishing House, 1998), 233.

[13]"Suicide Among Women in Nepal: Studying a Hidden Health Problem," *NHSSP* (2012), www.nhssp.org.np/pulse/Suicide%20Among%20Women%20Pulse%20Updates%204.pdf (22 April, 2017).

[14]Aleksandra Perczynska, "Child Marriage as a Health Issue-Nepal Case Study," OHCHR, *http://www.ohchr.org/documents/issues/children/study/righthealth/herturn.pdf* (26 April 2017).

[15]Shree Prasad Devkota & Shiba Bagale, "Education and Women in Nepal," *The Rising Nepal* http://therisingnepal.org.np/news/2234 (20 April 2017).

[16]"Empowering Adolescent Girls and Women: Promoting Equitable Education, Literacy and Life Long Learning,http://www.unesco.org/new/en/kathmandu/education/empowering-adolescent-girls-and-women-promoting-equitable-education-literacy-and-lifelong-learning/ (22 April 2017).

[17]Rana, *Contemporary Nepal*, 224.

[18]Rana, *Contemporary Nepal*, 224.

[19]"Unpaid Work, Poverty and Women's Rights," OHCHR, 1, http://www.ohchr.org/Documents/Issues/Poverty/UnpaidWork/CaritasNepal.pdf (20 April 2017).

[20]"Unconscious," *Merriam Webster Dictionary,*https://www.merriam-webster.com/dictionary/unconscious (1 May 2017).

[21]John A. Bargh and Ezequiel Morsella, "The Unconscious Mind," *Perspect Psychological Science* 3, no. 1 (Jan., 2008), 73.

[22]Calvin S. Hall and Gardner Lindzey, *Theories of Personality* (New York: John Wiley & Sons, 1957), 80.

[23]Winfield Bevins, *Discovering the Holy Spirit* (n.p: Winfield Bevins, 2010), 21.

[24]Wade C. Graber, *The Mission of the Holy Spirit* (Collierville, TN: Innovo Publishing, 2010), 80.

²⁵Millard J. Erickson in *Introducing Christian Doctrines*, 2nd ed., L. Arnold Hustad, ed. (Grand Rapids: Baker Academic, 2001), 278–279.

²⁶Bal Krishna Sharma, "Pentecostal Interaction with Religions: A Nepali Reflection," in Wonsuk Ma, ed., *Pentecostal Mission and Global Christianity: Edinburgh Centenary Series*, 20 (Oxford: Regnum, 2014), 241–254.

²⁷Williams A. Clebsch and Charles R. Jaekle, *Pastoral Care in Historical Perspective* (Upper Saddle River, NJ: Prentice Hall, 1964), 33.

²⁸L. K. Graham, "Healing," Rodney J. Hunter, ed., *Dictionary of Pastoral Care and Counseling* (Bangalore: Theological Publications in India, 2005), 497.

Chapter 12

¹This is an adaptation of the sermon preached at Oral Roberts University chapel on 19 Nov 2017.

²Scriptural quotations are taken from the New International Version unless stated otherwise.

³Robin McKie, "Onset of Puberty in Girls Has Fallen by Five Years Since 1920," *The Guardian*, 20 Oct 2012, https://www.theguardian.com/society/2012/oct/21/puberty-adolescence-childhood-onset.

⁴Eleanor Barkhorn, "Getting Married Later Is Great for College-Educated Women," *The Atlantic*, 15 March 2013, https://www.theatlantic.com/sexes/archive/2013/03/getting-married-later-is-great-for-college-educated-women/274040/.

⁵John Philip Jenkins, "Pornography – in Sociology," *Encyclopaedia Britannica*, www.britannica.com/topic/pornography, accessed 25 Feb 2019.

⁶David Kinnaman and Roxanne Stone, "Porn in the Digital Age: New Research Reveals 10 Trends," 6 April 2016, https://www.barna.com/research/porn-in-the-digital-age-new-research-reveals-10-trends/.

⁷Arina O. Grossu and Sean Maguire, "The Link Between Pornography, Sex Trafficking and Abortion," Issue Analysis IS17401 (Washington, DC: Family Research Council, Nov. 2017), 6.

⁸Jane Randel and Amy Sanchez, "Parenting in the Digital Age of Pornography," *HuffPost The Blog*, 26 Feb 2017, https://www.huffingtonpost.com/jane-randel/parenting-in-the-digital-age-of-pornography_b_9301802.html.

⁹Kim Painter, "Teenagers Do Listen: Parents Who Set Boundaries Find Their Influence Pays Off," *USA Today*, 8 Feb 2010, https://www.pressreader.com/usa/usa-today-us-edition/20100208/284515814438045.

¹⁰Painter, "Teenagers Do Listen."

¹¹Painter," Teenagers Do Listen."

Chapter 13

[1] In scripture, emotions are part of a rich human response, and they inform. But they never direct, except as part of stories of brokenness. Reference Cain's anger (Gen 4); Esau's hunger (Gen 25); etc. Compare Christ's temptation (Matt 4) and Passion (Psalm 22, Matt 26). Thus, rightly ordered, our bodies bear trustworthy witness, and our feelings follow—to respond, inform, enrich—rather than lead.

Chapter 14

[1] Deborah L. Tollman and Lisa M. Diamond, *APA Handbook of Sexuality and Psychology* (Alexandria, VA: APA Books, 2014), 633.
[2] Malay spelling of Sharia, which is the Islamic religious law that has jurisdiction over every Muslim living in Malaysia.
[3] Pang Khee Teik in Michele Tam, "Activists: Legalizing gay marriage in Asia won't solve Malaysia's LGBT issues," July 29, 2013; https://wlww.thestt;ar.com.my/news/nation/2013/07/29/gay-marriage-lgbt-rights-malaysia-thailand-vietnam/.
[4] Pang Khee Teik.
[5] Dominique Mosbergen, "Malaysia Staunchly Opposes LGBT Rights," October 16, 2015, https://www.huffingtonpost.com/entry/lgbt-malaysia_us_5615359 ae4b0cf9984d7cfae (a partnership site of *The Huffington Post* and *Berggruen Institute*).
[6] Ida Lim and Melissa Chi, "Same-Sex Marriage in Malaysia?" June 30, 2015, https://www.malaymail.com/news/malaysia/2015/06/30/same-sex-marriage-in-malaysia-advocates-say-even-basic-rights-still-in-shor/924273.
[7] Ethan Cole, "Malaysian Pastor Vows to Open First Gay-Friendly Church," August 25, 2007, https://www.christiantoday.com/article/malaysian.pastor.vows.to.open.first.gay.friendlychurch/12625.htm.
[8] Hannah Soo Park, "Gay Pastor Throws Wedding Reception in Malaysia," August 6, 2012, https://www.theknot.com/content/gay-pastor-throws-wedding-reception-in-malaysia.
[9] Kevin DeYoung, *What Does the Bible Teach about Homosexuality?* (Wheaton, Illinois: Crossway, 2015), 36.
[10] DeYoung, *What Does the Bible Teach*, 42.
[11] Wayne Grudem, "Bible and Homosexuality," Accessed June 25, 2018 https://world.wng.org/2013/04/the_bible_and_homosexuality?
[12] DeYoung, *What Does the Bible Teach*, 49.
[13] DeYoung, *What Does the Bible Teach*, 50–57.
[14] James M. Childs, Jr., ed., *Faithful Conversation: Christian Perspectives on Homosexuality* (Minneapolis: Fortress Press, 2003), 31.
[15] Greg L. Bahnses, *Homosexuality: A Biblical View* (Grand Rapids, Michigan:

Baker, 1978), 134.

[16] Ed Shaw, *Same-Sex Attraction and the Church: The Surprising Plausibility of the Celibate Life* (Downers Grove, Illinois: InterVarsity Press, 2015), 135–51.

[17] Shaw, *Same-Sex Attraction*, 153–162.

[18] http://pluc.org.my, accessed February 2, 2019.

[19] Tryphena Law, "From Struggling Pastor to Pastoring Strugglers," June 2012, http://pluc.org.my/wp-content/uploads/2012/06/Journeying-to-Freedom-through-Christ.pdf.

[20] "Ex-gay Groups: PLUC Against the Tide in Malaysia," September 10, 2012, http://www.psa91.com/pluc2.htm.

[21] Tryphena Law, Personal Testimony, https://youtu.be/fC9k3Jh2kfM.

Chapter 15

[1] For example, Robert Gagnon, *The Bible and Homosexual Practice: Texts and Hermeneutics* (Nashville, TN: Abingdon, 2001).

[2] This chapter is a reduced and revised version of my master's thesis. Megan Williamson, "A Macchian Pentecostal Pneumatological Framework for Ministry to Gay Celibate Christians in the Church" (Master's thesis, Continental Theological Seminary, Brussels, Belgium, 2015).

[3] Major works include Frank D. Macchia, *Baptized in the Spirit: A Global Pentecostal Theology* (Grand Rapids, MI: Zondervan, 2006); *Justified in the Spirit: Creation, Redemption, and the Triune God* (Grand Rapids, MI: Eerdmans, 2010); *Jesus the Spirit Baptizer: Christology in Light of Pentecost* (Grand Rapids, MI: Eerdmans, 2018).

[4] Wesley Hill, *Washed and Waiting*, rev. ed. (Grand Rapids, MI: Zondervan, 2016), Kindle.

[5] Hill, *Washed and Waiting*, 133.

[6] Hill, *Washed and Waiting*, 135.

[7] Hill, *Washed and Waiting*, 139.

[8] Hill, *Washed and Waiting*, 139.

[9] Hill, *Washed and Waiting*, 139–140.

[10] Hill, *Washed and Waiting*, 141.

[11] Eve Tushnet, *Gay and Catholic: Accepting My Sexuality, Finding Community, Living My Faith* (Notre Dame, IN: Ave Maria, 2014), 88.

[12] Tushnet, *Gay and Catholic*, 88–89; Alan Bray, *The Friend* (London: University of Chicago Press, 2003), 25.

[13] Alan Chambers, "The New Homosexuality," *Charisma Magazine*, March 10, 2009, http://www.charismamag.com/life/culture/3971-the-new-homosexuality (accessed January 06, 2015), quoted in Tushnet, *Gay and Catholic*, 101. Tushnet acknowledges that Chambers has changed many of his views on homosexuality

and admits she does not know if he still holds to this opinion today.
[14]Steve Summers, "Friends and Friendship," in *The Oxford Handbook of Theology, Sexuality, and Gender*, ed. Adrian Thatcher (Oxford: Oxford University Press, 2015), 698.
[15]Tushnet, *Gay and Catholic*, 104–105.
[16]Hill, *Washed and Waiting*, 142.
[17]Macchia, *Baptized*, 169.
[18]Hill, *Washed and Waiting*, 30.
[19]Macchia, *Baptized*, 174–175.
[20]Macchia, *Baptized*, 174–175. Miroslav Volf, *Exclusion and Embrace: A Theological Exploration of Identity, Otherness, and Reconciliation* (Nashville, TN: Abingdon, 1996), 66.
[21]Macchia, *Baptized*, 174.
[22]Macchia, *Baptized*, 174.
[23]Philip Yancey, *What's So Amazing about Grace?* (Grand Rapids, MI: Zondervan, 1997), 175.
[24]For example, Francis MacNutt, *Can Homosexuality Be Healed?* (Grand Rapids, MI: Chosen Books, 2006) argues that homosexuality can be healed through prayer.
[25]Some examples include singer-songwriter Dennis Jernigan and author and pastor Ron Citlau. Dennis Jernigan, *Sing Over Me* (Collierville, TN: Innovo, 2014); Adam T. Barr and Ron Citlau, *Compassion Without Compromise: How the Gospel Frees Us to Love Our Gay Friends Without Losing the Truth* (Bloomington, MN: Bethany House, 2014).
[26]James D. G. Dunn, *Romans 1–8*, Word Biblical Commentary 38A (Dallas, TX: Word Books, 1988), 477; Douglas Moo, *The Epistle to the Romans*, New International Commentary on the New Testament (Grand Rapids, MI: Eerdmans, 1996), 523.
[27]Dunn, *Romans 1–8*, vol. 38A, 477.
[28]Russell P. Spittler, "Glossolalia," *Dictionary of Pentecostal and Charismatic Movements*, eds. S. M. Burgess and G. B. McGee (Grand Rapids, MI: Zondervan, 1988), 341.
[29]Frank D. Macchia, "Sighs Too Deep for Words: Towards a Theology of Glossolalia," *Journal of Pentecostal Theology* 1 (1992), 68.
[30]Macchia, "Sighs," 69.
[31]Macchia, "Sighs," 66–67.
[32]Macchia, "Sighs," 65.
[33]Mark Yarhouse and Stanton L. Jones did a longitudinal study to counter the American Psychological Association's claim that a homosexual orientation is an immutable condition and attempts to change it could be harmful. They set out to answer the questions: (1) can a homosexual orientation be "healed" by religious means? and (2) is that attempt harmful? Their study showed that there is a possibility of change, though this is not true for every case, and that this

attempt to change is generally not harmful. Their subjects were participants in Exodus International, which at the time was an umbrella organization for many other ministries that used many different methods. For those subjects that did experience harm, it is possible that it was due to "inept, harsh, punitive or otherwise ill-conceived" methods. It is possible that the study included both those who experienced a change in sexual orientation and those who experienced change in sexual identity. Stanton L. Jones and Mark A. Yarhouse, *Ex-Gays: A Longitudinal Study of Religiously Mediated Change in Sexual Orientation* (Downers Grove, IL: InterVarsity, 2007).

[34] For an overview of reparative therapy theory, see Joseph Nicolosi and Linda Nicolosi, *A Parent's Guide to Preventing Homosexuality* (Downers Grove, IL: IVP Books, 2002); Elizabeth R. Moberly, *Homosexuality: A New Christian Ethic* (Cambridge, UK: Lutterworth, 1997).

[35] Some theologians who do this include: James V. Brownson, *Bible, Gender, Sexuality: Reframing the Church's Debate on Same-Sex Relationships* (Grand Rapids, MI: Eerdmans, 2013); David T. Gushee, *Changing our Mind: A Landmark Call for Inclusion of LGBTQ Christians and Response to Critics*, 3rd ed. (Canton, MI: Read the Spirit Books, 2017); Justin Lee, *Torn: Rescuing the Gospel from the Gay-vs.-Christians Debate* (New York: Jericho, 2012); Matthew Vines, *God and the Gay Christian: The Biblical Case in Support of Same-Sex Relationships* (New York: Convergent, 2014).

[36] Melody D. Palm, "Desires in Conflict: Hope and Healing for Individuals Struggling with Same-Sex Attraction," *Enrichment Journal* 15 no. 4 (Fall 2010), 94.

[37] Melinda Selmys, *Sexual Authenticity: An Intimate Reflection on Homosexuality and Catholicism* (Huntington, IN: Our Sunday Visitor Publishing, 2009), 67.

[38] Hill, *Washed and Waiting*, 31.

[39] Hill, *Washed and Waiting*, 61–62; Barr and Citlau, *Compassion without Compromise*, 104–105.

[40] Hill, *Washed and Waiting*, 171; Barr and Citlau, *Compassion without Compromise*, 106.

[41] Hill, *Washed and Waiting*, 160, takes his definition from Dallas Willard, *The Divine Conspiracy: Rediscovering Our Hidden Life in God* (San Francisco: Harper San Francisco, 1997), 165.

[42] Hill, *Washed and Waiting*, 162.

[43] Hill was heavily influenced by C. S. Lewis' essay, "The Weight of Glory." C. S. Lewis, *The Weight of Glory and Other Addresses* (1949; repr., New York: HarperCollins, 2001), 34, 36, 38–39.

[44] Hill, *Washed and Waiting*, 164–165.

[45] Hill, *Washed and Waiting*, 166.

[46] Hill, *Washed and Waiting*, 171.

[47] Macchia, *Justified*, 252.

[48] Macchia, *Justified*, 252.
[49] Macchia, *Justified*, 253.
[50] Macchia, *Justified*, 206.
[51] Andrew Marrin, *Love Is an Orientation: Elevating the Conversation with the Gay Community* (Downers Grove, IL: InterVarsity, 2009), 46–47.
[52] Micah J. Murray, "Why I Can't Say 'Love the Sinner/Hate the Sin' Anymore," *Huffington Post* blog, entry posted Dec. 31, 2013, http://www.huffingtonpost.com/micah-j-murray/why-i-cant-say-love-the-sinner-hate-the-sin-anymore_b_4521519.html (accessed January 19, 2015).
[53] Macchia, *Baptized*, 177.
[54] Hill, *Washed and Waiting*, 174.
[55] Martin Hallett, "Sexuality – a gift from God?" *True Freedom Trust*, June 2000, 4, https://secure.truefreedomtrust.co.uk/book/export/html/69 (accessed January 22, 2015).
[56] Hallett "Sexuality — a gift from God?" 2.
[57] Martin Hallett, "Homosexuality: Handicap and Gift," in *Holiness and Sexuality: Homosexuality in a Biblical Context*, ed. David Peterson (Carlisle, UK: Paternoster, 2004), 124, 139, cited in Hill, *Washed and Waiting*, 150.
[58] Tushnet, *Gay and Catholic*, 70–72.
[59] Tushnet, *Gay and Catholic*, 1.
[60] Tushnet, *Gay and Catholic*, 75.
[61] Tushnet, *Gay and Catholic*, 75–76.
[62] "[This clothing with power is] a consciousness wholly taken up with God so that one feels especially inspired to give of oneself to others in whatever gifting God has created within. It is essentially an experience of self-transcendence motivated by the love of God. Experience is certainly culturally mediated and will vary in nature from person to person, from context to context. But I simply cannot imagine this clothing with power unless some kind of powerful experience of the divine presence, love, and calling is involved, one that loosens our tongues and our hands to function under the inspiration of the Spirit." Macchia, *Baptized*, 14.
[63] Macchia, *Baptized*, 147.

Chapter 16

[1] Leland Ackerson, "Korean Confucianism," available at http://pusanweb.com/Exit/Jun97/CONFUSED.htm, accessed March 18, 2018.
[2] Yung Chung Kim, *Women of Korea: A History from Ancient Times to 1945* (Seoul: Ewha Woman University Press, 1976), 53.
[3] Don Baker, *Dimensions of Asian Spirituality: Korean Spirituality* (Honolulu, HI: University of Hawaii Press, 2008), 46. See also, X. Yao, *An Introduction to*

Confucianism (Cambridge: Cambridge University Press, 2000), 115.

[4] Baker, *Dimensions of Asian Spirituality*, 42.

[5] Baker, *Dimensions of Asian Spirituality*, 42–43.

[6] Donald Clark, *Culture and Customs of Korea* (Westport, CT: Greenwood Press, 2000), 158.

[7] Baker, *Dimensions of Asian Spirituality*, 43.

[8] Baker, *Dimensions of Asian Spirituality*, 44.

[9] Baker, *Dimensions of Asian Spirituality*, 43.

[10] Clark, *Culture and Customs of Korea*, 158.

[11] Clark, *Culture and Customs of Korea*, 157.

[12] Clark, *Culture and Customs of Korea*, 157.

[13] Clark, *Culture and Customs of Korea*, 159.

[14] Clark, *Culture and Customs of Korea*, 159.

[15] Angella Son, "Confucianism and the Lack of the Development of the Self among Korean American Women," *Pastoral Psychology* 54, no. 4 (2006), 325.

[16] Son, "Confucianism and the Lack of the Development," 325–335.

[17] Baker, *Dimensions of Asian Spirituality*, 44–45.

[18] Baker, *Dimensions of Asian Spirituality*, 45.

[19] Clark, *Culture and Customs of Korea*, 160.

[20] Clark, *Culture and Customs of Korea*, 160.

[21] Martina Deuchler, *The Confucian Transformation of Korea* (Cambridge, MA: Harvard University Press, 1992), 231–281.

[22] Karen Hurston, *Growing the World's Largest Church* (Springfield, MO: Gospel Publishing House, 1995), 22.

[23] Hurston, *Growing the World's Largest Church*, 22.

[24] Hurston, *Growing the World's Largest Church*, 22.

[25] A couple of American Assembles of God missionaries provided financial support. And the new location, Saedaemoon, is a city area which provides access to the city center.

[26] Hurston, *Growing the World's Largest Church*, 25–27.

[27] Church Growth International, *Church Growth Manual*, No. 7 (Seoul, South Korea: Church Growth International, 1998), 45.

[28] Wonsuk Ma, "Korean: Characteristics," in *Encyclopedia of Pentecostal and Charismatic Christianity*, ed. Stanley M. Burgess (New York: Routledge, 2006), 279.

[29] Sunghoon Myung and Younggi Hong, eds., *Charis and Charisma: David Yonggi Cho and the Growth of Yoido Full Gospel Church* (Eugene, OR: Wipf & Stock, 2003), 4–5.

[30] Hurston, *Growing the World's Largest Church*, 82–83.

[31] Hurston, *Growing the World's Largest Church*, 83–84.

[32] Hurston, *Growing the World's Largest Church*, 84.

[33] Hurston, *Growing the World's Largest Church*, 85.

[34] Hurston, *Growing the World's Largest Church*, 84–85. See also Young-hoon

Lee, *The Holy Spirit Movement in Korea: Its Historical and Theological Development* (Oxford: Regnum Books, 2009), 96.

[35] Susan C. Hyatt, "Spirit-Filled Women," in *The Century of the Holy Spirit: 100 Years of Pentecostal and Charismatic Renewal, 1901–2001*, ed. Vinson Synan (Nashville, TN: Thomas Nelson, 2001), 233–262.

[36] Hurston, *Growing the World's Largest Church*, 85.

[37] Philip D. Douglass, "Yonggi Cho and the Korean Pentecostal Movement: Some Theological Reflection," *Presbyterion* 17, no. 1 (1991), 16–34. See also Hurston, *Growing the World's Largest Church*, 85.

[38] Lee, *The Holy Spirit Movement in Korea*, 106. See also his article, "The Life and Ministry of D. Yonggi Cho and Yoido Full Gospel Church," *Asian Journal of Pentecostal Studies* 7, no. 1 (2004), 10, 16.

[39] John W. Hurston and Karen L. Hurston, *Caught in the Web* (Anaheim, CA: Church Growth International, 1981), 29–30.

[40] Joel Comskey, "Rev. Cho's Cell Groups and Dynamics of Church Growth," in *Charis and Charisma: David Yonggi Cho and the Growth of Yoido Full Gospel Church*, eds. Sunghoon Myung and Yonggi Hong (Eugene, OR: Wipf & Stock, 2003), 143–157.

[41] Lee, "The Life and Ministry," 8. Also see his book, *The Holy Spirit Movement in Korea*, 106–107.

[42] Hurston, *Growing the World's Largest Church*, 89–90.

[43] Hurston, *Growing the World's Largest Church*, 89–90.

[44] Myung and Hong, *Charis and Charisma*, 95–96.

[45] Hurston, *Growing the World's Largest Church*, 75.

[46] Hurston & Hurston, *Caught in the Web*, 39–40.

[47] Hurston, *Growing the World's Largest Church*, 76.

[48] Hurston, *Growing the World's Largest Church*, 76.

[49] Hurston, *Growing the World's Largest Church*, 76.

[50] Hurston & Hurston, *Caught in the Web*, 38.

[51] Hurston, *Growing the World's Largest Church*, 93.

[52] Hurston & Hurston, *Caught in the Web*, 49–50.

[53] Hurston & Hurston, *Caught in the Web*, 49–50.

[54] Hurston, *Growing the World's Largest Church*, 94.

[55] Hurston, *Growing the World's Largest Church*, 94.

[56] Hurston, *Growing the World's Largest Church*, 94.

[57] Hurston, *Growing the World's Largest Church*, 95.

[58] Hurston & Hurston, *Caught in the Web*, 57–58.

[59] MBN News, June 1, 2017.

[60] Julie C. Ma, "Changing Images: Women in Asian Pentecostalism," in *Women in Pentecostal-Charismatic Leadership*, eds. Estrelda Alexander and Amos Yong (Eugene, OR: Pickwick Pub., 2009), 203–214. See also Ma's article "The Role of Christian Women in the Global South" *Transformation: An International Journal of Holistic Mission Studies* 31:3 (2014), 194–206.

Postscript

[1] *Theology of the Body* is a series of 129 lectures that Pope John Paul II delivered to live audiences on Wednesdays from Sept., 1979 through Nov., 1984. The original record is housed in the Vatican, in *L'Osservatore Romano*, the newspaper of the Holy See. The English version is printed weekly by The Cathedral Foundation, Baltimore, MD. It is widely available through Catholic universities, Bishops and media outlets, such as https://www.ewtn.com/library/PAPALDOC/JP2TBIND.HTM

[2] Timothy Tennent, "Marriage, Human Sexuality and the Body," www.timothytennent.com (Oct-Dec, 2015); Christopher West, *Theology of the Body Explained* (2007).

[3] Timothy Tennent, "United Methodists' Document and the Local Option (Pt. V): Are We Now Facing a New Gnosticism in the Church," December 04, 2017, http://timothytennent.com (accessed August 15, 2018).

[4] For example, Pope John Paul, *Theology of the Body* Lecture Series, The Vatican, Rome, 1979–1984; Christopher West, *Theology of the Body Explained* (Leominster: Gracewing, 2014); Theology of the Body Institute, Philadelphia; Dietrich Von Hildebrand, *In Defense of Purity* (Steubenville, OH: Hildebrand Press,1927); Alexander Pruss, *One Body: An Essay in Christian Sexual Ethics* (Notre Dame: University of Notre Dame Press, 2013); Dennis Kinlaw, *Let's Start with Jesus* (Wilmore, KY: Francis Asbury Press, 2005).

[5] Theologian Randy Alcorn affirms what many readers, including myself, infer from the grammatical structure of Gen 3:8, that this verse indicates God's walking with Adam and Eve in the cool of the day was a pattern, not a one-off on the day the human pair first sinned. See www.epm.org.

[6] Kelly James, LPC, trauma counselor, ORU faculty, personal conversation, 7 Feb 2017.

[7] Helen Keller, *Optimism, My Key of Life* (New York: T.Y. Crowell, 1903).

[8] Atula Walling Prince and Brainerd Prince, "Sexuality, Gender, and Marriage: Pentecostal Theology of Sexuality and Empowering the Girl-Child in India," *Spiritus: ORU Journal of Theology* 3, no. 2 (2018), 109.

[9] National Sexual Violence Resource Center, "Sexual Revictimization Research Brief," published 2012, accessed Jan. 4, 2019 at www.nsvrc.org.

[10] https://www.nwahomepage.com/news/special-report-sex-trafficking-real-in-nwa-and-on-rise/ (accessed Nov. 19, 2018).

[11] Paul Strand, "Sweden's Secret Weapon in the Fight Against Sex Trafficking and Why It's So Effective," www.cbn.com, Feb., 2018 (accessed Nov. 17, 2018).

[12] Mark Regenerus, "Queering Science," Dec., 2018, www.firstthings.com, (accessed Nov. 21, 2018 — in an odd reversal of time, apparently due to the digital format and First Things being ahead of publication schedule).

[13] Mark Yarhouse and Erica Tan, *Sexuality & Sex Therapy* (Downers Grove, IL:

IVP Academic, 2014), 83.

[14] Judith Balswick and Jack Balswick, *Authentic Human Sexuality* (Downers Grove, IL: IVP Academic, 2008), 90.

[15] Balswick and Balswick, *Authentic Human Sexuality*, 68.

[16] William M. Struthers, "The Consequences of a Pornified Culture: Navigating the Neurological, Psychological and Clinical Minefields" (lecture, Asbury United Methodist Church, Tulsa, October 26, 2018).

Contributors

Joshua H. K. Banda is pastor and bishop of Northmead Assembly of God in Lusaka, Zambia. He previously served for two terms as Chair of the National AIDS Council Board of Zambia. He is Chancellor of City University of Science and Technology and sits on the Senate of Lusaka Apex Medical University.

Edwardneil Benavidez, a Filipino Pentecostal, serves as Dean for Religious Education at Bethel Bible College, Valenzuela City, Philippines. He is an adjunct faculty member of Asian Seminary of Christian Ministries, Makati City and a pastor of Precious Cross Christian Church, Makati City, Philippines.

Doreen Benavidez is a Filipina Pentecostal serving as the Head of the Research Department at Asian Seminary of Christian Ministries, Makati City, Philippines. She leads Mindoro Missions Team, a mission organization ministering to the Mangyan tribes in the Philippines. She is married to Edwardneil.

Teresa Chai, an ordained minister of the Assemblies of God Malaysia, now serves as Academic Dean at Asia Pacific Theological Seminary, Baguio, Philippines. She was the President at Alpha Omega College in Malaysia. She is also the Book Review Editor of *Asian Journal of Pentecostal Studies*.

Clayton Coombs is Academic Dean of Planetshakers College and an ordained minister of Planetshakers Church, a large multi-campus Pentecostal church based in Melbourne, Australia. In addition to a Fortress Press monograph, Clayton has published articles in Pentecostal theology and Greek philology.

Megan Grondin serves as Registrar and an adjunct professor at The King's University, Southlake, Texas. She earned her Bachelor of Divinity and Master of Theology from Continental Theological Seminary in Brussels, Belgium. She enjoys traveling, cooking, and spending time with her husband Tony.

Mark R. Hall is Professor of English and Dean of the College of Arts and Cultural Studies at Oral Roberts University, Tulsa, Oklahoma. Along with his studies in English, he also studied Theological and Historical

Studies, and Biblical Literature and has written on biblical topics as well as C. S. Lewis and the Inklings.

Annamarie Hamilton is completing her master's in counseling at Oral Roberts University. She was a youth-ministry volunteer for thirty years while, along with her husband, raising their own five children. With a bachelor's in music from Asbury University in Wilmore, Kentucky, she is also a worship flutist.

Tryphena Law, an ordained minister with the Assemblies of God Malaysia, serves as Executive Director of Pursuing Liberty Under Christ, a ministry to those with gender issues. Her own journey out of same-sex attraction has enabled her to work with others who want to experience freedom in Christ. Her testimony is in a booklet entitled *A Struggling Pastor to Pastoring Struggler* as well as in a DVD entitled *The Lady* produced by Sarawak Chinese Annual Conference.

Julie C. Ma is Associate Professor of Missiology and Intercultural Studies at Oral Roberts University, Tulsa, Oklahoma. Previously, she served as a Korean missionary in the Philippines (1981-2006) and Research Tutor of Missiology at Oxford Centre for Mission Studies, Oxford, United Kingdom. She also served the Edinburgh 2010 as a general (and executive) council member.

Wonsuk Ma, a Korean Pentecostal, serves as Dean and Distinguished Professor of Global Christianity at Oral Roberts University, Tulsa, Oklahoma. He previously served as a missionary in the Philippines and Executive Director of Oxford Centre for Mission Studies, Oxford, United Kingdom.

Michael McClymond is Professor of Modern Christianity at St Louis University, St. Louis, Missouri. He previously held teaching or research appointments at Wheaton College, Westmont College, the University of California–San Diego, Emory University, Yale University, and University of Birmingham (UK). An Anglican layperson, he has been a leader in Global Day of Prayer, Habitat for Humanity, and Stepping Into the Light (a substance abuse recovery ministry in St. Louis). He has written many publications that have received numerous awards.

Lian Sian Mung is a Burmese Pentecostal serving as Old Testament Instructor at Judson Bible College and as the senior pastor of Chicago Zomi Community Church in Wheaton, Illinois. He formerly taught Hebrew and Old Testament at Asia Pacific Theological Seminary, Baguio, Philippines.

Philippe Ouédraogo is executive director of Evangelical Association for Support and Development and Senior Pastor of Boulmiougou Assemblies of God Church in Ouagadougou, Burkina Faso. He is the author of *Female Education and Mission: A Burkina Faso Experience.*

Atula Walling Prince is Director of Shiksha Rath, Delhi, India, an afterschool holistic education for slum children. Previously, she has taught in a Bible college in Assam, worked with new church plants in Delhi, Christian AIDS/HIV National Alliance, and in Matthew Arnold School, Oxford, United Kingdom for special needs students.

Brainerd Prince, along with his wife Atula, founded Touch India Trust, Delhi, India, a charity working with Hindu communities through various projects. He presently is a Research Fellow with the Oxford Centre for Hindu Studies, Oxford, United Kingdom. He is also Visiting Tutor with Oxford Centre for Mission Studies, while directing Samvada, which trains university students to do research in international universities.

Kathaleen Reid-Martinez is the Provost and Chief Academic Officer of Oral Roberts University, Tulsa, Oklahoma. She also served as a Co-Chair of the Scholars Consultation of Empowered21. Her academic interests and research focus on developing leadership in emerging nations, and the impact and advancement of technologies influencing higher education.

Bal Krishna Sharma is Principal of Nepal Theological College in Kathmandu, Nepal. He also serves as a member of the Executive Board of the Assemblies of God of Nepal, Chairman of Nepal Christian Society, Nepal Bible Society, Association for Theological Education in Nepal and Theological Education by Extension Nepal.

Karuna Sharma teaches full-time at Nepal Theological College. She completed her Masters of Theology in Christian Counselling at Union Biblical Seminary. Her expertise is often called upon in the field of Christian ministry, particularly in counseling and women issues. She worked with United Mission to Nepal in the area of peace and reconciliation, as well as HIV/AIDS. She is the daughter of Bal Sharma.

Joseph Suico is Academic Dean of Pneuma School of Missions in Davao City, Philippines, while serving as the lead pastor of the Holy Ground Family Fellowship, Davao City. Previously, he served as a faculty member and Director of Research and Development at Asia Pacific Theological Seminary, Baguio, Philippines.

Lulu Suico has her MA in Theology and Development through Oxford Centre for Mission Studies, Oxford, United Kingdom. Her thesis was on sexual exploitation of children and the role of the Evangelical churches in the Philippines. She now serves as children's pastor of Holy Ground Family Fellowship in Davao City, Philippines. She is married to Joseph.

Timothy C. Tennent is President of Asbury Theological Seminary, Wilmore, Kentucky. Previous work includes Professor of World Missions and Indian Studies at Gordon-Conwell Theological Seminary, and pastor of churches in the states of Georgia and New England. He has taught at several institutions in Asia, Africa and Europe.

William M. Wilson is President of Oral Roberts University, Tulsa, Oklahoma and Chair and Executive Director of Empowered21. He organized and managed the Centenary Celebration of the Azusa Street Revival, and directed the International Center for Spiritual Renewal in Cleveland, Tennessee.

Select Bibliography

Ambrosiaster, Commentaries on Romans and 1–2 Corinthians. Translated by Gerald L. Bray. Ancient Christian Texts. Downers Grove, IL: IVP Academic, 2009.
Anderson, Ryan T. When Harry Became Sally: Responding to the Transgender Moment. New York: Encounter Books, 2018.
Bahnses, Greg L. Homosexuality: A Biblical View. Grand Rapids, MI: Baker, 1978.
Bailey, J. Michael. The Man Who Would be Queen: The Science of Gender-Bending and Transsexualism. Washington, DC: Joseph Henry Press, 2003.
Baker, Don. Dimensions of Asian Spirituality: Korean Spirituality. Honolulu, HI: University of Hawaii Press, 2008.
Bird, Phyllis A. Missing Persons and Mistaken Identities. Minneapolis: Fortress Press, 1997.
Bray, Alan. The Friend. London: University of Chicago Press, 2003.
Brock, Colin and Nadine Cammis. "Factors Affecting Female Participation in Education in Seven Developing Countries." 2nd ed. Education Papers 9. London: Dept. for International Development, 1997.
Brodbeck, Simon and Brian Black. "Introduction." In Gender and Narrative in the Mahabharata. Edited by Simon Brodbeck and Brian Black. London: Routledge, 2007: 10–11.
Brownson, James. Bible, Gender, Sexuality: Reframing the Church's Debate on Same-Sex Relationships. Grand Rapids, MI: Eerdmans, 2013.
Childs, James M. Jr., Ed. Faithful Conversation: Christian Perspectives on Homosexuality. Minneapolis: Fortress Press, 2003.
Chrysostom, John. Homilies on the Epistle to the Romans. Nicene and Post Nicene Fathers. Vol. 11. Grand Rapids: Eerdmans, 1989.
Clark, Donald. Culture and Customs of Korea. Westport, CT: Greenwood Press, 2000.
Clebsch, Williams A. and Charles R. Jaekle. Pastoral Care in Historical Perspective. Upper Saddle River, NJ: Prentice Hall, 1964.
Corbin, Juliet and Anselm Strauss. Basics of Qualitative Research: Techniques and Procedures for Developing Grounded Theory. London: SAGE, 2008.
Costa, Lee Ray and Andrew Matzner. Male Bodies, Women's Souls: Personal Narratives of Thailand's Transgendered Youth. New York: The Haworth Press, 2007.
Davidson, Richard M. Flame of Yahweh: Sexuality in the Old Testament. Peabody, MA: Hendrickson, 2007.
Dearman, Andrew. "Marriage in the Old Testament." In Biblical Ethics and

Homosexuality. Edited by Robert L. Brawley. Louisville, KY: Westminster John Knox Press, 1996: 53–68.

Dempster, Murray, Bryon Klaus and Douglas Petersen, eds. Globalization of Pentecostalism. Eugene, OR: Wipf and Stock, 1999.

DeYoung, Kevin. What Does the Bible Teach about Homosexuality? Wheaton, IL: Crossway, 2015.

Ennew, Judith. The Sexual Exploitation of Children. New York: St. Martins Press, 1986.

Fee, Gordon. The First Epistle to the Corinthians. New International Commentary on the New Testament. Grand Rapids: Eerdmans, 1987.

Garland, David. 1 Corinthians. Baker Exegetical Commentary on the New Testament. Grand Rapids: Baker Academic, 2003.

Graham, L. K. "Healing." Dictionary of Pastoral Care and Counseling. Edited by Rodney J. Hunter. Bangalore: Theological Publications in India, 2005.

Green, Edward C. and Allison H. Ruark. AIDS, Behaviour and Culture: Understanding Evidence-based Prevention. Walnut Creek, CA: Left Coast Press, 2011.

_____. "Paradigm Shift and Controversy in AIDS Prevention." Journal of Medicine and the Person 4:1 (2006): 23–33.

Grudem, Wayne. The Bible and Homosexuality. https://world.wng.org/2013/04/the_bible_and_homosexuality

Hill, Wesley. Washed and Waiting. Rev. Ed. Grand Rapids, MI: Zondervan, 2016.

Hurtley, James B. Man and Woman in Biblical Perspective. Grand Rapids, MI: Zondervan, 1981.

Hyatt, Susan C. "Spirit-Filled Women." In The Century of the Holy Spirit: 100 Years of Pentecostal and Charismatic Renewal, 1901–2001. Edited by Vinson Synan. Nashville, TN: Thomas Nelson, 2001: 233–262.

Ireland, Kevin. "Sexual Exploitation of Children and International Travel and Tourism." Child Abuse Review 2:4 (1993): 263–270.

Jeffreys, Sheila. Gender Hurts: A Feminist Analysis of the Politics of Transgenderism. Abingdon, UK: Routledge, 2014.

Jernigan, Dennis. Sing Over Me. Collierville, TN: Innovo, 2014.

Joshua Kembo, Joshua. "Changes in Sexual Behavior and Practice and HIV Prevalence Indicators among Young People Aged 15–24 Years in Zambia: An In-depth Analysis of the 2001–2002 and 2007 Zambia Demographic and Health Surveys." Sahara Journal 10:3–4 (2013):150–162.

Kilbourne, Phyllis and Marjorie McDermid, eds. Sexually Exploited Children: Working to Protect and Heal. Monrovia, CA: MARC, 1998.

Kuby, Gabrielle. The Global Sexual Revolution: Destruction of Freedom in the Name of Freedom. Translated by James Patrick Kirchner. Kettering, OH: Angelico Press/Lifesite, 2015.

Lee, Young-hoon. The Holy Spirit Movement in Korea: Its Historical and Theological Development. Oxford: Regnum Books, 2009.

Lewis, C. S. The Weight of Glory and Other Addresses. Repr., New York: HarperCollins, 2001.

Longenecker, Richard N. The Epistle to the Romans: A Commentary on the Greek Text. New International Greek Testament Commentary. Grand Rapids: Eerdmans, 2016.

Luitel, Samira. "The Social World of Nepalese Women." Occasional Papers in Sociology and Anthropology 7 (2001): 101–114.

Ma, Julie C. "Changing Images: Women in Asian Pentecostalism." In Women in Pentecostal-Charismatic Leadership. Edited by Estrelda Alexander and Amos Yong. Eugene, OR: Pickwick, 2009: 203–214.

Macchia, Frank D. Baptized in the Spirit: A Global Pentecostal Theology. Grand Rapids, MI: Zondervan, 2006.

_____. Justified in the Spirit: Creation, Redemption, and the Triune God. Grand Rapids, MI: Eerdmans, 2010.

_____. "Sighs Too Deep for Words: Towards a Theology of Glossolalia." Journal of Pentecostal Theology 1 (1992): 47–73.

Mayer, Lawrence S. and Paul R. McHugh. "Sexuality and Gender: Findings from the Biological, Psychological, and Social Sciences." The New Atlantis: A Journal of Technology and Society 50 (Fall 2016): 7–58.

Meredith, Martin. The State of Africa: A History of Fifty Years of Independence. London: Free Press, 2005.

Merry, Sally Engle. "Women, Violence, and the Human Rights System." Women, Gender, and Human Rights: A Global Perspective. Edited by Marjorie Agosin. Jaipur: Rawat Publications, 2003: 83–98.

Moo, Douglas. The Epistle to the Romans. The New International Commentary on the New Testament. Grand Rapids: Eerdmans, 1996.

Nakonz, Jonas and Angela Wai Yan Shik. "And All Your Problems Are Gone: Religious Coping Strategies among Philippine Migrant Workers in Hong Kong." Mental Health, Religion and Culture 12:1 (2009): 25–38.

Namaste, Viviane K. Invisible Lives: The Erasure of Transsexual and Transgendered People. Chicago: University of Chicago, 2000.

Narayanan, Vasudha. "Gender in a Devotional Universe." In The Blackwell Companion to Hinduism. Edited by Gavin Flood. New York: John Wiley and Sons, 2008: 569–587.

O'Grady, Ron. Tourism in the Third World: Christian Reflections. Maryknoll, NY: Orbis Books, 1982.

Origen, Homilies on Joshua. Edited by Cynthia White. Translated by Barbara Bruce. The Fathers of the Church. Vol. 105. Washington, DC: Catholic University of America Press, 2002.

Ouédraogo, Philippe. Female Education and Mission: A Burkina Faso Experience. With Forward by Prime Minister Tertius Zongo. Oxford: Regnum Books, 2014.

_____. "Transforming Communities through Education." In Good News from

Africa: Community Transformation through the Church. Edited by Brian E. Woolnough. Oxford: Regnum Books, 2013: 81–90.

Ricoeur, Paul. Oneself as Another. Translated by Kathleen Blamey. Chicago: University of Chicago Press, 1992.

_____. Time and Narrative. Vol. 3. Translated by Kathleen Blamey and David Pellauer. Chicago: University of Chicago Press, 1988.

Sepulveda, Juan. "Pentecostal Theology in the Context of the Struggle for Life." In Faith Born in the Struggle for Life. Edited by Dow Kirkpatrick. Grand Rapids: Eerdmans, 1988: 298–318.

Shaw, Ed. Same-Sex Attraction and the Church: The Surprising Plausibility of the Celibate Life. Downers Grove, IL: InterVarsity Press, 2015.

Sharma, Bal Krishna. "Pentecostal Interaction with Religions: A Nepali Reflection," In Pentecostal Mission and Global Christianity. Edited by Wonsuk Ma, et al. Regnum Edinburgh Centenary Series 20. Oxford: Regnum, 2014: 241–254.

Singal, Jesse. "When Children Say They Are Trans." The Atlantic, https://www.theatlantic.com/magazine/archive/ 2018/07/when-a-child-says-shes-trans/561749/.

Strachan, Owen and Gavin Peacock. The Grand Design: Male and Female He Made Them. Fearn, Ross-shire, UK: Christian Focus, 2016.

Tarwater, John K. Marriage as Covenant: Considering God's Design at Creation and the Contemporary Moral Consequences. Lanham, MD: University Press of America, 2006.

Thoits, Peggy A. "Patterns in Coping with Controllable and Uncontrollable Events." In Life-span Developmental Psychology: Perspectives on Stress and Coping. Edited by E. Mark Cummings, Anita L. Greene and Katherine H. Karrakar. Hillsdale, NJ: Psychology Press, 1991: 235–258.

Tillich, Paul. "Reason and Revelation, Being and God." Systematic Theology. Vol. 1. Chicago: University of Chicago Press, 1973.

Tennent, Timothy. "Marriage, Human Sexuality and the Body." Oct-Dec, 2015. https://timothytennent.com.

Tertullian, De Anime. Corpus Christianorum Series Latina. Vol. 2. Tornhout, Belgium: Brepols, 1954.

Thiselton, Anthony C. The First Epistle to the Corinthians: A Commentary on the Greek Text. The New International Greek Testament Commentary. Grand Rapids: Eerdmans, 2000.

Towner, Philip H. The Letters of Timothy and Titus. The New International Commentary on the New Testament. Grand Rapids: Eerdmans, 2006.

Turner, R. Jay and Patricia Roszell. "Psychosocial Resources and the Stress Process." In Stress and Mental Health: Contemporary Issues and Prospects for the Future. Edited by William R. Avison and Ian H. Gotlib. New York: Plenum, 1994: 179–210.

Tushnet, Eve. Gay and Catholic: Accepting My Sexuality, Finding Community, Living My Faith. Notre Dame, IN: Ave Maria, 2014.

Volf, Miroslav. Exclusion and Embrace: A Theological Exploration of Identity, Otherness, and Reconciliation. Nashville, TN: Abingdon, 1996.

Yong, Amos. Hospitality and the Other: Pentecost, Christian Practices and the Neighbour. New York: New York University, 2008.

Scripture Index

Old Testament
Genesis
  1:2 *15*
  1:26–31 *10, 11, 14, 21,*
    93, 112, 231, 241,
    248, 285, 286
  2:16–26 *10, 11, 12, 13,*
    14, 21, 32, 226, 241,
    287
  3:1–7, 15, 16, 21–24 *14,*
    215, 244, 287, 288
  4:1 *231*
  19 *242*
  38:14–39 *16, 19, 241*
  39:9 *16, 21*
  41:25–39 *15, 16*
Exodus
  18:13–26 *276*
  22:22–24 *141*
Leviticus
  18:22 *29, 35,*
    242, 243
  19:29 *241*
  20:10–26 *29, 35, 218,*
    220, 241, 242
Deuteronomy
  6:4–9 *140*
  24:17 *142*
  29:23 *242*
Judges
  4:31 *17*
  13: 5–7 *17*
  13:25 *17*
  14:6 *17*
  14:19 *17*
  15:14 *17, 18*
  16:1–3 *18, 19*
  16:4–21 *18*

Joshua
  11:19–20 *43*
1 Samuel
  16:13–14 *19, 20*
II Samuel
  8:15 *20*
  11:1–4 *20, 21*
  11:6–25, 27 *21*
  23:34 *20*
  23:39 *20*
Ruth
  1:14–16 *13*
Psalm
  82:2–3 *139*
Proverbs
  5:17–20 *221*
Song of Solomon
  86, 87, 221
  1:5 *86*
  5:3 *44*
  14:23–26 *27*
Isaiah
  191
  1:9–10 *242*
  11:2 *15*
  13:19 *242*
Jeremiah
  241
  2:23–25 *88*
  23:14 *242*
  49:18 *242*
  50:40 *242*
Lamentations
  4:6 *242*
Ezekiel
  16:50–58 *242*
  18:22 *242*
  20:13 *242*

Joel
  3:3 *140*
Amos
  2:7, 42–46 *140*
  4:11 *242*
Zephaniah
  2:9 *242*
Malachi
  2:15 *13*
New Testament
Matthew
  5:3, 13–16 *142, 263*
  8:5–13 *244*
  10:14, 15 *242*
  11:23, 24 *242*
  18:1–9 *140, 141*
  19:1–29 *13, 14, 141,*
    231, 233, 241
Mark
  1:25–26, 29–31, 40–42
    142
  6:30–40 *142*
  9:33–7, 42 *141*
  10:13–29 *141*
  12:25 *233*
  12:31 *93*
Luke
  2:25, 52 *141, 287*
  4:18–19 *141, 149, 191*
  7:1–10 *245*
  9:46–48 *141*
  10:10–12 *242*
  14:26 *13*
  17:26–30 *242*
  18:15–29 *141*
John
  3:16–17 *287*
  5:44 *261*

Acts
1:8 *22*
2:42–46 *276*
10, 10:15 *262, 263*

Romans
1:18 *39*
1:23–32 *25, 27–32, 46, 242, 243*
2:16, 29 *261*
3:21–26 *261*
5:5, 5–12 *253, 287*
8:17–27 *254, 258, 261, 262*
10:10, 11 *262*
11:4, 24 *29*
12:2 *147, 245*
16:3–5 *276*

I Corinthians
3: 16–17 *49*
4:5 *261*
5:9–11 *39*
6:1–11 *28*
6:9–10 *25, 27, 28, 33–36, 42–48, 235, 237*
6:11 *38–42, 44, 47, 48*
7:5 *235*
10:18, 23 *40*
11:2 *44*
16:16 *277*

II Corinthians
1:22 *22*
4:16–17 *254*
10:18 *261*
12:21 *28*

Galatians
3:27–28 *244*
5:5 *261*
5:16–18 *22*
5:19–23 *22, 26, 28, 36, 41*
5:24, 25 *36*

Ephesians
1:4, 13–14 *4, 22, 261*
2:3 *41*
4:12–13 *258*
5:28 *227*
6:1–4 *140*

Philippians
2:12–15 *287*

Colossians
3:9 *44*
4:15 *276*

I Thessalonians
4:3–7 *215*

I Timothy
1:9–10 *25, 26, 27, 29, 33, 34*
6:3–5 *26*

II Timothy
2:15 *26*
3:2–5 *26*

I Peter
1:17 *261*

II Peter
1:5–7 *26*

I John
5:4 *287*

Titus
2:11–14 *45*
3:1–7 *26, 43, 46*

Philemon
1–2 *276*

Hebrews
4:12 *2229*
13:4 *215*

James
1:27 *139*
2:11 *241*
3:13–18 *26*

Jude
7 *242*

Revelation
16:15 *30*
21:1–5 *287*

www.ingramcontent.com/pod-product-compliance
Lightning Source LLC
Chambersburg PA
CBHW071259110526
44591CB00010B/721